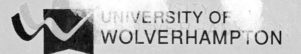

Mechanisms of Action of
Chemical Biocides

THEIR STUDY AND
EXPLOITATION

A complete list of titles in the Society for
Applied Bacteriology Technical Series appears at
the end of this volume

THE SOCIETY FOR APPLIED BACTERIOLOGY
TECHNICAL SERIES NO 27

Mechanisms of Action of Chemical Biocides

THEIR STUDY AND

EXPLOITATION

Edited by

S.P. DENYER

Department of Pharmaceutical Sciences
University of Nottingham

W.B. HUGO

618 Wollaton Road
Nottingham

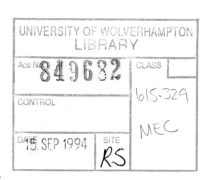
OXFORD

BLACKWELL SCIENTIFIC PUBLICATIONS

LONDON EDINBURGH BOSTON

MELBOURNE PARIS BERLIN VIENNA

© 1991 by the Society for Applied Bacteriology
and published for them by
Blackwell Scientific Publications
Editorial offices:
Osney Mead, Oxford OX2 0EL
25 John Street, London WC1N 2BL
23 Ainslie Place, Edinburgh EH3 6AJ
3 Cambridge Center, Cambridge,
    Massachusetts 02142, USA
54 University Street, Carlton
    Victoria 3053, Australia

Other editorial offices:

Arnette SA
2, rue Casimir-Delavigne
75006 Paris
France

Blackwell Wissenschaft
Meinekestrasse 4
D-1000 Berlin 15
West Germany

Blackwell MZV
Feldgasse 13
A-1238 Wien
Austria

First published 1991

Set by Setrite Typesetters, Hong Kong
Printed and bound in Great Britain by
The Alden Press, Oxford

DISTRIBUTORS

Marston Book Services Ltd
PO Box 87
Oxford OX2 0DT
(*Orders*: Tel: 0865 791155
    Fax: 0865 791927
    Telex: 837515)

USA
Blackwell Scientific Publications, Inc.
3 Cambridge Center
Cambridge, MA 02142
(*Orders*: Tel: 800 759−6102)

Canada
Oxford University Press
70 Wynford Drive
Don Mills
Ontario M3C 1J9
(*Orders*: Tel: (416) 441−2941)

Australia
Blackwell Scientific Publications
(Australia) Pty Ltd
54 University Street
Carlton, Victoria 3053
(*Orders*: Tel: (03) 347−0300)

British Library
Cataloguing in Publication Data

Mechanisms of action of chemical biocides.
    1. Antimicrobials
    I. Denyer, S.P.   II. Hugo, W.B. (William Barry)
    1920−
    615.329

    ISBN 0-632-02928-5

Library of Congress
Cataloging in Publication Data

Mechanisms of action of chemical biocides: their
    study and exploitation/edited by S.P. Denyer,
    W.B. Hugo.
            p.   cm.−(Technical series/The
    Society for Applied Bacteriology; no. 27)
        Includes bibliographical references and index.
        ISBN 0-632-02928-5
        1. Bactericides−Mechanism of action.
    I. Denyer, S.P.   II. Hugo, W.B. (William
    Barry)   III. Series: Technical series
    (Society for Applied Bacteriology); no. 27.
    QR97.B32M43   1991
    589.9′024−dc20

Contents

Effect of Biocides on DNA, RNA and Protein Synthesis 225
T. EKLUND AND I.F. NES

Biocide-Induced Enzyme Inhibition 235
S.J. FULLER

Mechanisms of Chemical Reactions with Biomolecules 251
R.D. WAIGH AND P. GILBERT

Intracellular Delivery of Biocides 263
S.P. DENYER, D.E. JACKSON AND M. AL-SAGHER

Microbial Adherence and Biofilm Production 271
S.P. GORMAN

Contributors

M. AL-SAGHER, *Department of Pharmaceutical Sciences, University of Nottingham, University Park, Nottingham NG7 2RD, UK*

JILL BARBER, *Department of Pharmacy, University of Manchester, Oxford Road, Manchester M13 9PL, UK*

A.E. BEEZER, *Chemical Laboratory, University of Kent, Canterbury CT2 7NH, UK*

E.G. BEVERIDGE, *Department of Pharmaceutics, Sunderland Polytechnic, Sunderland SR2 7EE, UK*

SALLY F. BLOOMFIELD, *Chelsea Department of Pharmacy, King's College, University of London, Manresa Road, London SW3 6LX, UK*

I. BOYD, *Department of Pharmaceutics, Sunderland Polytechnic, Sunderland SR2 7EE, UK*

I. CHOPRA, *Department of Microbial Biochemistry and Genetics, American Cyanamid Co., Lederle Laboratories, Pearl River, NY 10965, USA*

B.N. DANCER, *School of Pure and Applied Biology, University of Wales College of Cardiff, Cardiff CF1 3NX, UK*

S.P. DENYER, *Department of Pharmaceutical Sciences, University of Nottingham, Nottingham NG7 2RD, UK*

I. DEW, *Department of Pharmaceutics, Sunderland Polytechnic, Sunderland SR2 7EE, UK*

T. EKLUND, *Norwegian Dairies Association, POB 9051 Vaterland, N−0134 Oslo 1, Norway*

J. FORD, *Department of Pharmacy, Liverpool Polytechnic, Byrom Street, Liverpool L3 3AF, UK*

S.J. FULLER, *Sterling-Winthrop Research Centre, Willowburn Avenue, Alnwick, Northumberland NE66 2JH, UK*

P. GILBERT, *Department of Pharmacy, University of Manchester, Oxford Road, Manchester M13 9PL, UK*

L. GLEDHILL, *Department of Pharmaceutical Sciences, University of Nottingham, University Park, Nottingham NG7 2RD, UK*

S.P. GORMAN, *School of Pharmacy, Medical Biology Centre, The Queen's University of Belfast, Belfast BT9 7BL, UK*

G.W. HANLON, *Department of Pharmacy, Brighton Polytechnic, Moulsecoomb, Brighton, E. Sussex BN2 4GJ, UK*

M. HASWELL, *Electron Microscopy Unit, Sunderland Polytechnic, Sunderland SR2 7EE, UK*

N.A. HODGES, *Department of Pharmacy, Brighton Polytechnic, Moulsecoomb, Brighton, E. Sussex BN2 4GJ, UK*

W.B. HUGO, *618 Wollaton Road, Nottingham NG8 2AA, UK*

D.E. JACKSON, *Department of Pharmaceutical Sciences, University of Nottingham, University Park, Nottingham NG7 2RD, UK*

S.A.A. JASSIM, *Department of Pharmaceutical Sciences, University of Nottingham, University Park, Nottingham NG7 2RD, UK*

R.G. KROLL, *Department of Microbiology, AFRC Institute of Food Research, Reading Laboratory, Shinfield, Reading RG2 9AT, UK*

P.A. LAMBERT, *Pharmaceutical Sciences Institute, Department of Pharmaceutical Sciences, Aston University, Aston Triangle, Birmingham B4 7ET, UK*

P.N. LEVETT, *University of the West Indies, Faculty of Medical Sciences, Queen Elizabeth Hospital, St Michael, Barbados*

C.W.G. LOWE, *Department of Pharmaceutics, Sunderland Polytechnic, Sunderland SR2 7EE, UK*

I.F. NES, *Laboratory of Microbial Gene Technology NLVF, POB 51, N-1432, ÅS-NLH, Norway*

R.A. PATCHETT, *Department of Microbiology, AFRC Institute of Food Research, Reading Laboratory, Shinfield, Reading RG2 9AT, UK*

MARY K. PHILLIPS-JONES, *Department of Molecular Biology and Biotechnology, Biochemistry Section, University of Sheffield, Sheffield S10 2TN, UK*

E.G.M. POWER, *Welsh School of Pharmacy, University of Wales College of Cardiff, Cardiff CF1 3XF, UK*

MURIEL E. RHODES-ROBERTS, *Department of Biological Sciences, University College of Wales, Aberystwyth, Dyfed SY23 3DA, UK*

A.D. RUSSELL, *Welsh School of Pharmacy, University of Wales College of Cardiff, Cardiff CF1 3XF, UK*

W.G. SALT, *Microbiology Unit, Department of Chemistry, Loughborough University of Technology, Loughborough, Leicestershire LE11 3TU, UK*

G.S.A.B. STEWART, *Department of Applied Biochemistry and Food Science, School of Agriculture, University of Nottingham, Sutton Bonington, Loughborough, Leicestershire LE12 5RD, UK*

R.D. WAIGH, *Department of Pharmacy, University of Manchester, Oxford Road, Manchester M13 9PL, UK*

P. WILLIAMS, *Department of Pharmaceutical Sciences, University of Nottingham, University Park, Nottingham NG7 2RD, UK*

D. WISEMAN, *Postgraduate School of Studies in Pharmacy, University of Bradford, Bradford BD7 1DP, UK*

Preface

This volume, the 27th in the Society for Applied Bacteriology Technical Series, is based on demonstrations held at a meeting of the Society at the AFRC Institute of Food Research, Reading Laboratory, on 19 October 1988.

There have been studies on the killing of bacteria and the evaluation of antimicrobial agents dating back to the 18th Century, and even before bacteria were identified empirical experiments were reported. With the advance of the science of biochemistry, however, papers began to appear, especially in Germany, on studies to understand how disinfectants worked and in 1872 Ritthausen reported the interaction of phenol with proteins. Meyer in 1901 made distribution studies. Reichel in 1909 studied uptake and this was extended by Cooper in 1913 working in England. Experiments initiated in Quastel's laboratory in Cambridge University in 1925 investigated the action of disinfectants on enzyme systems exploiting the methylene blue technique of Thunberg. Shoup and Kimler found the first hint of action on membrane function in 1934 and Hotchkiss, working in the USA, reported effects on membrane integrity in 1944. These were some of the early and fundamental studies which led to the development of many methods for investigating the action of antimicrobial agents, an academic approach which has borne much fruit in the design of new antibiotics.

In the context of this Technical Series volume, emphasis has been placed on antimicrobial agents largely employed for the control of contamination rather than the treatment of infection (although some medically useful chemical agents are discussed). As such, the biocides referred to are principally of the non-antibiotic type and include agents used for preservation and disinfection in a wide variety of areas including the pharmaceutical, food, cosmetic, environmental, service, construction, manufacturing and engineering industries. Their current usage is widespread and extensive, representing a considerable financial investment as well as an important potential toxicological and environmental consideration.

A major review of methods for assessing damage to bacteria induced by both chemical and physical agents appeared in 1973 written by Russell, Morris and Allwood (*Methods in Microbiology*, 8, pp. 95–182, London, Academic Press) and the reader's attention is drawn to this paper which gives a comprehensive account of general laboratory methodologies. This Technical Series reviews the current status of these methods and how they may be applied in a programme to determine how an antimicrobial agent acts. It concentrates on antibacterial mechanisms of action but many of the methods can be extended to the study of antifungal effects. The topic can be considered under the main headings of whole cell studies, structural and biochemical effects, and then some more general effects. Mode of action studies, if intelligently assessed and applied, can lead to the design or selection of novel biocides or combinations of biocides, an understanding of resistance mechanisms, and give direction to toxicological studies.

We wish to thank all the demonstrators for the presentation of their exhibits on the 19 October 1988 and in the preparation of their chapters in this book. Their efforts on the day were greatly helped by the local organizer, Dr Rohan Kroll, and by Dr Susan Passmore, the Society's Meetings Secretary.

S.P. Denyer
W.B. Hugo

Methods for Assessing Antimicrobial Activity

SALLY F. BLOOMFIELD

*Chelsea Department of Pharmacy, King's College,
University of London, Manresa Road, London SW3 6LX, UK*

In any study of mechanisms of antibacterial action, quantitative assessment of activity under appropriate conditions forms an essential part of the initial investigation. Antibacterial agents may exert any number of different effects on the structure and functioning of bacterial cells. Identification of those effects which occur at concentrations producing antimicrobial action may play a vital part in delineating primary lesions from secondary effects.

In carrying out biochemical studies with whole cells or cell fractions it is inevitable that these studies will be performed under conditions which may differ significantly from those used to determine antimicrobial action. The implications of these alterations in reaction conditions must be carefully assessed, and experiments planned to reduce these differences to a minimum.

In this chapter methods used for the assessment of antimicrobial activity in relation to mechanism of action studies are considered. These methods are also described by Reybrouk (1982) and Hugo & Russell (1987).

Bacteriostatic and Bactericidal Effects

Antibacterial action may be either bacteriostatic or bactericidal.

Bacteriostasis is the term used to describe the prevention or inhibition of growth by an agent when measured under conditions where growth would normally occur. The effect is reversible such that if the agent is removed or neutralized, the cells will recommence growth and cell division.

Bactericidal effects occur when bacterial cells exposed to an agent are not recoverable (i.e. do not recommence growth) after removal or neutralization of the agent. This is due to an irreversible lethal process taking place in the cell.

Under laboratory conditions, where the behaviour of populations rather than individual cells is investigated, differences between bacteriostatic and bactericidal effects may be difficult to distinguish in a situation where some cells may be dividing and others dying, i.e. a dynamic situation.

Mechanisms of Action of
Chemical Biocides

Mechanism of action studies indicate that some antimicrobial agents are primarily bactericidal (e.g. chlorine and iodine) whilst others may be mainly bacteriostatic (although where bacteriostasis is maintained death will inevitably result). Some agents may also exert bacteriostatic or bactericidal effects according to their concentration. In studying mechanisms of action it is important to consider that although cell damage may result in bacteriostasis, it is the inability of the cells to make good this damage which produces a bactericidal effect. Thus, for example, with membrane-active antibacterial agents such as phenols and chlorhexidine, although loss of metabolites through the damaged membrane inhibits cell growth, it is the extent of the membrane damage and the inability of the cells to make good this loss on neutralization of the agent, which ultimately produces bactericidal effects.

Dynamics of Antibacterial Action

1   In order to establish the bacteriostatic effect of an antibacterial agent, the dynamics of growth in the absence of inhibitors must first be considered. The typical growth curve (Fig. 1a) for a batch culture obtained under optimal growth conditions usually consists of:

a   a lag phase in which cells may be metabolically active but show no increase in cell numbers;
b   an exponential phase during which cell division occurs following an exponential relationship;
c   a stationary phase where little or no further growth is observed. This can be due to a number of factors including exhaustion of nutrients or oxygen, pH changes and accumulation of toxic metabolites.

Bacteriostasis may be seen as an increase in the lag phase together with a decrease in growth rate which may be partial (as in Fig. 1b) or total (as in Fig. 1c).

2   The dynamics of bactericidal action are usually assessed from time-survivor curves in which customarily the log number of viable cells is plotted as a function of time. The typical death curve (Fig. 1d) is also sigmoidal in shape and may comprise a number of phases:

a   an initial lag or shoulder which may be a function of the rate of penetration of the agent to its site of action within the cell. It is also consistent with the idea that antibacterial resistance is not constant within a bacterial population but is distributed about an average value such that some cells die more or less rapidly than the average;
b   a linear phase in which the rate of kill follows an exponential relationship and is consistent with first-order chemical reaction kinetics;
c   a 'tailing' effect which represents the death of residual cells of above average resistance within the population or those for which biocide access has been slow.

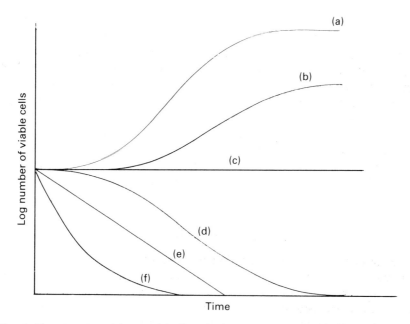

FIG. 1. Bacteriostatic and bactericidal effects as determined from time-survivor curves. (a) A typical growth curve; (b, c) growth inhibitory and bacteriostatic effect, respectively; (d, e, f) bactericidal effects.

Experimental investigations with antibacterial agents suggest that curves of type e and f (Fig. 1) may also be obtained but it is suggested that these are usually associated with rapid rates of kill where initial 'shoulder' and 'tailing' effects may go undetected. The significance of the tailing effect is discussed in more detail by Cerf (1977).

Quantitative Assessment of Growth and Death of Microbial Populations

For quantitative assessment, growth rates may be determined for the exponential phase of the growth curve using the following equation:

$$\text{Growth rate constant } (K_1) = \frac{2.303}{t} \log_{10} \left(\frac{N}{N_0}\right),$$

where t is the time taken for the number of organisms to increase from N_0 to N. The value of K_1 can be used for quantitative comparison of growth inhibitory activity under varying conditions.

A similar approach may be used for quantitative assessment of time-survivor curves whereby death rates are determined from the linear portion of the curve using the following equation:

$$\text{Death rate constant } (K_2) = \frac{2.303}{t} \log_{10} \left(\frac{N_0}{N} \right),$$

where N_0 is the initial number of organisms, N is the final number of organisms and t is the time taken for the viable count to fall from N_0 to N.

Sensitivity to bactericidal agents may also be expressed by the decimal reduction value (D-value). This is defined as the time taken to achieve a 90% reduction in viable cells (i.e. a 1-log reduction). Calculation of D-values assumes a linear type E survival curve (Fig. 1) and the data must therefore be carefully interpreted where deviations from linearity are observed.

Whereas standard European tests for disinfectant activity are tending to adopt a standard 5-log reduction to represent satisfactory activity, in the case of mechanism of action studies, where the sensitivity of biochemical and other assays will rarely allow detection of less than 1% of the original activity, then a 1–2-log reduction in survivors is probably more appropriate.

In some situations considerable insight into mechanisms of action can also be gained from observations on the length of the lag phase before onset of rapid killing, which may indicate changes in the rate of penetration of an agent to its site of action. The nature of the tailing effect should also be considered.

Factors Affecting Antibacterial Activity

As mentioned previously, although assessment of antimicrobial activity in relation to biochemical and other observations may play a vital role in identifying primary lesions, it is almost inevitable that, in practice, activity and mechanism of action studies are carried out under different experimental conditions. Accurate interpretation of the results will therefore depend on a clear understanding of the factors which may affect the activity of an agent in relation to biochemical effects. In many cases these factors are deliberately exploited for elucidating mechanisms of action. The activity of antimicrobial agents against micro-organisms depends on two major factors – the nature of the physical environment and the condition of the organism. Three main aspects require consideration. These various aspects are comprehensively reviewed by Russell (1982) and only practically issues are summarized here.

Pretreatment factors

The structure and functioning of bacterial cells and their sensitivity to antibacterial agents may be profoundly affected by the conditions under which they are grown (Gilbert 1988). Thus, for mechanism of action studies, it is important that the conditions used for cultivation and those involved in the preparation of test suspensions, be identical and rigorously controlled.

Factors during treatment

Any number of environmental factors may affect the activity of an antibacterial agent. This may involve effects on the bacterial cell itself or alternatively (or possibly additionally) may result from direct effects on the agent. Only those factors which are well known and have been most extensively studied are summarized below. They serve to stress the importance of rigorous control of experimental conditions for mechanism of action studies.

Concentration of antibacterial agent

The activity of antibacterial agents may be profoundly affected by relatively minor changes in concentration. The concentration exponent (η), used for quantitative assessment of the relationship between activity and concentration, is calculated from the equation:

$$\eta = \frac{\log t_2 - \log t_1}{\log c_1 - \log c_2}$$

where t_1 and t_2 are the times taken to produce a given reduction in survivors with antibacterial concentrations c_1 and c_2, respectively.

Concentration exponents for antibacterial agents may range from 1 for formaldehyde, quaternary ammonium and mercury compounds up to 6 for phenols and 10 for alcohols. To a certain extent, the concentration exponent may be indicative of the mechanism of action (Hugo & Denyer 1987).

Temperature

The activity of antibacterial agents usually increases geometrically with increasing temperature. Temperature effects may be calculated from the following formula:

$$\theta^{(T_2 - T_1)} = \frac{k_2}{k_1}$$

where k_2 and k_1 are the death rate constants at temperatures T_2 and T_1, respectively. The temperature coefficient (θ) refers to the effect of temperature per 1°C rise and for a 10°C rise Q_{10} is used. Q_{10} values can vary from 1.0 to nearly 300 (Berry & Michaels 1950; Bean 1967; Hugo & Russell 1987).

Number of organisms

In general the activity of an antibacterial agent decreases as the inoculum size increases. The extent of this effect varies with different antibacterial agents but it is important that studies of antibacterial activity are carried out with inocula which are similar in size to those used for biochemical and other studies. Problems associated with the use of large inocula for studying bacteriostasis are discussed later.

Environmental pH

Environmental pH can affect antimicrobial activity in a number of ways:
1 It may affect the activity of the antimicrobial agent. Many antibacterial agents are weak acids or weak bases. Experience has shown that the majority of agents are more active in their unionized form. Activity of these agents will therefore depend on their pK_a in relation to the pH of the suspending medium. The interaction of chemically reactive agents such as chlorine and glutaraldehyde with cell constituents may also be affected by pH.
2 It may produce changes in the charge distribution of the bacterial cell surface thereby affecting uptake of charged antibacterial agents.

Other constituents of the suspending medium

All constituents of the suspending medium should be considered in terms of possible effects on antibacterial activity. Neutralizing effects of organic matter on the activity of disinfectant formulations have been widely studied. Surface active agents which are common formulation components in pharmaceuticals, cosmetic and other formulations may also affect activity. In general, it would seem that at concentrations of surface active agent below the critical micelle concentration (CMC), activity of the antibacterial agent is potentiated due to effects of the surfactant on the cell surface which increase permeability. At concentrations above the CMC, interaction and micellization produce a reduction in the aqueous phase concentration of 'free' antibacterial agent causing reduced activity. Metal cations and chelators such as EDTA can also have a marked effect on activity.

Other factors

Mechanism of action studies are usually carried out with aqueous suspensions of test organisms. Experimental observations with pharmaceutical and other formulations show that where a solid or non-miscible liquid phase is introduced, loss of activity may occur as a result of adsorption or partitioning. For mechanism of action studies which are invariably carried out *in vitro*, the possibility of interaction with glass or other container surfaces must be considered. Laboratory investigations suggest that loss of activity can result from adsorption of agents on container surfaces. Reduced sensitivity to antibacterials may also be associated with growth of organisms as biofilms on glass or PVC surfaces. Experiments by Hugo *et al.* (1986) indicated that adsorption of *Pseudomonas cepacia* on to the surface of glass containers enabled cells to survive in the presence of 0.05% (w/v) chlorhexidine. The organisms were firmly attached to the glass and colonized glass slides could be used to infect uncontaminated chlorhexidine solutions.

Neutralization and recovery of organisms

In quantifying antibacterial activity, assessment of viability is usually based on organisms' ability to grow and divide, producing visible turbidity or surface colonies. It must be borne in mind, however, that a cell may recover to initiate growth under one set of conditions but not under another; the viability of a population is never an 'absolute' value, but relates to the conditions under which it was determined. Another factor, sometimes overlooked in mechanism of action studies, is that viability is usually assessed from the ability of cells to initiate growth after neutralization of the agent and the results are then interpreted in conjunction with biochemical assays in which the agent is maintained in contact with the cells throughout the study.

For evaluation of antibacterial activity two aspects of recovery must be considered.

Neutralization of antibacterial agents

For accurate assessment of surviving organisms following contact with anti-bacterial agents, activity must be arrested at the moment of sampling. It is also important that concentrations of agents which might inhibit the growth of survivors are not transferred to recovery media. This is usually achieved by means of inactivating agents which overcome the activity of inhibitory agents. The inactivator must itself be non-toxic to the bacteria and any product resulting from neutralization must also be non-toxic. Where appropriate, inactivators may be added directly to reaction mixtures. Alternatively, they may be added to diluents and/or recovery media as appropriate.

Examples of suitable inactivating agents are shown in Table 1. Non-ionic detergents such as polysorbate 80 (Tween 80) may be used alone at high concentration (up to 10%) or at a lower concentration (3%) mixed with lecithin (0.3%) to inactivate quaternary ammonium compounds, chlorhexidine, phenols and hexachlorophene. Egg lecithin or soya bean lecithin (90% purity) should be used. Lecithin is insoluble in water but may be dispersed by mixing with the warm detergent before making solutions up to volume. Lecithin produces cloudiness in the medium which may interfere with detection of growth.

Sodium thiosulphate inactivates chlorine and iodine but may be inhibitory

TABLE 1. *Inactivating agents for some antimicrobial agents*

Antimicrobial agent	Inactivating agent
Phenols and cresols	Dilution Tween 80
p-hydroxybenzoates	Dilution Tween 80
Chlorine and iodine	Sodium thiosulphate Sodium sulphite Nutrient broth
Glutaraldehyde Formaldehyde	Glycine Dimedone and morpholine
Quaternary ammonium compounds and chlorhexidine	Lubrol and lecithin Tween 80 and lecithin
Mercury compounds	Thioglycollic acid
Bronopol	Cysteine

to staphylococci, hence the suggestion that the concentration in the recovery medium should not exceed 0.1% (w/v) (Kayser & Van der Ploeg 1965; Gross *et al.* 1973). Sulphite (0.1%) may be less toxic than thiosulphate to bacteria (Green & Litsky 1974). Low concentrations of chlorine and iodine may be adequately inactivated by protein material in nutrient media (MacKinnon 1974).

Formaldehyde and glutaraldehyde are difficult to inactivate because excess sodium bisulphite will inhibit growth of bacteria and germination of spores. Mixtures of dimedone and morpholine may be used for formaldehye (Nash & Hirch 1954), and glycine (1–2% w/v) for inactivation of glutaraldehye (Gorman & Scott 1976; Cheung & Brown 1982). Inactivation of bronopol by 0.1% (w/v) cysteine is described by Moore & Stretton (1978).

Antibacterial agents such as phenols with high dilution coefficients may be inactivated by dilution. For phenols, inactivation is usually achieved by dilution to less than 0.01% (w/v).

All evaluations must include controls to demonstrate the efficacy and non-toxicity of neutralization systems. This can be done by mixing antibacterial agents at appropriate concentrations with neutralization systems followed by addition of known numbers of viable cells. Suspensions are then diluted and plated to establish that there is no reduction in the number of recoverable organisms. It is possible, however, that a greater number of organisms may be recovered under these conditions than from test samples where antibacterial agents interact with bacterial cells before contact with neutralizing agents (e.g.

phenols and quats) where recovery on plating from a series of dilutions may increase with increasing dilution (e.g. plates may show 200 colonies at 10^{-1} dilution, but 50 at 10^{-2} dilution). This may occur despite the fact that control tests indicate satisfactory neutralization at 10^{-1} dilution.

Laboratory investigations by El-Khouly & Youssef (1974) and Leak (1983) suggest that optimum concentrations of inactivators such as Tween/lecithin and thioglycollate for recovery of organisms following treatment with p-hydroxybenzoic acid esters and chlorhexidine or mercurial compounds, respectively, may be different for different bacterial species.

An alternative approach to neutralization involves membrane filtration. Samples of reaction mixtures are filtered through membrane filters which are washed *in situ* to remove traces of the antibacterial agent. The membrane is transferred to the surface of an appropriate nutrient agar medium. Nutrients diffusing through the membrane support growth of colonies arising from surviving organisms.

Conditions for initiation of growth of micro-organisms

Where dilution of suspensions is required for viable counting, either water, quarter-strength Ringer solution, 0.9% saline, peptone water or nutrient broth may be used. Laboratory observations suggest that the composition of the diluent may profoundly affect subsequent recovery of damaged bacteria. Recovery of bacteria may likewise be affected by the composition of the growth medium and the time and temperature of incubation. In some cases, optimum conditions for recovery of injured microbes are quite different from those used for cultivation; Harris (1963) showed that the optimum temperature for growth of phenol-damaged bacteria was 28°C.

Methods for recovery and revival of injured micro-organisms are discussed in more detail by Russell *et al.* (1979) and Russell (1981).

Tests for Determining Bacteriostatic Activity

In determining the minimum growth inhibitory concentration (MIC) of a bacteriostatic agent, the organisms is introduced into the system which contains the antimicrobial agent but which also provides optimum nutrients and environmental conditions for growth. Following an incubation period (usually 18–24h) the culture is examined either visually or by other means to assess whether there is an increase in numbers of viable cells.

In relating the results of MIC determinations to biochemical studies, two major problems are encountered:

1 Whereas biochemical or other studies are usually carried out with aqueous, saline or buffered suspensions, for MIC determinations, nutrient materials

which may range from simple salts to undefined bacteriological media constituents such as meat extract and peptone, must be included. As mentioned
previously both the growth media and growth environment (e.g. incubation
temperature) may affect activity.

2   Experimental investigations show clearly that MIC values will depend on
inoculum size, MICs increasing with increasing inoculum size. For mode of
action studies, the sensitivity of many biochemical assays dictates the use of
suspensions containing about $1-5 \times 10^9$ organisms/ml ($c.$ 1 mg dry weight
organic material per ml), whereas MICs are normally determined with inoculum
sizes of 10^3-10^5 organisms/ml, which in batch culture will grow to a maximum
of about 5×10^8 organisms/ml, as determined by availability of nutrients and
oxygen, the production of toxic metabolites and other inhibitory factors.
Investigations by Hugo & Bloomfield (1971) have shown that it is possible
with organisms such as *Staphylococcus aureus* and *Escherichia coli* to observe
growth, and thus determine MICs, with inocula as high as 3×10^9 or 4×10^9
organisms/ml using washed suspensions introduced into fresh media under
conditions of forced aeration.

In the laboratory, bacteriostatic assays generally involve either agar diffusion
techniques in which inhibition zones are used for assessment of activity or
serial dilution methods in which the MIC is determined.

Agar diffusion techniques

These tests are relatively simple and may be either 'qualitative' (i.e. simple
screening for activity against a range of micro-organisms) or 'quantitative' (i.e.
determination of the concentrations of antibacterial agent required to inhibit
growth).

For qualitative assay, as shown in Fig. 2, a nutrient agar plate is inoculated
with micro-organisms either by adding the organisms to the agar before it is
poured, or by streaking the organisms across the surface of the plate. For
seeded plates a solution of the antibacterial is introduced into cups which can
be cut into the surface of the plate using a sterile cork borer or impregnated
on sterile filter paper discs which are then placed on the agar surface. For
streak plates the antibacterial solution is pipetted into a trough cut into the
agar at right angles to the streaks or again impregnated on a filter paper strip
which is placed on the agar surface. One of the advantages of using filter
paper discs or strips is that the paper can be dried before placing on the agar
surface. This is useful for low-water-soluble antibacterial agents. These can
be dissolved in organic solvents which can be evaporated off to avoid any toxic
effects which may occur from the solvent itself. Evaporation of solvents from
filter paper discs is usually done using an infra-red lamp bulb. It must be
borne in mind however, that agents which low water solubility may show

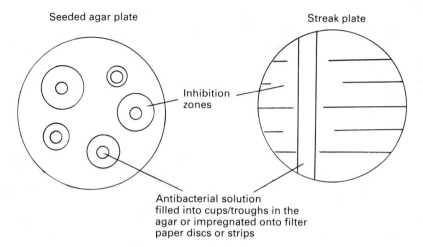

FIG. 2. Qualitative assay of antibacterial agents by agar diffusion methods.

limited agar diffusion. Following storage for a short period (2–3 h) to allow diffusion of the antibacterial agent into the agar without microbial growth, plates are then incubated and the radius of the inhibition zone measured. Zone diameters may be used to give a measure of the relative activity against a range of micro-organisms. Since the size of the diffusion zone depends on the rate of diffusion, quantitative assessment of MICs by this method requires a knowledge of the diffusion rate of the compound under investigation.

In order to use diffusion methods in quantitative estimations of antibacterial activity, the equation of Eversole & Doughty (1935) is applied:

$$M_t = M_o \exp^- \left(\frac{x^2}{4Dt}\right), \tag{1}$$

or

$$x^2 = 4Dt \ln \left(\frac{M_o}{M_t}\right). \tag{2}$$

This refers to a solution of constant concentration (M_o) consisting of neutral particles in contact with an infinite column of pure water or agar, which at zero time is free from solute: as diffusion takes place into this column, at a time t the concentration (M_t) at a distance x from the original junction is given by equation (1); D is the diffusion coefficient which is the amount of solute which would diffuse across a unit area under a concentration gradient of unity in unit time if the rate were constant during that time.

In practice, a solution of the antibacterial substance of concentration M_o is placed on the surface of seeded agar in a tube or in a cup cut into a plate of seeded agar; after incubation a zone of inhibition is observed extending for a distance x from the edge of the tube or cup (Fig. 3).

Under experimental conditions the inoculum, temperature, medium and incubation times can be kept constant and thus $4Dt$ will be constant. The equation can then be written as:

$$\ln M_o = \text{constant} \times x^2 + \ln M_t.$$

Thus $\ln M_o$ is proportional to the square of the length of the inhibition zone (x) and on plotting x^2 against $\ln M_o$ (as shown in Fig. 3) a straight line is obtained, intercepting the concentration axis at $\ln M_t$.

The value of M_t obtained from the graph is known as the critical concentration and this is usually 2−4 times greater than the minimum inhibitory concentration as found by broth dilution methods.

Diffusion assays are used routinely for assay of antibiotics, vitamins, etc., in situations where chemical assays are not appropriate. These assays involve a comparison of inhibition zones for solutions of unknown potency with a standard solution of known potency. From regression plots of $\ln M_o$ against x^2, the potency ratio is determined and can be used to calculate the potency of the unknown solution. Investigations in relation to antibiotic assays suggest that accuracy depends on a number of factors (Lees & Tootill 1955).

A useful modification of the agar diffusion assay which allows direct

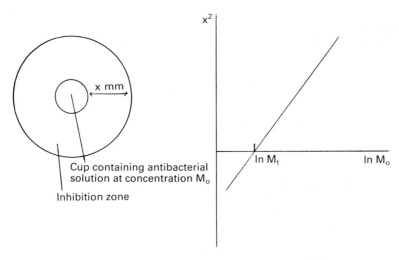

FIG. 3. Quantitative assay of antibacterial agents by agar diffusion methods.

determination of MICs is the gradient plate method (Fig. 4). For this assay, square Petri dishes (y cm across) are required. The plates are tilted and molten agar (10 ml) containing a known concentration (C µg/ml) of antibacterial agent is added. The agar is allowed to set in the form of a wedge and the plates are then laid flat. A second 10-ml volume of molten agar is added and allowed to set. Plates are then stored to allow for diffusion to occur giving a concentration gradient across the plate from C to 0 µg/ml. A number of test organisms can then be streaked on the surface of the gradient or alternatively the plate can be overlaid with $2-3$ ml molten agar seeded with a simple test organism. Following incubation the zone of inhibition (x) is measured and the MIC calculated from the equation:

$$\text{MIC (µg/ml)} = \frac{y - x}{y} \times C \,\text{µg/ml}.$$

Serial dilution methods

For determination of MICs by serial dilution methods, graded concentrations of the agent are added to nutrient broth or nutrient agar. For achieving the required concentration range of water-soluble compounds, concentrated solution may be added to double- or triple-strength broth and made up to volume with water as appropriate. For compounds of low water solubility, intermediary solvents may be required to achieve the desired concentration range in which case the system must be checked to ensure that the quantity of solvent added is not inhibitory. Laboratory experience suggests that volumes of $50-100$ µl per 10 ml broth of solvents such as chloroform, acetone, methyl and ethyl alcohol are satisfactory, although the sensitivity to these solvents may vary from one species to another and should be checked. Mode of action studies with the chlorinated phenolic compound Fentichlor (Hugo & Bloom-

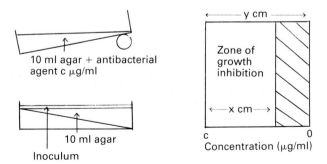

FIG. 4. Gradient plate method for determination of minimum growth inhibitory concentration (MIC).

field 1971) indicated that for compounds of low water solubility, antibacterial activity may continue to increase at concentrations above saturation.

For determining MICs, media are then inoculated with test organisms, incubated and the MIC determined as the lowest concentration which inhibits visible growth. One of the advantages of using agar as opposed to broth dilution is that a number of test organisms can be inoculated on to a single series of plates. Although serial dilution provides a direct quantitative assessment of active concentrations, it must be remembered that, in effect, the MIC is a concentration which lies between the observed maximum inhibitory concentration and the minimum inhibitory concentration. Thus the accuracy of the end-point will depend on the range of concentrations used. In practice, for initial screening it is usual to employ a series of 10-fold or doubling concentrations, e.g. 0.001, 0.01, 0.1, 1.0, ..., 10% (w/v), or 0.01, 0.02, 0.04, 0.08, ... % (w/v). Once the approximate MIC is known, an arithmetical series of initially not less than eight dilutions is employed, e.g. 0.1, 0.2, 0.3, 0.4, ... % (w/v). In practice the choice of dilutions should take into account the concentration exponent of the agent under consideration.

Bacteriostatic assays — determination of end-point

For the majority of methods described so far, identification of MICs depends on visible growth. Laboratory observations would suggest that the lower level of visible detection for bacterial growth in nutrient media is of the order of $1-5 \times 10^8$ organisms/ml. In practice, as described previously, a compound may show partial inhibition whereby an inoculum of 10^3-10^5 may undergo a number of generations without visible detection. Experience has shown that the sensitivity of detection of opacity can to a certain extent be increased by the use of instrumentation such as the biophotometer. Mode of action studies involving continuous optical density monitoring are described by Brown & Richards (1964) and Brown & Winsley (1971). For detection of very low levels of viable organisms, counting procedures as described for bactericidal tests are usually employed.

Tests for Determining Bactericidal Activity

Essentially all determinations of bactericidal activity comprise three main phases:
1 Bacterial suspension is added to a solution of the antibacterial agent at a given concentration.
2 At measured contact times samples of cells are removed and the agent neutralized by suitable means.
3 A sample of the neutralized suspension is transferred to nutrient medium and its viability assessed.

Methods for quantifying bactericidal action generally fall into two groups as illustrated in Fig. 5. These may be either extinction time (end-point) methods or viable counting methods.

Extinction time methods

Extinction time methods can be of three types:

1 Determination of the time taken to kill a fixed inoculum using a given concentration of antibacterial agent (mean death time, MDT).

2 Determination of the minimum concentration required to produce total kill within a given time period (minimum bactericidal concentration, MBC).

3 Determination of the time required to reduce the number of surviving organisms to one using a given concentration of antibacterial agent (mean single survivor time, MSST).

The method for MDT determination is best illustrated from a set of results as given in Fig. 5. A standard inoculum is added to a solution of the antibacterial agent. Samples are taken at intervals, and transferred to recovery medium which is incubated and examined for growth. The extinction time is determined for a number of replicate samples from which the MDT can be calculated. A similar approach is used to determine the MBC for a fixed death time where the concentration rather than the contact time is varied.

Experience has shown a number of variations in relation to the design and interpretation of such tests. These can be illustrated by comparing the results of MDT determinations with time-survivor curves (Fig. 5).

1 *Distribution of resistance of test organisms.* Variation in MDT or MBC determinations can be partly explained on the basis of variation in antibacterial sensitivity within the population: if several replicate tests are performed over the initial period, the viable population is usually of the order of $10^2 - 10^7$ cells/sample. In this situation the death rate will reflect the average resistance of the population. In the latter stages of the time-survivor curve, the number of survivors will be small $(1 - 10$ organisms/sample) and the death rate will be determined by the resistance of individual cells. Thus a different end-point may be obtained in replicate tests, the end-point depending on the recovery of one or a few atypical cells within the population.

2 *Sampling errors.* Variation may occur as a result of errors which arise from sampling a small volume from the total reaction mixture. If an MDT determination is performed and a number of samples are removed from a single reaction mixture, up to the point where there is more than 1 organism per sample (point x, Fig. 5) then all samples will be positive. Between points x and y (after y all samples will be negative) where the number of survivors is less than 1 per sample, the frequency with which positive or negative samples are obtained will follow the Poisson distribution, $p = e^{-N}$, where p is the proportion of negative samples and N is the number of viable organisms per sample.

In an attempt to avoid the problems associated with sampling errors, Berry & Bean (1954) developed an alternative method in which Poisson distribution theory was developed to allow estimation of the MSST. The theory is similar to that used for most probable number counts and is illustrated in Fig. 5.

From Poisson distribution:

$$p = e^{-N},$$

$$N = \frac{-\ln p}{\ln e}$$

but $\ln e = \ln 2.718 = 1$.

Converting to natural logarithms (as shown in Fig. 5):

$$\ln N = \ln (- \ln p).$$

If we plot a time-survivor curve of $\ln (-\ln p)$ against time (t) a straight line will result where

$$\ln (- \ln p) = 0, N = 1.$$

Thus, if we determine the time at which $\ln (- \ln p)$ intercepts the time axis (i.e. $\ln (- \ln p) = 0$), then this is the MSST.

This method has the advantage that a more precise estimate of the time required to achieve a specific level of kill is obtained, but this precision will depend on performing a substantial number of estimates (>20). The method also requires a preliminary knowledge of the extinction zone.

Viable counting methods

Tests described above depend essentially on determining an end-point at which there is a single or undetectably low number of survivors. Although this approach gives information regarding the time at which survivors are reduced to an undetectable level, it gives little information on the time course of the bactericidal action and in view of the non-linear nature of time-survivor curves, end-point determinations taken in isolation can be misleading.

Viable counting methods again involve inoculating standard numbers of cells into a solution of the antibacterial agent. At standard time intervals samples are withdrawn and the number of viable organisms determined by colony counting procedures.

As with all methods, the number of recoverable organisms depends on a number of factors. It is important that, at the moment of sampling, the action of the agent is immediately arrested, otherwise continuing mortality or bacteriostasis may occur. Where the original suspension contains large numbers of organisms (say 10^6-10^8 organisms/ml) the sample of suspension must be

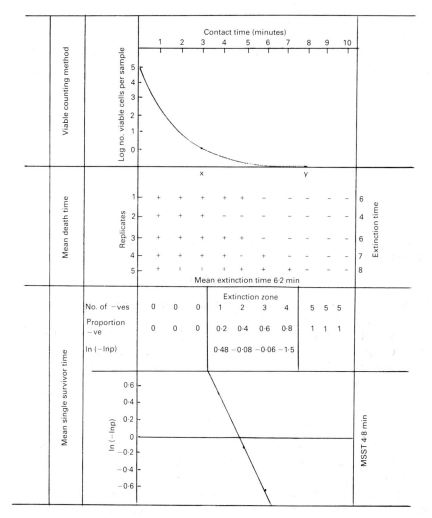

FIG. 5. Methods used for the determination of bactericidal activity.

diluted such that the sample plated contains a countable number of colonies. Laboratory observations indicate that the nature of the neutralizer, the dilution fluid and the medium and incubation conditions used for colony counting can profoundly affect the number of cells which retain viability and form colonies on plating. All of these aspects are discussed in the earlier section on 'Neutralization and recovery of organisms'.

For colony counting, any of the standard methods may be used. For the pour plate method, the suspension is added to molten agar at 45°C. For the surface viable count method, standard volumes of suspension are dropped on to the surface of a nutrient agar plate which has been surface dried in a 30−37°C incubator or laminar flow cabinet for 2−3 h.

For accurate counting, it is suggested that 2−3 replicate plates should be prepared, each containing 50−200 colonies. After incubation of plates, colonies are counted and, based on the assumption that each colony arose from a single recoverable cell, the viability of the neutralized sample can be calculated. Serious errors can, however, occur in situations where the agent causes clumping of cells. If the clumping is serious then one colony may represent not one single organism but a clump of, for instance, 100 cells. This occurs most frequently with agents such as the quaternary ammonium compounds and chlorhexidine. The bacterial cell surface bears a negative charge and where this becomes neutralized by positively charged molecules then clumping may occur. In this situation alternative methods based on a most probable number estimate, such as the mean single survivor time method, have been used (Hugo & Longworth 1964).

An alternative method of preparing surface viable count plates is provided by the spiral plater. Although the instrument requires considerable financial outlay, this automated method for the preparation of plates represents a considerable saving in time and materials. The spiral plater is designed to deposit a known volume of sample on a rotating agar plate in an ever decreasing amount in the form of an Archimedian spiral. After incubation, different colony densities are apparent on the surface of the plate. A modified counting grid is provided which relates the area of the plate to the volume of the sample. By counting an appropriate area of the plate, the number of bacteria in the sample is estimated. Counting of plates can be done manually or by means of a laser counter. The fact that for the spiral plater (compared with traditional pour plate and surface viable methods) the colonies are spread evenly over the central area of the plates increases the accuracy of the laser counting technique. Statistical comparisons of the results of spiral plating compared with traditional methods is given by Gilchrist *et al.* (1973) and Jarvis *et al.* (1977).

The Use of Rapid Methods for Evaluation of Antimicrobial Activity

Over the past few years increasing attention has been paid to the development of rapid methods for estimation of microbial viability. The fundamental principle of all these methods is that they can be used for early detection of much smaller populations (10^3-10^5 organisms/ml) of bacteria compared with conventional methods which require at least 18−24 h growth to give about 10^8

organisms/ml. A number of different methods are available including electrical methods, microcalorimetry, 'direct epifluorescent' filtration techniques (DEFT), adenosine-5'-triphosphate (ATP), bioluminescence and radiometry. Each of these methods has its particular advantages and limitations. The various methods and their applications and limitations are reviewed in detail by Leech (1988).

At present the main application of these methods is in quality control of manufactured products such as food, beverages, pharmaceuticals and cosmetics, where early detection of growing microbial populations has obvious commercial advantages. The use of rapid methods to facilitate economic and rapid screening of biocides for use as preservatives, disinfectants and so on is also under investigation.

Although attractive in principle, there are a number of problems. In using these methods to assess antibacterial activity it is important to realize that the methods are indirect and depend on the detection of metabolic activities such as breakdown of nutrients, ATP-ase, production of heat, etc. Quantitative evaluation of viable populations presupposes a constant relationship between metabolic activity and viability. In contact with antimicrobial agents this relationship will vary from one agent to another according to its mode of action. For mechanism of action studies, it is obvious therefore that these methods may find application not as a method of viable counting but to facilitate studies of the effects of antimicrobial agents on cell function.

Factors affecting the Accuracy of Bacteriostatic and Bactericidal Assays

In evaluating the activity of antibacterial agents, the accuracy of the estimate obtained will depend on three factors:
1   experimental design;
2   rigorous control of experimental conditions;
3   the number of replicate tests performed.
Factors which can affect the activity of an antibacterial agent have already been discussed and they indicate the need for rigorous control of experimental conditions. Laboratory experience and deliberately planned experiments have shown that even quite minimal differences such as batch-to-batch variation of standard laboratory media and slight adjustments in laboratory techniques can have a significant effect on the results obtained.

Over the years a number of standard tests have been introduced for application to disinfectant formulations. Results of collaborative trials with these tests both within and between laboratories can be used to give some idea of the accuracy of the various methods described in this chapter.

For standard end-point tests such as the Rideal−Walker and Chick−Martin tests where sampling errors represent a particular problem, it is estimated that the between-laboratory reproducibility is of the order of 30% (Croshaw 1981). Obviously, the MSST test, in which the end-point is estimated from a much larger number of replicates, may be used to improve the reproducibility of estimates.

In an attempt to improve the repeatability and reproducibility of standard disinfectant tests, various European countries have developed a quantitative suspension test in which the concentration required to produce a given 'anti microbial effect' (usually a 5-log reduction) is determined. These tests are reviewed by Reybrouk (1982). Statistical evaluations of repeatability and reproducibility as determined from collaborative trials are described by Van Klingeren et al. (1977), Reybrouk et al. (1979) and Van Klingeren et al. (1981).

References

BEAN, H.S. 1967. Types and characteristics of disinfectants. *Journal of Applied Bacteriology* **30**, 6–16.

BERRY, H. & BEAN, H.S. 1954. The estimation of bactericidal activity from extinction time data. *Journal of Pharmacy and Pharmacology* **6**, 649–655.

BERRY, H. & MICHAELS, I. 1950. The evaluation of the bactericidal activity of ethylene glycol and some of its monoalkyl ethers against *Bacterium coli*. *Journal of Pharmacy and Pharmacology* **2**, 243–249.

BROWN, M.R.W. & RICHARDS, R.M.E. 1964. The effect of Tween 80 on the resistance of *Pseudomonas aeruginosa* to chemical inactivation. *Journal of Pharmacy and Pharmacology* **16**, 51–55.

BROWN, M.R.W. & WINSLEY, B.E. 1971. Synergism between Polymixin and Polysorbate 80 against *Pseudomonas aeruginosa*. *Journal of General Microbiology* **68**, 367–373.

CERF, O. 1977. Tailing of survival curves of bacterial spores. *Journal of Applied Bacteriology* **42**, 1–20.

CHEUNG, H.Y. & BROWN, M.R.W. 1982. Evaluation of glycine as an inactivator of glutaraldehyde. *Journal of Pharmacy and Pharmacology* **34**, 211–214.

CROSHAW, B. 1981. Disinfectant testing with particular reference to the Rideal-Walker and Kelsey-Sykes Tests. In *Disinfectants: their Use and Evaluation of Effectiveness*, ed. Collins, C.H., Allwood, M.C., Bloomfield, S.F. & Fox, A. pp. 1–16. Society for Applied Bacteriology Technical Series No. 16. London: Academic Press.

EL-KHOULY, A.E. & YOUSSEF, R.T. 1974. Antibacterial effectiveness of mercurials. *Journal of Pharmaceutical Science* **63**, 681–685.

EVERSOLE, W.G. & DOUGHTY, E.W. 1935. The diffusion coefficients of molecules and ions from measurements of undisturbed diffusion in a stationary medium. *Journal of Physical Chemistry* **39**, 289–292.

GILBERT, P. 1988. Microbial resistance to preservative systems. In *Microbial Quality Assurance in Pharmaceuticals, Cosmetics and Toiletries*, ed. Bloomfield, S.F., Baird, R., Leak, R.E. & Leach, R. pp. 171–191. Chichester: Ellis Horwood.

GILCHRIST, J.E., CAMPBELL, J.E., DONNELLY, C.B., PEELER, J.T. & DELANEY, J.M. 1973. Spiral plate method for bacterial determination. *Applied Microbiology* **25**, 244–252.

GORMAN, S.P. & SCOTT, E.M. 1976. Evaluation of potential inactivators of glutaraldehyde in disinfection studies with *Escherichia coli*. *Microbios Letters* **1**, 197–204.

GREEN, B.L. & LITSKY, W. 1974. The use of sodium sulfite as a neutralizer for evaluating povidone–iodine preparations. *Health Laboratory Science* **11**, 188–194.

GROSS, A., COFONE, L. & HUFF, M.B. 1973. Iodine inactivating agent in surgical scrub testing. *Archives of Surgery* **106**, 175–178.

HARRIS, N.D. 1963. The influence of recovery medium and incubation temperature on the survival of damaged bacteria. *Journal of Applied Bacteriology* **26**, 387–397.

HUGO, W.B. & BLOOMFIELD, S.F. 1971. Studies of the mode of action of the phenolic antibacterial agent Fentichlor against *Staphylococcus aureus* and *Escherichia coli*. 1. The adsorption of Fentichlor by the bacterial cell and its antibacterial activity. *Journal of Applied Bacteriology* **34**, 557–567.

HUGO, W.B. & DENYER, S.P. 1987. The concentration exponent of disinfectants and preservatives (biocides). In *Preservatives in the Food, Pharmaceutical and Environmental Industries*, ed. Board, R.G., Allwood, M.C. & Banks, J.G. pp. 281–291. Society for Applied Bacteriology Technical Series No. 22. Oxford: Blackwell Scientific Publications.

HUGO, W.B. & LONGWORTH, A.R. 1964. Some aspects of the mode of action of chlorhexidine. *Journal of Pharmacy and Pharmacology* **16**, 655–662.

HUGO, W.B., PALLENT, L.J., GRANT, D.J.W., DENYER, S.P. & DAVIES, A. 1986. Factors contributing to the survival of a strain of *Pseudomonas cepacia* in chlorhexidine solution. *Letters in Applied Microbiology* **2**, 37–42.

HUGO, W.B. & RUSSELL, A.D. 1987. Evaluation of non-antibiotic antimicrobial agents. In *Pharmaceutical Microbiology*, 4th edn, ed. Hugo, W.B. & Russell, A.D. pp. 253–280. London: Academic Press.

JARVIS, B., LACH, V.H. & WOOD, J.M. 1977. Evaluation of the spiral plate maker for the enumeration of micro-organisms in foods. *Journal of Applied Bacteriology* **43**, 149–157.

KAYSER, A. & VAN DER PLOEG, G. 1965. Growth inhibition of staphylococci by sodium thiosulphate. *Journal of Applied Bacteriology* **28**, 286–293.

LEAK, R.E. 1983. Some factors affecting the preservative testing of aqueous systems. *PhD thesis*, University of London.

LEECH, R. 1988. New methodology for microbiological quality assurance. In *Microbial Quality Assurance in Pharmaceuticals, Cosmetics and Toiletries*, ed. Bloomfield, S.F., Baird, R., Leak, R.E. & Leech, R. pp. 195–216. Chichester: Ellis Horwood.

LEES, K.W. & TOOTILL, J.P.R. 1955. Microbiological assay on large plates. Part I. General consideration with particular reference to routine assay. *Analyst* **80**, 95–110.

MACKINNON, I.H. 1974. The use of inactivators in the evaluation of disinfectants. *Journal of Hygiene* **74**, 189–195.

MOORE, K.E. & STRETTON, R.J. 1978. A method for studying the activity of preservatives and its application to Bronopol. *Journal of Applied Bacteriology* **45**, 137–141.

NASH, T. & HIRCH, A. 1954. The revival of formaldehyde-treated bacteria. *Journal of Applied Chemistry* **4**, 458–463.

REYBROUK, G. 1982. The evaluation of the antimicrobial activity of disinfectants. In *Principles and Practice of Disinfection, Sterilization and Preservation*, ed. Russell, A.D., Hugo, W.B. & Ayliffe, G.A.J. pp. 134–157. London: Academic Press.

REYBROUK, G., BORNEFF, J., VAN DE VOORDE, H. & WERNER, H.P. 1979. A collaborative study on a new quantitative suspension test, the *in vitro* test for the evaluation of the bactericidal activity of chemical disinfectants. *Zentralblatt für Backteriologie, Parasitenkunde, Infektionskrankheiten und Hygiene, I. Abteilung Originale, Reihe B* **168**, 463–479.

RUSSELL, A.D. 1981. Neutralization procedures in the evaluation of bactericidal activity. In *Disinfectants: their Use and Evaluation of Effectiveness*, ed. Collins, C.H., Allwood, M.C., Bloomfield, S.F. & Fox, A. pp. 45–59. Society for Applied Bacteriology Technical Series No. 16. London: Academic Press.

RUSSELL, A.D. 1982. Factors influencing the efficacy of antimicrobial agents. In *Principles and Practice of Disinfection, Preservation and Sterilization*, ed. Russell, A.D., Hugo, W.B. & Ayliffe, G.A.J. pp. 107–133. London: Academic Press.

RUSSELL, A.D., AHONKHAI, I. & ROGERS, D.T. 1979. Microbiological applications of the inactivation of antibiotics and other antimicrobial agents. *Journal of Applied Bacteriology* **46**, 207–245.

VAN KLINGEREN, B., LEUSSINK, A.B. & PULLEN, W. 1981. *A European collaborative study on the repeatability and reproducibility of the standard suspension test for the evaluation of disinfectants in food hygiene*. National Institute of Public Health, Bilthoven, The Netherlands.

VAN KLINGEREN, B., LEUSSINK, A.B. & VAN, WIJNGAARDEN, L.J. 1977. A collaborative study on the repeatability and the reproducibility of the Dutch Standard-suspension-test for the evaluation of disinfectants. *Zentralblatt für Bakteriologie, Parasitenkunde, Infektionskrankheiten und Hygiene, I. Abteilung Originale, Reihe B* **164**, 521–548.

Effects of Chemical Agents on Bacterial Sporulation, Germination and Outgrowth

A.D. RUSSELL,[1] B.N. DANCER[2] AND E.G.M. POWER[1]

[1]Welsh School of Pharmacy; and [2]School of Pure and Applied Biology, University of Wales College of Cardiff, Cardiff CF1 3XF, UK

The bacterial spore is a complex entity which is resistant to many chemical and physical agents (Russell 1982, 1983, 1990a, b; Waites 1982, 1985). However, this resistance is lost during germination and/or outgrowth and is regained during the complex series of events comprising sporulation (Russell et al. 1989).

It is the purpose of this paper to consider some of the techniques available for studying the effects of chemical agents on the bacterial spore and its associated forms, and to discuss how the agents act and how resistance may arise.

Determination of Sporostatic Activity

Theoretical aspects

The minimum growth inhibitory concentration (MIC) of an antibacterial agent is the lowest concentration which inhibits bacterial growth. In the present context, it is used to refer to the lowest concentration preventing germination and/or outgrowth. As pointed out by Russell (1982), there is a close relationship between the MIC of a substance against Gram-positive non-spore-forming bacteria and the MIC of that substance against vegetative cell development from spores (Table 1). General methods for laboratory assessment of antibacterial activity are given by Spooner & Sykes (1972) and by Bloomfield (this book).

Practical considerations

Sporostatic activity can be determined in a manner similar to that used for measuring bacteriostatic potency. In essence, experiments are of two types:

Mechanisms of Action of
Chemical Biocides

23

TABLE 1. *Inhibitory and lethal concentrations of some antibacterial agents* against sporulating and non-sporulating Gram-positive bacteria*

Antibacterial agent[†]	Inhibitory concentration (% w/v)		Lethal concentration (% w/v)	
	Bacteriostatic	Sporostatic	Bactericidal	Sporicidal[‡]
Chlorocresol	0.02	0.02	0.1	>0.4
Cresol	0.08	0.1	0.3	>0.5
Phenol	0.2	0.2	0.5	>5
BZK	0.0004	0.0005		
CPC	0.0005	0.00025	0.002	>0.05
CHA	0.0001	0.0001	0.002	>0.05
PMN	0.00001	0.00002	0.002	>0.02
Glutaraldehyde			<0.1	2.0
Formaldehyde			<1	8.0
Hypochlorite			$1-2$ parts/10^6	$50-100$ parts/10^6

* Lethal effect may depend on pH, temperature and period of treatment.
[†] BZK, benzalkonium chloride; CPC, cetylpyridinium chloride; CHA, chlorhexidine diacetate; PMN, phenylmercuric nitrate.
[‡] In some instances, agents are ineffective at their maximum solubility.

1　Liquid medium: 5-ml volumes of double-strength nutrient medium (e.g. nutrient broth) are made up to 10 ml with appropriate volumes of inhibitor and sterile glass-distilled water (Water for Injections, BP) and inoculated with an appropriate dilution of spore inoculum. After incubation at, usually, 37°C for 24 and 48 h, the presence or absence of growth is noted. The MIC is the lowest concentration preventing growth.
2　Solid medium: 10-ml volumes of double-strength nutrient medium (e.g. nutrient agar) are made up to 20 ml with appropriate volumes of inhibitor and sterile water. After being allowed to set and harden, the surface is inoculated (streak, spot) with an approriate dilution of spore inoculum. Plates are incubated and the MIC determined.

Methods (1) and (2) provide initial information about the sporostatic activity of a test chemical but do not demonstrate the site (germination and/or outgrowth) at which the agent acts.

A problem with some antibacterial compounds is the fact that they interact with broth or agar media. This is true with chlorhexedine and quaternary ammonium compounds (QACs) but the concentrations at which this occurs are considerably higher than the MICs against spores, and many non-sporulating bacteria. Glutaraldehyde is a particular problem, however, since it interacts strongly with $-NH_2$ groups in peptones leading to a darkening of media with a possible interference with the interpretation of results. It is recommended that other procedures be used when this disinfectant is being studied (see page 28).

A third procedure involves a microsopical examination of the effect of antibacterial agents by slide culture. Not only does this procedure give an MIC value but it also provides information as to whether germination or outgrowth is affected.

Determination of Sporicidal Activity

Theoretical aspects

The principles of assessing sporicidal activity are essentially the same as for determining bactericidal activity. The main difference is that a treated spore has to pass through complex stages (germination and outgrowth) before a vegetative cell is formed and eventually a colony on, or in, a solid medium is produced. Thus, to obtain an accurate 'end-point' at the time of sampling and to ensure that surviving spores can adequately express themselves, it is essential to ensure that recovery conditions are such to enable viable but damaged spores the opportunity to revive. This topic has been well reviewed by Gould (1984), but it must be pointed out that most available information relates to the recovery and revival of spores damaged by physical processes rather than by chemical agents (Foegeding & Busta 1981; Waites & Bayliss 1984). The revival of damaged organisms of various types has been considered in detail (Andrew & Russell 1984).

Practical considerations

Evaluation of sporicidal activity (Table 1) usually takes the form of addition of spores to disinfectant with removal of spores at different times, the quenching of residual agent to prevent carry-over into recovery medium and the counting of colonies in/on an appropriate recovery agar medium. Quenching of activity can be carried out by three methods; these were considered in detail by Russell (1981), with theoretical concepts discussed by Russell et al. (1979), and will thus be listed only briefly here: (a) dilution to a subinhibitory level; (b) chemical neutralization; (c) membrane filtration with or without washing with an appropriate neutralizer (see Chiori et al. 1965; Prince & Ayliffe 1972; Russell et al. 1985).

To relate this procedure of evaluating sporicidal activity to the theoretical aspects considered above, and in particular to the concept of providing optimum conditions for the revival of damaged spores, it may be necessary to prolong the incubation period well beyond the normal 48 h at (usually) 37°C and to examine possible specific revival procedures. Some of these are listed in Table

TABLE 2. *Revival of spores injured by chemical agents*

Sporicide	Post-treatment revival procedure[*][†]	Reference
Formaldehyde	Heat activation (60–90°C), plating	Spicher & Peters (1981)
Glutaraldehyde	1 UDS ± sonication, incubation in GML, plating in TSA	Gorman *et al.* (1983)
	2 Heat (50–90°C), dilution in GM or GML, plating in TSA	Gorman *et al.* (1983)
	3 NaOH *or* KOH, plating	Dancer *et al.* (1989)[‡]
Povidone–iodine	Incubation in GML, plating in TSA	Gorman *et al.* (1983)

* Only a small proportion of treated spores may be revived.
† UDS, urea + dithiothreitol + sodium lauryl sulphate; GM, germination medium; GML, germination medium + lysozyme; TSA, tryptose-soy agar.
‡ Other treatments ineffective: see text.

2. For example, it has been claimed that subjecting formaldehyde-treated spores of *B. subtilis* to a post-treatment heat shock at temperatures of 60–90°C enables most of the supposedly killed spores to revive. A very small proportion of glutaraldehyde-exposed spores of *B. subtilis* can be revived when the spores are subsequently exposed to alkali (Dancer *et al.* 1989). To determine whether the effect of alkali was to relieve the strain imposed on germination (page 28) or outgrowth (page 31), the following experiments were carried out (Dancer *et al.* 1989; Power *et al.* 1989): glutaraldehyde-treated spores were washed with 2% (w/v) glycine (as an aldehyde inactivator), treated with sodium hydroxide (optimal concentration 20–50 mmol/l) and then transferred to a germination medium consisting of L-alanine (2 mmol/l) and D-glucose (5 mmol/l) in phosphate buffer (0.06 mol/l, pH 7.2). Spores similarly treated, except for NaOH exposure, acted as controls. The results indicated that; (a) the decrease in OD_{600} (optical density) in germination medium (i.e. extent of germination: see page 28) decreased as the aldehyde pretreatment concentration increased, and (b) that NaOH exposure after glutaraldehyde treatment increased the subsequent degree of germination, although this depended on the concentration of glutaraldehyde to which the spores had originally been exposed. In other experiments, spores were allowed to germinate and then were exposed to low concentrations of glutaraldehyde, glycine and NaOH as described above. They were resuspended in nutrient broth at 37°C and outgrowth monitored from the rise in OD_{600}. Sodium hydroxide was found to exert its effect at the germination level rather than at the outgrowth level. To

determine whether alkali induced protein release, *B. subtilis* NCTC 8236 spores (1 mg dry wt/ml) were treated with the dialdehyde, neutralized with glycine and washed several times with quarter-strength Ringer solution. They were exposed to 20 mmol/l NaOH for 10 min, centrifuged in a microfuge and the supernatant fluid assayed by the method of Spector (1978) for the release of protein: only 1 μg was released by alkali treatment.

Other methods of reviving glutaraldehyde-treated spores have been un-successful. These have included the following: various coat-removal pro-cedures, heat treatment, lysozyme treatment, and lysozyme following alkali (Power *et al.* 1989), and acid treatment and protease treatment (Dancer *et al.* 1989).

Methods of producing spores for sporicide studies are described by Waites & Bayliss (1980)

Inhibition of Germination

Theoretical concepts

Activation is a treatment resulting in a spore which is poised for germination but which still retains most spore properties; it is thus responsible for the breaking of dormancy in spores but is reversible. Germination itself is an irreversible process and is defined as a change of activated spores from a dormant to a metabolically active state within a short period of time.

The first biochemical step in germination is termed a biological trigger reaction. Specific chemical agents trigger the rapid germination of bacterial spores. This initiation process can be induced by metabolic or non-metabolic means, although it is now generally believed that the trigger reaction is allosteric in nature rather than metabolic, because the inducer does not need to be metabolized to induce germination. The most widely studied nutrient germinant is L-alanine, whereas calcium dipicolinate (CaDPA) is an example of a non-nutrient germinant. Initiation of germination is followed rapidly by various degradative changes in the spore, leading within a short period of time to outgrowth.

Inhibition and control of spore germination are of great importance in many fields, not least in food preservation (Smoot & Pierson 1982).

Practical considerations

Inhibition

The germination of bacterial spores can be demonstrated experimentally in various ways (Gould 1971). These include:

1 loss of heat resistance (an early event in germination);

2   loss of heat resistance accompanied by changes in staining properties (spores are difficult to stain by conventional techniques), decrease in refractility whereby phase-bright cells become phase-dark, and decrease in dry weight;
3   release of DPA;
4   decrease in optical density (OD).

For the sake of convenience, method (4) is usually employed for studying antibacterial agents (see Fig. 1), although it must be pointed out that OD changes are considered (Stewart *et al.* 1981) to be a comparatively late event in germination and might thus not be a suitable method for studying the effects of inhibitors on the trigger mechanism. Nevertheless, the OD method has proved to be of value in examination of the overall effects of antibacterial compounds on germination (and on outgrowth) as well as in determining whether any inhibition is or is not reversible.

For this purpose, a suitable spectrophotometer, set at an appropriate wavelength, e.g. 500 nm, is employed. A suitable germination medium is a nutrient broth, or alternatively a very simple medium consisting of L-alanine (2 mmol/l) and D-glucose (5 mmol/l) in phosphate buffer (0.06 mol/l, pH 7.2). Media should be pre-equilibrated at the desired temperature, inoculated with spores to give an OD reading of *c.* 0.3−0.4 and changes in OD monitored during subsequent incubation. A problem with glutaraldehyde is its interaction with broth constituents and with L-alanine. In this instance, therefore, it is recommended (Dancer *et al.* 1989) that spores are pretreated with

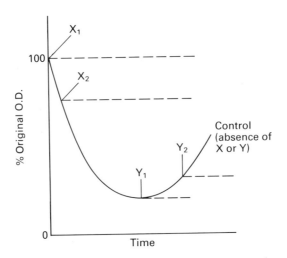

FIG. 1. Effects of antibacterial (*X*,*Y*) on germination and outgrowth as measured by changes in optical density (OD). *X* or *Y* can be added at different times as indicated (*X₁*, *X₂*, *Y₁*, *Y₂*). *X* inhibits germination and *Y* inhibits outgrowth. Examples of antibacterial agents are given in Table 3.

the aldehyde for an appropriate period of time, washed with a neutralizer (2% w/v glycine) and then placed in the germination medium.

The changes in OD can be related to structural changes in the cells as observed microscopically. A microscopical technique using slide agar cultures in the presence of different concentrations of an antibacterial compound can also be used for observing its action on germination (or on outgrowth).

Reversibility of inhibition

Three methods can be adopted for studying the reversibility of inhibition of germination, in each case followed by incubation and the measurement of OD changes.

1 Centrifugation and resuspension of cells in inhibitor-free germination medium.

2 Addition of a non-toxic agent (neutralizer, antidote) that quenches the action of the inhibitor.

3 Membrane filtration (a 0.45-μm pore size filter is suitable) to remove antibacterial agent and transfer of the membrane to fresh, inhibitor-free germination medium. With some agents, however, membrane filtration must be combined with washing with a neutralizer to ensure removal of antibacterial agent from the cells, e.g. quaternary ammonium compounds (Chiori et al. 1965; Russell et al. 1985).

Inhibition of trigger action

It was pointed out above that a simple germination medium consisting of L-alanine + D-glucose in phosphate buffer could be used in inhibition studies. A similar medium can be employed to study the effect of inhibitors of the L-alanine-induced trigger action. Yasuda & Tochikubo (1984) used L-alanine (1 mmol/l) and D-glucose (5 mmol/l) in 0.05 mol/l KH_2PO_4/Na_2HPO_4 buffer (pH 7.2) in their studies on B. subtilis spores; glucose was shown to have a stimulative effect on the binding affinity of L-alanine. Germination was started by the addition of a small volume of a dense spore suspension, to give a final cell density of c. 2×10^8/ml, to the above germination medium containing a test inhibitor or D-alanine (0–0.05 mmol/l). In some experiments, the medium contained D-alanine (0–0.5 mmol/l), L-alanine (0.01–10 mmol/l) and test inhibitor, and the germination rate (%/min) calculated from OD readings or by loss of heat resistance during incubation at 37°C. D-alanine acts as a competitive inhibitor of the binding of L-alanine. The results obtained with a combination of D-alanine and hydrophobic test inhibitors were used to obtain information about the effect of these inhibitors on the binding affinity of D-alanine.

A somewhat similar approach was employed by Sofos *et al.* (1986) in their investigation into the effect of sorbic acid on the commitment to germination of *Cl. botulinum* and *B. cereus* spores. The spores were exposed to 100 mmol/l L-alanine at pH 7 for specified time intervals and were then transferred into an excess of D-alanine (1.8 mol/l) with or without sorbate at pH 7. Commitment to germinate in L-alanine occurred rapidly (<0.5 min) but was complete only after 22.5 min of exposure. It was stated that if sorbate inhibited binding of L-alanine to the trigger site the combined effect of the two inhibitors (D-alanine plus sorbate) should have been identical to the effect of D-alanine used alone. However, sorbate in D-alanine solution produced a greater degree of inhibition than D-alanine alone, from which it was concluded that sorbate did not compete with L-alanine for a common binding site. Unfortunately, details of the method for measuring germination were not provided in this paper, although a microscopical procedure is believed to have been used.

The concept of using an OD technique for studying commitment to germination, i.e. the trigger reaction, has been criticized by Stewart *et al.* (1981). Working with a sporogenic strain of *B. megaterium* KM, these authors found that the rate of commitment to germinate after short exposure to L-alanine increased exponentially from the time of addition of the amino acid. They demonstrated that the decrease in OD was a late event in germination and was thus an unsuitable parameter for studying germination-triggering reactions. Stewart *et al.* (1981) determined the time necessary for spores to become committed to germinate after exposure to L-alanine by quenching and rapidly removing L-alanine from germinating suspensions with an excess of D-alanine and then observing the ability of these spores to continue germinating. Commitment by this method was found to occur much more rapidly than germination measured by loss of ^{45}Ca or decrease in OD.

From experiments already described, we believe that glutaraldehyde is able to act at a very early stage in germination, although this has yet to be proved conclusively. Experiments are currently under way to examine this contention further. It would also be instructive to consider the influence of various food and pharmaceutical preservatives, as well as disinfectants, on the trigger mechanism since little is known about their mechanism of action at this level.

The L-alanine-induced commitment to germination is sometimes referred to as metabolic activation. Non-metabolic activation may be achieved with some spores by using calcium dipicolinate or sodium hydroxide. These, and other agents (Russell 1982) might be of use in studying further the effects of antibacterial agents on the trigger mechanism. Germination (Ger) mutants of *B. subtilis* 168 (Moir *et al.* 1979; Sammons *et al.* 1981) might also be of value in this context.

Inhibition of Outgrowth

Theoretical concepts

Outgrowth is defined as the development of a vegetative cell from a germinated spore. It takes place in a synchronous and orderly manner when germination is carried out in a medium that supports vegetative growth. After germination, germinated spores become swollen and shed their coats to allow the young vegetative cells to emerge, elongate and divide. There is a sequential alteration in the structure of the cortex and in the inner and outer spore coats. Of the macromolecular biosynthetic processes occurring after germination, RNA synthesis is the first, closely followed in *Bacillus* spp. by the onset of protein synthesis, with DNA synthesis occurring some time later. During outgrowth, all types of RNA are synthesized. Cell wall synthesis commences after RNA and protein syntheses but before DNA synthesis and coincides with the swelling of the germinated spore.

In temperature-sensitive mutants of *B. subtilis* affected in outgrowth, outgrowth proceeds at the permissive temperature (35°C) — both in terms of cytological changes and of RNA, protein and DNA syntheses — whereas at the non-permissive temperature (47°C), RNA and protein syntheses are reduced and DNA synthesis cannot be detected.

Practical considerations

Complex synthetic media have been formulated for studying outgrowth. In our hands, adequate results have been obtained by using a nutrient broth. If broth has also been used for studying germination this obviates the need for changing the environment. Under such circumstances, it is possible to monitor both germination and outgrowth continuously using a spectrophotometer. Outgrowth is indicated by a rise in OD following the decrease occurring during germination (Fig. 1). An antibacterial agent under test can be added at any point desired, e.g. as demonstrated in Fig. 1 which shows that X inhibits germination and Y outgrowth.

Again, however, there is a problem with glutaraldehyde because of its interaction with the constituents of nutrient media. This has been overcome by allowing spores to germinate, e.g. in L-alanine + glucose + phosphate buffer (see page 28), centrifuging, resuspending the cells in sterile glass-distilled water (Water for Injections, BP) exposing to glutaraldehyde for the desired period, neutralizing the aldehyde (with 2% w/v glycine), washing and resuspending the cells in Nutrient Broth (Oxoid) prewarmed to 37°C. Changes in OD can then be monitored in the usual manner.

It must be added, however, that although these methods demonstrate the effect of an antibacterial agent on outgrowth, clearly they do little to explain exactly how such a compound achieves its effect. Information on this aspect is sadly lacking for the majority of non-antibiotic compounds. Antibiotics added during outgrowth have a sequential effect depending on whether they inhibit mRNA (e.g. actinomycin D), DNA (e.g. mitomycin C), protein (e.g. chloramphenicol, tetracycline) or cell wall (e.g. β-lactams) syntheses (see Russell 1982). It is noteworthy that for some bacilli, the antibiotic they produce during sporulation is thought to act to delay outgrowth, e.g. in *B. brevis*. The effects of non-antibiotic agents on such biosynthetic processes, on interaction with nucleic acids or on leakage of intracellular materials from outgrowing cells appear to have been given scant attention, although it would be expected that much useful information could be obtained. Temperature-sensitive mutants affected in outgrowth might be of value in studying antibacterial action.

Reversibility of the action of inhibitors of outgrowth has been little studied, but this can be done experimentally in a manner similar to that described earlier for examining the reversibility of action of germination inhibitors.

Examples of antibacterial agents known to prevent germination or outgrowth are presented in Table 3.

Effects of Antibacterial Agents on the Sporulation Process

Theoretical aspects

Sporulation is a multi-phase process leading to the production of a spore from a vegetative cell. In brief, these stages are as follows: Stage 0 is the vegetative cell, Stage I the preseptation phase in which DNA is present in the axial filament form. Stage II is the septation phase in which assymetric cell formation occurs. In Stage III, engulfment of the fore-spore occurs. Cortex formation between the inner and outer fore-spore membranes commences in Stage IV, with synthesis of spore coats, dipicolinic acid (DPA) and uptake of Ca^{2+} in Stage V. Spore maturation occurs in Stage VI, the coat material becoming more dense and refractility increasing. In Stage VII, there is lysis of the mother cell and liberation of the mature spore.

Obviously, then, there are several stages where antibacterial agents could act or conversely where resistance to such agents could arise. The latter aspect is undoubtedly of significance and is being increasingly studied because of its importance in food and medical microbiological contexts and elsewhere. Sporulation (Spo^-) mutants which are unable to develop beyond a genetically determined point are clearly of value in correlating structural changes, biochemical characteristics and sensitivity or resistance. Other types of mutants

TABLE 3. *Inhibitors of the trigger mechanism, spore germination and outgrowth* *

	Inhibitors of:	
Trigger mechanism	Germination	Outgrowth[†]
Alcohols?	Phenols	Nisin
Sorbate?	Cresols	QACs
Glutaraldehyde?	Parabens	Chlorhexidine
Chlorocresol?	Alcohols	Ethylene oxide
	Sodium thioglycollate	Chlorine compounds
	Glutaraldehyde	Glutaraldehyde
	Hg^{2+}	PMN
	Formaldehyde	

* An antibacterial agent may act at more than one stage.
[†] QACs, quaternary ammonium compounds; PMN, phenylmercuric nitrate.
? Action here unproven.

are considered elsewhere (pages 37 and 38). Useful information on Spo⁻ mutants is provided by Jenkinson (1981, 1983) and Hill (1983).

Disinfectant-induced structural changes in fully developed spores have been described (Kulikovsky *et al.* 1975) but these have not been adequately related to the biochemical effects of disinfectants on sporulating cells, so that the mechanisms of action of many of these antibacterial agents on spores and on sporulating forms are often poorly described. This is an area which might yield considerable information if experiments (depending on the agent under test) could be devised for relating changes in structure in developing spores before and after treatment, leakage of intracellular constituents, uptake, cortex and coat development to the lethal effects of test chemical bactericidal or sporicidal agents. Useful markers for monitoring the development of resistance during sporulation are toluene (resistance is an early event), heat (intermediate event) and lysozyme (late event).

Practical considerations

Wild-type strain

Spore development from a vegetative cell is best observed by using a 'step-down' procedure, the principle of which is that cells growing in a rich culture medium are inoculated into a poor medium which is then incubated. Details of the technique and for determining sensitivity to antibacterial agents are considered below. *Bacillus subtilis* 168 is widely employed in such studies.

Spo⁻ mutants

Table 4 lists some Spo⁻ mutants of *B. subtilis* 168 which we have found to be
of use in examining the effects of antibacterial agents on the sporulation
process. A suitable step-down procedure is as follows: bacteria from a single
colony on a fresh nutrient agar plate are grown at 37°C overnight in a
hydrolysed casein medium. The culture is diluted in the same medium to give
an absorbance at 600 nm of *c.* 0.1 and is incubated at 37°C in a shaking
water bath to an absorbance at 600 nm of 0.7−0.8 (*c.* 0.25 mg dry wt/ml).
The culture is centrifuged and the cells are resuspended in the same volume
of a nutritionally very poor medium (resuspension medium) and incubation is
continued at 37°C. The time of resuspension is referred to as t_0 and subsequent
periods (1 h, 2 h, etc.) as t_1, t_2, etc.

Antibacterial sensitivity

Spore samples (wild type, *B. subtilis* 168) are removed at intervals, exposed to
the test chemical (or to moist heat, e.g. at temperatures of 80−90°C) for a
relevant period of time, the antibacterial agent neutralized in an appropriate
manner and survivor counts determined as usual. Such studies with a wild-
type strain (168) of *B. subtilis* (Table 4) involving the development of resistance to
chemicals have employed 10% toluene (exposure time 2 min), chlorhexidine
diacetate (200 μg/ml, 10 min), lysozyme (250 μg/ml 10 min) and glutaraldehyde (2% alkaline, 10 min) as well as moist heat (80°C, 10 min), as described
by Power *et al.* (1988) and Shaker *et al.* (1988a). The results of these studies
have shown that resistance to chlorhexidine occurs later than to toluene but at
about the same time as to heat resistance, whereas glutaraldehyde resistance is
a very late event, occurring after the development of lysozyme resistance
(Table 5).

With the Spo⁻ mutants, the cells are allowed to attain their full point of

TABLE 4. *Examples of sporulation mutants (Spo⁻) of* B.subtilis *used
in sporicidal studies*

Strain	Genotype	Sporulation phenotype
168	*trp* C2	Wild-type (Spo⁺)
23.1	*trp* C2 rif *spo* IVC 23	Stage IV
92	*leu spo* IVD 92	Stage IV
89	*trp* C2 *spo* VA89	Stage V
91	*trp* C2 *spo* VB91	Stage V
156	*trp* C2 *leu spo* VD156	Stage V
513	*trp* C2 *spo* VIA513	Stage VI

TABLE 5. *Onset of resistance to antibacterial agents during the sporulation process*

Agent	Sporulation stage:	
	At which resistance develops	Where resistance is fully developed
Toluene	Late Stage III	Early Stage IV
Chlorhexidine	Stage IV	Stage V
Heat	Stage V	Stage VI
Lysozyme	Middle of Stage V	Stage VI
Glutaraldehyde	Late Stage V	Stage VI completed

development and are then exposed to chemical or physical treatments as described for the wild-type strain.

Mechanisms of Bacterial Spore Resistance

Theoretical concepts

Bacterial spores are among the most resistant of cell forms to antibacterial agents. The mechanisms whereby this resistance occurs are not fully understood, although they often, but not necessarily, appear to be associated with the inner and outer spore coats. The cortex has also been suggested as being a contributory factor in spore resistance expressed to some agents (Imae & Strominger 1976a, b). It must also be noted that different factors may be involved for the resistance of different types of spores to the same agent (Waites & Bayliss 1979).

Generally, permeation of the outer layers of the spore is necessary for an antibacterial agent to bring about the desired effect, namely a sporicidal action. Little is known, however, about the manner in which this permeation is achieved and indeed in at least one case (ethylene oxide), the role of the spore coats in resistance is equivocal (Dadd & Daley 1982).

Practical considerations

Development of resistance during sporulation

Useful information can be obtained by undertaking experiments to correlate resistance development with structural changes that occur in a sporulating cell. Wild-type cultures, e.g. *B. subtilis* 168, and Spo⁻ mutants can be employed, as previously described.

Some 12 or so polypeptides are found in the spore coat of *B. subtilis* which are synthesized at different times and which are incorporated into the spore at Stages V and VI (Jenkinson 1981, 1983; Jenkinson *et al.* 1980, 1981). Extraction of these spore coat proteins by shaking the spores with glass beads in a Braun tissue disintegrator, treatment of the insoluble fraction with lysozyme followed by extensive washing and subsequent solubilization of the proteins is described by Jenkinson (1983). The coat proteins can then be analysed by SDS–PAGE. It has been suggested (Jenkinson 1981) that one polypeptide (mol. wt 36 000, 36 K), which is formed very late in sporulation, may have a direct role in conferring lysozyme resistance upon the spores. Studies in our laboratory suggest that the development of glutaraldehyde resistance is unlikely to be due to the deposition of specific core coat proteins because of the highly reactive nature of the dialdehyde molecule (Power *et al.* 1988). Nevertheless, generally the idea of attempting to correlate resistance with a specific component of the spore coats is an attractive one. It is unfortunate that this aspect has not been considered further.

Removal of spore coats

Coatless spores remain viable. This statement therefore provides a clue as to another approach to the solving of the mechanism(s) of spore resistance presented to chemical agents. There are various methods for removing the inner and/or outer spore coats, but not all are equally effective. Spore coats may be extracted by employing 2-mercaptoethanol (ME), sodium lauryl (dodecyl) sulphate (SLS), dithiothreitol (DTT) and urea, as described below. Methods are described by Nishihara *et al.* (1980, 1981) and Gorman *et al.* (1984).

1 UDS spores: exposure of spores to 8 mol/l urea, 0.05 mol/l DTT and 1% SLS (pH 10.3) for 180 min at 37°C.

2 UDT spores: exposures of spores to 8 mol/l urea and 0.05 mol/l DTT (pH 10.5) for 180 min at 37°C.

3 UME spores: exposures of spores to 8 mol/l urea and 10% ME for 60 min at 60°C.

4 SD spores: exposures of spores to 0.05% SLS, 0.01 mol/l DTT and 0.1 mol/l NaCl in 100 mol/l borate buffer (pH 10) for 120 min at 38°C.

5 UMS spores: as for UME with the addition of 1% (w/v) SLS.

Of these treatments, UDS is usually considered to be the most satisfactory.

A comparison can then be made of the reactions of intact spores and of coatless spores to the antibacterial agent, and the role of the coats in determining spore response assessed. Susceptibility to antibacterial agents can be determined by various means, e.g. viable counting procedures and spectrophotometric methods for detecting whether cell lysis occurs. Both lysozyme and nitrous acid/sodium nitrite induce lysis of coatless spores, but pretreatment of these forms with glutaraldehyde reduces considerably the extent of this lysis.

Table 6 depicts the sensitivity of UDS spores to various types of antibacterial agent, and demonstrates that many chemicals are considerably less active against normal than against coatless spores, implying that the coats have an important role to play in intrinsic spore resistance.

Conditional cortexless mutants

In conditional spore cortexless mutants of *B. sphaericus* deficient in the synthesis of *meso*-diaminopimelic acid (Dap), the muramic lactam (and hence cortex) content increases with an increase in the external concentration of Dap (Imae & Strominger 1976a, b). These mutants would thus appear to be useful tools in studying the role of the cortex in expressing resistance to disinfectants and other compounds. Indeed, it was found that characteristic spore properties were associated with different amounts of cortex, e.g. *c*. 25% of maximum cortex content was necessary to show octanol resistance, but *c*. 90% was necessary to show heat resistance.

Spores of this organism with varying cortical contents can thus be obtained by growth in media containing different Dap concentrations. Following harvesting and washing, the spores can then be exposed to various antibacterial compounds for appropriate periods, the numbers of survivors determined in the usual manner and the sporicidal effect related to the cortical content. Unfortunately, this is altogether too simplistic an approach, because (as pointed out by Waites 1982) other changes in the spore may also occur which are not taken into account.

TABLE 6. *Mechanisms of spore resistance to antibacterial agents*

Antibacterial agent	Spore component responsible	Comment*
Alkali	Cortex	⎫
Lysozyme	Coat(s)	⎪
Hypochlorites	Coat(s)	⎬ UDS spores highly
Glutaraldehyde	Coat(s)	sensitive
Iodine	Coat(s)	⎭
Hydrogen peroxide	Coat(s)	Varies with strain
Chlorhexidine	Coat(s)	UDS spores rather more sensitive
Ethylene oxide	Coat(s)?	Exact relationship unclear
Octanol	Cortex	⎱ Dap⁻ mutants of
Xylene	Cortex	⎰ *B.sphaericus* used

* UDS, urea + dithiothreitol + sodium lauryl sulphate.

State of protoplast (core)

The water content of the protoplast is undoubtedly of considerable importance in the response of bacterial spores to heat (Gould 1984). However, there is less information about the role of the protoplast in expressing chemical resistance (Waites 1985), although there is some evidence to suggest that conditions within the protoplast may be important (Waites 1982). Thus, a mutant of *B. subtilis* which did not synthesize dipicolinic acid (DPA) during sporulation was less resistant to phenol (Balassa *et al.* 1979). Other examples, particularly with *Cl. bifermentans*, where protoplast structure may be important in determining resistance to disinfectants, are provided by Waites (1982).

Obviously, this is an area which has been little investigated but which could produce useful information. Again, however, possible changes elsewhere in the spore would have to be taken into consideration in any hypothesis.

Mechanisms of Sporicidal Action

Theoretical concepts

This is an important field of study. However, the complex structure of the bacterial spore in relation to a non-sporulating or vegetative bacterial cell has inevitably meant that progress has been slow. The spore presents several sites at which interaction with an antibacterial agent is possible, e.g. the inner and/or outer spore coats, cortex, spore membranes, core. It does not necessarily mean, however, that such an interaction is associated with the death of the spore or that there is only one site or target in the spore which must be inactivated.

This section will describe some of the methods which have been used to examine the effects of chemicals on bacterial spores and will consider their implications in terms of the mechanism of action of these compounds.

Practical considerations

Binding to intact spores

The binding of an antibacterial agent to intact spores requires, usually, a fairly dense suspension of spores and an appropriate, usually chemical, assay system for the antibacterial compound. If a radio-labelled compound is being used, then the amount of radioactivity remaining unbound to the spore can easily be measured. Most often, however, an unlabelled compound is employed and the spores have to be removed after treatment for an assay of unbound substance to be carried out. Spores can be removed by centrifugation, although allowance should be made for the contact between cells and drug during centrifugation. An alternative procedure is membrane filtration, although a major problem here is the clogging of the filter with the large number of spores present and possible binding of the drug to the filter.

We have studied the uptake of glutaraldehyde to *B. subtilis* spores and to non-sporulating bacteria (Power & Russell 1989). Equal volumes of a suitable spore suspension (2 mg dry wt/ml) and glutaraldehyde solutions are mixed and samples removed and centrifuged at high speed to remove the dialdehyde, the concentration of which in the supernatant solution is determined by a hydroxylamine assay, as previously reported (Power & Russell, 1988). Rates of uptake and adsorption isotherms can then be plotted, from which information about the type of uptake can be obtained. Similar procedures can be adopted with other antibacterial agents, spores can be produced in different ways (e.g. growth on different media to yield varying sensitivities to sporicides, Waites & Bayliss 1980), or alternatively Spo⁻ mutants can be employed.

It must be emphasized, however, that uptake merely provides data of a preliminary nature and that it should be regarded as only one experimental tool in considering the activity of a sporicidal agent. Furthermore, sporostatic agents may also be bound, and uptake cannot therefore be used as a means of assessing sporicidal activity, although we have shown that spores of *B. subtilis* take up less glutaraldehyde than do cells of *Escherichia coli* or *Staphylococcus aureus* (Power & Russell 1989).

Surface changes in spores

Surface changes can be measured by various techniques. These include:
1 the use of microelectrophoresis to measure the mobility of cells treated with various concentrations of an antibacterial compound;
2 hydrophobicity studies with appropriate hydrophobic solvents, usually hydrocarbons (although octanol is also suitable). Bacterial spores are only slightly hydrophobic but changes occur during germination and outgrowth (Shaker *et al.* 1988b) and when cells are exposed to agents such as glutaraldehyde and chlorhexidine.

Spore coats

Some disinfectants themselves affect the spore coat(s). For example, chlorine will itself remove coat protein (Waites & Bayliss 1979): one method of detecting this is to determine whether chlorine-treated spores undergo germination-like changes when exposed to lysozyme. Hydrogen peroxide also removes protein (presumably from the coat) in *Cl. bifermentans*. Likewise, sublethal levels of peroxide increase the germination rate in this organism. Foegeding &

Busta (1983) used a polyacrylamide gel system to examine the protein removed by hypochlorite treatment of *Cl. botulinum* spores.

Isolated spore coats can also be prepared and their interaction with an antibacterial agent examined (Gorman *et al.* 1984). This technique does not appear to have been widely studied.

Effects on cortex

The interaction of an antibacterial agent with the spore cortex may be inferred from a knowledge of the chemical properties of the agent, of the cortex and of the effects of the compound, e.g. glutaraldehyde (Russell 1982) on spores. A useful method with the dialdehyde is to prepare coatless forms, pretreat with acid or alkaline glutaraldehyde, wash with glycine to remove the agent and then expose to peptidoglycan-affecting agents such as lysozyme or sodium nitrite. An alternative technique is to prepare cortical fragments (Gorman *et al.* 1984), expose to glutaraldehyde, wash with glycine to remove the chemical and then determine the amount of hexosamine released on exposure to lysozyme or nitrite. Interestingly, Gorman *et al.*, (1984) found that a period of 2 days was necessary for cortical fragments to take up a comparable amount of glutaraldehyde as intact spores. In practice, therefore, this latter procedure may not be very satisfactory.

Effects on core

Fitz-James (1971) has described a method of producing spore protoplasts. In this technique, coats are first removed (DTT + SLS treatment: see earlier) and the coatless spores are then suspended in appropriate hypertonic solutions (e.g. 0.14 mol/l sodium chloride or buffered 0.3 mol/l sucrose or 0.45 mol/l succinate) containing two essential cations, and subjected to lysozyme digestion (usually $50-100$ µg/ml). Ca^{2+} ions (supplied as $CaCl_2$, $10-20$ mmol/l) are essential for membrane integrity, whilst Mg^{2+} ions (supplied as $MgSO_4$, 10 mmol/l) are essential for changes indicative of core hydration. Lysozyme was shown to digest both the cortex and the germ cell wall. The procedure was found to be most satisfactory with *B. megaterium* KM, but lysozyme had no effect on the germ cell wall of *B. cereus*, and *B. subtilis* protoplasts appeared to retain remnants of spore coat(s).

In buffered succinate, spore protoplasts increase in size and synthesize protein. They can thus be employed in this sytem to determine the effects of an antibacterial agent (e.g. glutaraldehyde: Gorman *et al.* 1984) or in a buffered sucrose system to measure bacteriolytic activity with, for example, membrane-active agents. This procedure could therefore be used not only to study effects on the protoplast membrane or core but also to provide information about the role of layers external to the core in spore resistance.

DPA leakage

The release of DPA is indicative of membrane damage. It has been studied most widely with spores subjected to high temperatures and as an event occurring during germination. Pretreatment of spores with alkaline glutaraldehyde, but not acid glutaraldehyde, reduces, but does not eliminate, leakage when the spores are subsequently exposed to high temperatures. Glutaraldehyde also reduces the loss of DPA during germination, which is inhibited by the dialdehyde (see earlier). In contrast, chlorhexidine increases DPA loss when spores are heated, but decreases the amount lost during germination of chlorhexidine-pretreated spores, although it predominantly inhibits outgrowth (Table 3). Spores exposed to hypochlorites leak DPA (Kulikovsky *et al.* 1975).

DPA leakage can be measured in the following ways:

1 by absorbance at 279 nm: unfortunately, this method is not necessarily specific because of possible interference by nutrient medium (if germination is being studied) or test antibacterial agent;

2 by a colorimetric method (Janssen *et al.* 1958): care must be taken to ensure that the test antibacterial compound does not interact with the chemicals used in the assay;

3 by means of a chelation procedure using ethylene-bis (β-aminoethyl ether)-N,N,N^1,N^1-tetraacetic acid (Scott & Ellar 1978).

Comments and Conclusions

In comparison with their effects on non-sporulating bacteria, the action of antibacterial agents on sporulating bacteria has been less well documented and comparatively little is known about the mechanisms of action of, and resistance to, sporicidal agents. This paper describes some of the more useful techniques currently available and also considers changes that occur in sporulation, germination and outgrowth in relation to sensitivity. It points to useful areas for further investigation.

Acknowledgement

We thank the Department of Health and Social Security for a research studentship to one of us, EGMP.

References

ANDREW, M.H.E. & RUSSELL, A.D. (eds) 1984. *The Revival of Injured Microbes.* Society for Applied Bacteriology Symposium No. 12. London: Academic Press.

BALASSA, G., MILHAUD, P., RAULET, E., SILVA, M.T. & SOUSA, J.C.F. 1979. A *Bacillus subtilis* mutant requiring dipicolinic acid for the development of heat-resistant spores. *Journal of General Microbiology* 110, 365–379.

42   A.D. RUSSELL *ET AL.*

Chiori, C.O., Hambleton, R. & Rigby, G.J. 1965. The inhibition of spores of *Bacillus subtilis* by cetrimide retained on washed membrane filters and on the washed spores. *Journal of Applied Bacteriology* **28**, 322–330.

Dadd, A.H. & Daley, G.M. 1982. Role of the coat in resistance of bacterial spores to inactivation by ethylene oxide. *Journal of Applied Bacteriology* **53**, 109–116.

Dancer, B.N., Power, E.G.M. & Russell, A.D. 1989. Alkali-induced revival of *Bacillus* spores after inactivation by glutaraldehyde. *FEMS Microbiology Letters* **57**, 345–348.

Fitz-James, P.C. 1971. Formation of protoplasts from resting spores. *Journal of Bacteriology* **105**, 1119–1136.

Foegeding, P.M. & Busta, F.F. 1981. Bacterial spore injury — an update. *Journal of Food Protection* **44**, 776–786.

Foegeding, P.M. & Busta, F.F. 1983. Proposed mechanism for sensitization by hypochlorine treatment of *Clostridium botulinium* spores. *Applied and Environmental Microbiology* **45**, 1374–1379.

Gorman, S.P., Hutchinson, E.P., Scott, E.M. & McDermott, L.M. 1983. Death, injury and revival of chemically treated *Bacillus subtilis* spores. *Journal of Applied Bacteriology* **54**, 91–99.

Gorman, S.P., Scott, E.M. & Hutchinson, E.P. 1984. Interaction of the *Bacillus subtilis* spore protoplast, cortex, ion-exchange and coatless forms with glutaraldehyde. *Journal of Applied Bacteriology* **56**, 95–102.

Gould, G.W. 1971. Methods for studying bacterial spores. In *Methods in Microbiology*, Vol. 6A, ed. Norris, J.R. & Ribbons, D.W. pp. 327–381. London: Academic Press.

Gould, G.W. 1984. Injury and repair mechanisms in bacterial spores. In *The Revival of Injured Microbes*, ed. Andrew, M.H.E. & Russell, A.D. pp. 199–220. Society for Applied Bacteriology Symposium No. 12. London: Academic Press.

Hill, S.H.A. 1983. spoVH and spoVJ — new sporulation loci in *Bacillus subtilis* 168. *Journal of General Microbiology* **129**, 293–302.

Imae, Y. & Strominger, J.L. 1976a. Relationship between cortex content and properties of *Bacillus sphaericus* spores. *Journal of Bacteriology* **126**, 907–913.

Imae, Y. & Strominger, J.L. 1976b. Conditional spore cortex-less mutants of *Bacillus sphaericus* 9602. *Journal of Biological Chemistry* **251**, 1493–1499.

Janssen, F.W., Lund, A.J. & Anderson, L.E. 1958. Colorimetric assay for dipicolinic acid in bacterial spores. *Science* **127**, 26–27.

Jenkinson, H.F. 1981. Germination and resistance defects in spores of a *Bacillus subtilis* mutant lacking a coat polypeptide. *Journal of General Microbiology* **127**, 81–91.

Jenkinson, H.F. 1983. Altered arrangement of proteins in the spore coat of a germination mutant of *Bacillus subtilis*. *Journal of General Microbiology* **129**, 1945–1958.

Jenkinson, H.F., Kay, D. & Mandelstam, J. 1980. Temporal dissociation of late events in *Bacillus subtilis* sporulation from expression of genes that determine them. *Journal of Bacteriology* **141**, 793–805.

Jenkinson, H.F., Sawyer, W.D. & Mandelstam, J. 1981. Synthesis and order of assembly of spore coat proteins in *Bacillus subtilis*. *Journal of General Microbiology* **123**, 1–16.

Kulikovsky, A., Pankratz, H.S. & Sadoff, H.L. 1975. Ultrastructural and chemical changes in spores of *Bacillus cereus* after action of disinfectants. *Journal of Applied Bacteriology* **38**, 39–46.

Moir, A., Lapperty, E. & Smith, D.A. 1979. Genetic analysis of spore germination mutants of *Bacillus subtilis* 168: the correlation of phenotype with map locations. *Journal of General Microbiology* **111**, 165–180.

Nishihara, T., Tomita, M., Yamanaka, N., Ichikawa, T. & Kondo, M. 1980. Studies on the bacterial spore coat. 7. Properties of alkali-soluble components from spore coat of *Bacillus megaterium. Microbiology and Immunology* **24**, 105–112.

NISHIHARA, T., YUTSODO, T., ICHIKAWA, T. & KONDO, M. 1981. Studies on the bacterial spore coat. 8. On the SDS–DTT extract from *Bacillus megaterium* spores. *Microbiology and Immunology* **25**, 327–331.

POWER, E.G.M. & RUSSELL, A.D. 1988. Assessment of "Cold Sterilog Glutaraldehyde Monitor". *Journal of Hospital Infection* **11**, 376–380.

POWER, E.G.M. & RUSSELL, A.D. 1989. Glutaraldehyde: its uptake by sporing and non-sporing bacteria, rubber, plastic and an endoscope. *Journal of Applied Bacteriology* **67**, 379–342.

POWER, E.G.M., DANCER, B.N. & RUSSELL, A.D. 1988. Emergence of resistance to glutaraldehyde in spores of *Bacillus subtilis* 168. *FEMS Microbiology Letters* **50**, 223–226.

POWER, E.G.M., DANCER, B.N. & RUSSELL, A.D. 1989. Possible mechanisms for the revival of glutaraldehyde-treated spores of *Bacillus subtilis* NCTC 8236. *Journal of Applied Bacteriology* **67**, 91–98.

PRINCE, J. & AYLIFFE, G.A.J. 1972. In-use testing of disinfectants in hospitals. *Journal of Clinical Pathology* **25**, 586–589.

RUSSELL, A.D. 1981. Neutralisation procedures in the evaluation of bactericidal activity. In *Disinfectants: Their Use and Evaluation of Effectiveness*, ed. Collins, C.H., Allwood, M.C., Bloomfield, S.F. & Fox, A. pp. 45–59. Society for Applied Bacteriology Technical Series No. 16. London: Academic Press.

RUSSELL, A.D. 1982. *The Destruction of Bacterial Spores*. London: Academic Press.

RUSSELL, A.D. 1983. Mechanisms of action of chemical sporicidal and sporistatic agents. *International Journal of Pharmaceutics* **16**, 127–140.

RUSSELL, A.D. 1990a. Chemical sporicidal agents. In *Disinfection, Sterilization and Preservation*, 4th edn, ed. Block, S.S. Philadelphia: Lea & Febiger.

RUSSELL, A.D. 1990b. Activity of chemical and physical agents on microorganisms. In *Topley and Wilson's Principles of Bacteriology, Virology and Immunology*, 8th edn, ed. Dick, H.M. & Linton, A.H., London: Edward Arnold.

RUSSELL, A.D., AHONKHAI, I. & ROGERS, D.T. 1979. Microbiological applications of the inactivation of antibiotics and other antimicrobial agents. *Journal of Applied Bacteriology* **46**, 207–245.

RUSSELL, A.D., DANCER, B.N., POWER, E.G.M. & SHAKER, L.A. 1989. Mechanisms of bacterial spore resistance to disinfectants. In *Proceedings of the Fourth Conference on Chemical Disinfection*. pp. 9–29. Binghamton, New York.

RUSSELL, A.D., JONES, B.D. & MILBURN, P. 1985. Reversal of the inhibition of bacterial spore germination and outgrowth by antibacterial agents. *International Journal of Pharmaceutics* **25**, 105–112.

SAMMONS, R.L., MOIR, A. & SMITH, D.A. 1981. Isolation and properties of spore germination mutants of *Bacillus subtilis* 168 deficient in the initiation of germination. *Journal of General Microbiology* **124**, 229–241.

SCOTT, I.R. & ELLAR, D.J. 1978. Study of calcium dipicolinate release during bacterial spore germination by using a new, sensitive assay for dipicolinate. *Journal of Bacteriology* **135**, 133–137.

SHAKER, L.A., DANCER, B.N., RUSSELL, A.D. & FURR, J.R. 1988a. Emergence and development of chlorhexidine resistance during sporulation of *Bacillus subtilis* 168. *FEMS Microbiology Letters* **51**, 73–76.

SHAKER, L.A., FURR, J.R. & RUSSELL, A.D. 1988b. Mechanism of resistance of *Bacillus subtilis* spores to chlorhexidine. *Journal of Applied Bacteriology* **64**, 531–539.

SMOOT, L.A. & PIERSON, M.D. 1982. Inhibition and control of bacterial spore germination. *Journal of Food Protection* **45**, 84–92.

SOFOS, J.N., PIERSON, M.D., BLOCHER, J.C. & BUSTA, F.F. 1986. Mode of action of sorbic acid on bacterial cells and spores. *International Journal of Food Microbiology* **3**, 1–17.

SPECTOR, T. 1978. Refinement of the Coomassie blue method of protein quantitation. *Analytical Biochemistry* **86**, 142–146.

SPICHER, G. & PETERS, J. 1981. Heat activation of bacterial spores after inactivation by formaldehyde. Dependence of heat activation on temperature and duration of action. *Zentralblatt für Bakteriologie, Parasitenkunde, Infektionskrankheiten und Hygiene, I. Abteilung Originale, Reihe B* **172**, 188–196.

SPOONER, D.F. & SYKES, G. 1972. Laboratory assessment of antibacterial activity. In *Methods in Microbiology*, Vol. 7B, ed. Norris, J.R. & Ribbons, D.W. pp. 213–276. London: Academic Press.

STEWART, G.S.A.B., JOHNSTONE, K., HAGELBERG, E. & ELLAR, D.J. 1981. Commitment of bacterial spores to germinate. A measure of the trigger reaction. *Biochemical Journal* **198**, 101–106.

WAITES, W.M. 1982. Microbial resistance to non-antibiotic antimicrobial agents: Resistance of bacterial spores. In *Principles and Practice of Disinfection, Preservation and Sterilisation*, ed. Russell, A.D., Hugo, W.B. & Ayliffe, G.A.J. pp. 207–220. Oxford: Blackwell Scientific Publications.

WAITES, W.M. 1985. Inactivation of spores with chemical agents. In *Fundamental and Applied Aspects of Bacterial Spores*, ed. Dring, G.J., Ellar, D.J. & Gould, G.W. pp. 383–396. London: Academic Press.

WAITES, W.M. & BAYLISS, C.E. 1979. The effect of changes in the spore coat on the destruction of *Bacillus cereus* spores by heat and chemical agents. *Journal of Applied Biochemistry* **1**, 71–76.

WAITES, W.M. & BAYLISS, C.E. 1980. The preparation of bacterial spores for evaluation of the sporicidal activity of chemicals. In *Microbial Growth and Survival in Extremes of Environment*, ed. Gould, G.W. & Corry, J.E.L. pp. 159–172. Society for Applied Bacteriology Technical Series No 15. London: Academic Press.

WAITES, W.M. & BAYLISS, C.E. 1984. Damage to bacterial spores by combined treatments and possible revival and repair processes. In *The Revival of Injured Microbes*, ed. Andrew, M.H.E. & Russell, A.D. pp. 221–240. Society for Applied Bacteriology Symposium No. 12. London: Academic Press.

YASUDA, Y. & TOCHIKUBO, K. 1984. Effect of glucose on the interaction of hydrophobic compounds with the alanine receptor field of *Bacillus subtilis* spores. *Microbiology and Immunology* **28**, 1203–1210.

Bacterial Resistance to Disinfectants, Antiseptics and Toxic Metal Ions

I. CHOPRA

Department of Microbiology, School of Medical Sciences,
University of Bristol, Bristol BS8 ITD, UK

The existence of antibiotic-resistant bacteria has been known for many years and has recently been comprehensively described (Foster 1983; Chopra 1988a). In contrast, less is known about the genetic and biochemical basis of resistance to other antibacterial agents such as disinfectants, antiseptics and toxic metal ions. Nevertheless, in recent years there has been a gradual increase in our knowledge of resistance mechanisms to non-antibiotic agents, and sufficient information has now been gathered to allow consideration of the topic as a separate issue from antibiotic resistance. Indeed, the principal objective of this chapter is to consider the biochemical basis of bacterial resistance to non-antibiotic inhibitors. Although the subject is of fundamental scientific interest, studies in this area may also have the practical outcome of suggesting ways of overcoming, or circumventing, resistance mechanisms. This could be beneficial since several of the agents to be described are used as disinfectants, antiseptics or preservatives (Hugo & Russell 1982; Russell & Hugo 1987).

There are two broad categories of resistance: intrinsic (or intrinsic insusceptibility) and acquired. The term 'intrinsic resistance' is used to imply that inherent features of the cell are responsible for preventing antimicrobial action and to distinguish this situation from acquired resistance, which occurs when resistant strains emerge from previously sensitive bacterial populations, usually after exposure to the inhibitor concerned. Acquired resistance can arise either by acquisition of plasmids and transposons or by chromosomal mutations. Because of space limitations this chapter will deal primarily with acquired resistance, but readers wishing to be informed on intrinsic resistance should consult the recent reviews of Hancock & Nicas (1984) and Chopra (1987).

* Present address: Department of Microbial Biochemistry and Genetics, American Cyanamid Co., Lederle Laboratories, Pearl River, NY 10965, USA.

Mechanisms of Action of
Chemical Biocides

Arsenicals

A diverse range of bacteria express resistance to arsenicals such as arsenate and arsenite (Trevors *et al.* 1985). In many cases the genes (*ars*) encoding resistance are plasmid-located (Foster 1983; Trevors *et al.* 1985) and, for determinants found in *Escherichia coli* and *Staphylococcus aureus*, expression of resistance involves an inducible resistance mechanism (Foster 1983). The basis of arsenical resistance has been extensively studied in *E. coli* and the subject reviewed in recent articles (Foster 1983; Rosen 1986; Chopra 1988b).

The *ars* operon is induced by arsenate, arsenite and antimony, each of the ions inducing resistance to all three inhibitors. Initial investigations into the biochemical basis of arsenical resistance in *E. coli* involved studies on arsenate accumulation. In *E. coli* arsenate is normally accumulated by phosphate transport systems (Fig. 1). *Escherichia coli* possesses two constitutive phosphate transport systems termed Pit (for 'Pi transport') and Pst (for 'Phosphate specific transport') (Fig. 1). The Pit system has a lower affinity for phosphate than does the Pst system, but both are responsible for arsenate uptake. Although possession of *ars* by a resistant cell results in decreased arsenate accumulation, the *ars* gene products do not interact directly with the Pst or Pit transport systems to influence arsenate uptake. Indeed, *ars*-mediated resistance to both arsenate and arsenite results from extrusion of the toxic anions from the cell (Rosen 1986; Rosen *et al.* 1988). The transport system is a primary anion pump requiring intracellular ATP for extrusion of arsenicals (Rosen 1986; Rosen *et al.* 1988) (Fig. 1).

Further insight into the molecular basis of *ars*-mediated resistance to arsenicals has been provided by gene cloning, nucleotide sequence analysis, and studies of gene expression in minicells. Three structural genes *ars*A, *ars*B and *ars*C are contained in a 4.3-kb region of the resistance determinant. A summary of the known, or predicted, properties and functions of the ArsA, ArsB and ArsC polypeptides is given in Table 1 and a model showing their possible roles in efflux of arsenate is included in Fig. 1.

Cadmium

Resistance to cadmium is a common plasmid-mediated character in *Staph. aureus* (Foster 1983). Two distinct resistance determinants have been identified, designated *cad*A and *cad*B (Foster 1983). The *cad*A determinant confers about a 100-fold increase in resistance to cadmium whereas *cad*B only confers low-level resistance. Some naturally occurring plasmids carry both *cad*A and *cad*B whereas others possess only *cad*A (Foster 1983). Both determinants are expressed constitutively and also confer resistance to zinc ions.

The nature of *cad*B-mediated resistance is unknown, but it has now been

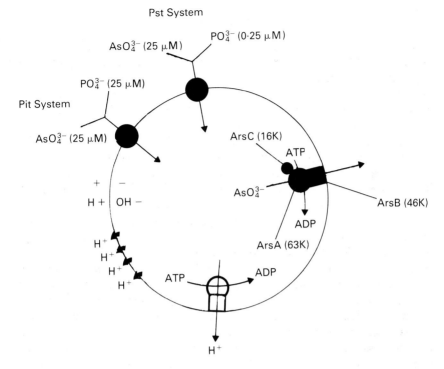

FIG. 1. Accumulation of phosphate and arsenate by *E. coli*. The upper left-hand-side of the diagram shows the Pst (Phosphate specific transport) and Pit (Pi transport) systems, both of which can accumulate phosphate and arsenate ions. The values of $0.25\,\mu M$ or $25\,\mu M$ where indicated are the K_m values for phosphate, or the K_i values for arsenate as a competitive inhibitor of phosphate transport. Beneath the Pit system is illustrated the electrogenic extrusion of protons, catalysed by the respiratory chain, which establishes the electrochemical proton gradient with the indicated polarity. The lower portion of the diagram shows the F_0F_1 proton translocating ATP-ase; above this the ATP-ase mediating arsenical efflux is illustrated. This is believed to consist of three polypeptides, ArsA, ArsB and ArsC. From Chopra (1988b).

established that *cad*A-mediated resistance results from an energy-dependent efflux system that excretes cadmium ions from resistant cells (Foster 1983; Chopra 1988b) (Fig. 2). Prior to efflux in staphylococci containing *cad*A, cadmium ions are transported into the cell by the energy-dependent manganese transport system (Fig. 2). This uptake system is highly specific for cadmium and manganese ions. The nature of the product(s) encoded by *cad*A is unknown and hence knowledge on this staphylococcal efflux system is more limited than that previously described for arsenical efflux mediated by staphylococcal plasmids.

TABLE 1. *Nature and function of ars-encoded polypeptides involved in expression of resistance to arsenicals in* E. coli. *(From Chopra 1988b.)*

Protein	Amino acid residues	Molecular weight	Isoelectric point	% non-polar residues	Proposed function
ArsA	583	63 169	6.1	46.7	Catalytic subunit of arsenical translocating ATP-ase
ArsB	429	45 577	9.8	61.5	Membrane-located anion translocating component of the arsenical pump
ArsC	141	15 811	5.9	43.3	Modifies ArsA and ArsB activity to allow recognition (efflux) of arsenate

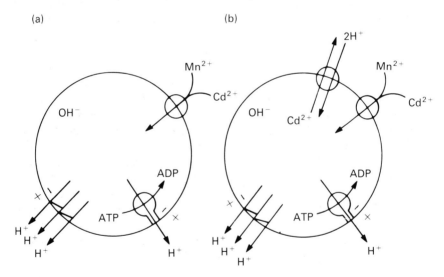

FIG. 2. Accumulation of manganese and cadmium ions by *Staph. aureus*. (a) illustrates cadmium and manganese co-transport into a cadmium-sensitive cell. (b) also illustrates transport of these cations, but in addition shows the *cad*A-encoded cadmium efflux protein in a cadmium-resistant cell, which promotes electroneutral cadmium/proton exchange. For other details see the text and the legend to Fig. 1. From Chopra (1988b).

Copper

Plasmid-determined resistance to copper has been reported in a number of bacterial species including *Staph. aureus*, *E. coli*, *Mycobacterium scrofulaceum* and plant pathogens (Groves & Young 1975; Ishihara *et al.* 1978; Tetaz & Luke 1983; Erardi *et al.* 1987; Cooksey 1987; Mellano & Cooksey 1988).

Cotter *et al.* (1987) studied the biochemical basis of copper resistance mediated by Rts1, a plasmid originally described by Ishihara *et al.* (1978). Resistance was ascribed to decreased accumulation of cupric ions by *E. coli*. However, resistant organisms still accumulate considerable quantities of copper ions and only a threefold drop in uptake was demonstrated when compared with sensitive organisms (Cotter *et al.* 1987). Since plasmid Rts1 confers at least a 150-fold increase in resistance (tolerance) to copper (Ishihara *et al.* 1978), the significance of decreased copper uptake as a resistance mechanism seems doubtful.

In *M. scrofulaceum* a high molecular weight plasmid confers the ability to remove copper from the culture medium by sulphate-dependent precipitation as copper sulphide (Erardi *et al.* 1987). This leads to the formation of a black, cell-associated precipitate during culture of resistant organisms. In addition, the 110-MDal plasmid confers a sulphate-independent copper resistance mechanism (Erardi *et al.* 1987). Tetaz & Luke (1983) isolated an *E. coli* strain from animal effluent that possessed a conjugative plasmid conferring copper resistance. The colonies of copper-resistant strains of *E. coli* carrying the plasmid were darkened suggesting sulphide formation. However, the authors did not determine whether copper sulphide was present. It is unclear whether sulphate-dependent or -independent resistance mechanisms are encoded by the plasmids described by other authors (Groves & Young 1975; Ishihara *et al.* 1978; Cooksey 1987; Mellano & Cooksey 1988). However, both resistance mechanisms may depend upon initial binding of copper to plasmid-encoded resistance proteins. In this context Mellano & Cooksey (1988) have identified possible copper-binding sites in proteins predicted to be encoded by the copper-resistance determinant from the plant pathogen *Pseudomonas syringae* pv. *tomato*. Two proteins have been implicated in resistance, both of which contain repeated sequences of the general structure Asp−His−X−X−Met−X−X−Met (Fig. 3). These regions may represent repeated copper-binding domains that could play a role in copper resistance.

Ethylenediamine Tetraacetate (EDTA)

The chelating agent EDTA affects the surface of Gram-negative bacteria and in many cases causes the outer membrane to become more permeable to

A	1295	Asp	His	Gly	Ser	Met	Asp	Gly	Met
	1395	Asp	Hiś	Ser	Lys	Met	Ser	Thr	Met
	1427	Asp	His	Gly	Ala	Met	Ser	Gly	Met
	1451	Asp	His	Gly	Ala	Met	Gly	Gly	Met
B	2113	Asp	His	Ser	Gln	Met	Gln	Gly	Met
	2137	Asp	His	Ser	Lys	Met	Gln	Gly	Met
	2161	Asp	His	Ser	Gln	Met	Gln	Gly	Met
	2185	Asp	His	Ser	Lys	Met	Gln	Gly	Met
	2209	Asp	His	Ser	Gln	Met	Gln	Gly	Met

FIG. 3. Predicted amino acid sequences of homologous repeated units in two proteins (A and B) thought to be involved in plasmid-encoded copper resistance in the plant pathogen *Pseudomonas syringae* pv. *tomato*. The numbers on the left indicate the positions (in base pairs) of the first codon of each repeating unit. Conserved amino acids are boxed. From Mellano & Cooksey (1988).

various molecules (Heppel 1968; Leive 1974). Mutational resistance to EDTA involving outer membrane changes has been reported in *Pseudomonas aeruginosa* (Hancock & Nicas 1980, 1984). Resistance is associated with enrichment of an outer membrane protein, termed H1, which is increased up to 24-fold in resistant bacteria. This is accompanied by a concomitant decrease in the outer membrane cation level. The mechanism by which protein H1 confers protection is unknown but it may replace outer membrane divalent cations at a site which can otherwise be attacked by EDTA. This mechanism of resistance has not been found in other organisms (Hancock & Nicas 1984).

Hexachlorophane

There is one report of plasmid-encoded resistance to hexachlorophane (Sutton & Jacoby 1978). In this case the plasmid conferred about a fivefold increase in resistance on the host organism, *Ps. aeruginosa*. The biochemical basis of the resistance mechanism is unknown.

Mercuric Ions and Organomercurials

Plasmid-encoded resistance to mercury or organomercurials has been found in a wide variety of bacterial species (Trevors *et al.* 1985). The genetic and biochemical basis of resistance has been extensively reviewed in recent years (Foster 1983, 1987; Trevors *et al.* 1985; Chopra 1987; Walsh *et al.* 1988) so only a brief summary is provided here, based upon information in the reviews.

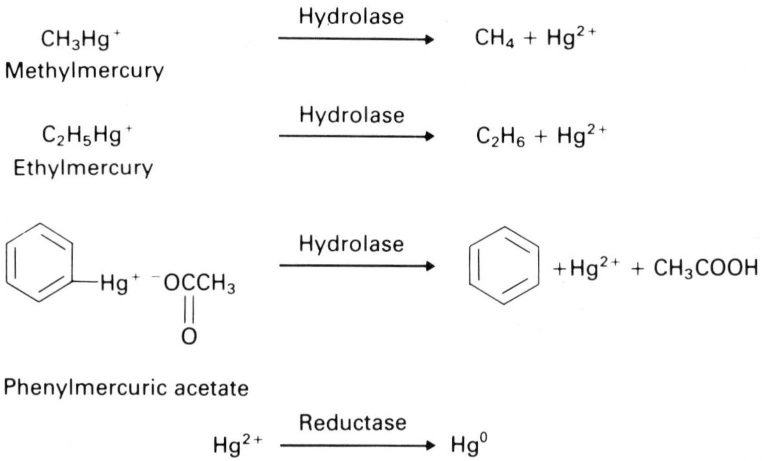

$$CH_3Hg^+ \xrightarrow{\text{Hydrolase}} CH_4 + Hg^{2+}$$

Methylmercury

$$C_2H_5Hg^+ \xrightarrow{\text{Hydrolase}} C_2H_6 + Hg^{2+}$$

Ethylmercury

$$\text{C}_6\text{H}_5\text{—Hg}^+\ ^-\text{OCCH}_3 \xrightarrow{\text{Hydrolase}} \text{C}_6\text{H}_6 + Hg^{2+} + CH_3COOH$$
(with $\|$ O below)

Phenylmercuric acetate

$$Hg^{2+} \xrightarrow{\text{Reductase}} Hg^0$$

FIG. 4. Enzymic basis of organomercurial-mercury volatilization mediated by bacterial plasmids. From Chopra (1987).

Resistance to the compounds frequently depends upon reduction of mercuric ions to metallic mercury (Fig. 4) which, due to its high vapour pressure, evaporates. A cytoplasmically located mercuric reductase reduces mercuric ions to metallic mercury, and for organomercurials this may be preceded by the action of one or more plasmid-encoded hydrolases (lyases) (also cytoplasmic) which break carbon–mercury bonds to release mercuric ions. The latter can then be reduced by the reductase (Fig. 4).

Since the plasmid-specified mercuric reductases and hydrolases are cytoplasmic enzymes there is a requirement for extracellular mercury and organomercurials to cross the cytoplasmic membrane to be detoxified. The resistance determinant (mer) of the E. coli plasmid R100 encodes a mercuric-ion-specific transport system (merT) which appears to direct mercuric ions through the cytoplasmic membrane to prevent them from encountering otherwise sensitive proteins. The R100-encoded mercuric reductase and merT probably interact indirectly through another mer-specified protein, merC (Fig. 5).

The nucleotide sequence of the R100-1-encoded merT gene has been determined. This allows prediction of the primary amino acid sequence of the merT protein. It contains 116 amino acids, many of which are hydrophobic. Figure 6 displays the hydropathy plot (Kyte & Doolittle 1982) of the R100-1-encoded merT protein. Most of the protein is probably embedded within the lipid bilayer of the cytoplasmic membrane with a few short hydrophilic regions that are likely to project out of the membrane. Since cysteine residues are

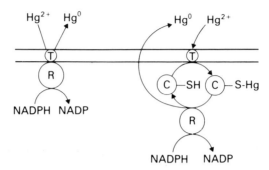

FIG. 5. Mechanism of resistance to mercuric ions mediated by the *mer* determinant of plasmid R100. Two possible mechanisms for detoxification of mercuric ions are shown. The parallel lines represent the cytoplasmic membrane. The diagram on the left indicates that the reductase protein (R) interacts directly with the membrane-bound transport protein (T). On the right it is suggested that another *mer* operon specified protein (*mer*C:C) is required to bind the incoming Hg in the form of an adduct and transport it to cytoplasmic reductase (R) molecules. From Chopra (1987).

likely candidates for mercuric ion binding sites, it is interesting to note that a pair of cysteine residues (positions 24 and 25) occurs within a membrane-spanning region (Fig. 6). This arrangement suggests a model for mercuric ion transport during its detoxification. Mercuric ions might initially be sequestered by binding to the *mer*T thiol groups of the cysteine residues at positions 24 and 25. A series of redox exchange reactions might then pass the ions to further thiol groups in the *mer*C protein and finally to the mercuric reductase (see Fig. 5).

Organic Cations: Quaternary Ammonium Compounds, Propamidine, Chlorhexidine, Crystal Violet, Acriflavine and Ethidium

Plasmid-determined resistance to several organic cations has been reported in *Staph. aureus* (Lyon & Skurray 1987; Chopra 1988b; Yamamoto *et al.* 1988). In some cases concomitant resistance to a number of these compounds occurs which include euflavine and proflavine (the components of acriflavine) (Ac), ethidium bromide (Eb), amidines such as propamidine isothionate (Pi), chlorhexidine (Ch) and diamidinodiphenylamine dihydrochloride (Dd), and quaternary ammonium compounds (Qa) such as cetyltrimethylammonium bromide (cetrimide) and benzalkonium chloride. The structures of these compounds are shown in Fig. 7 from which it can be seen that they are all cationic. Genetic studies on plasmid-determined resistance to these compounds in *Staph. aureus* has identified three distinct resistance determinants designated *qac*A, *qac*B and *qac*C (Lyon & Skurray 1987; Chopra 1988b; Yamamoto *et al.* 1988).

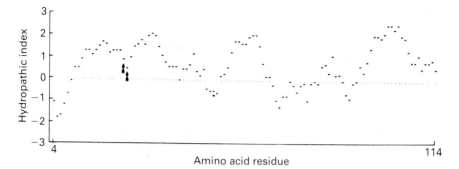

FIG. 6. Hydropathic profile of the R100-encoded *mer*T protein. Hydropathy was calculated according to Kyte & Doolittle (1982) with a moving segment of seven amino acids. The portions above the mid-point line (positive values) indicate hydrophobic regions, the regions below (negative values) indicate hydrophilic regions. The pattern proceeds from the N-terminus on the left to the C-terminus on the right. Cysteine residues at positions 24 and 25 are indicated by arrows (see text for discussion). From Chopra (1987).

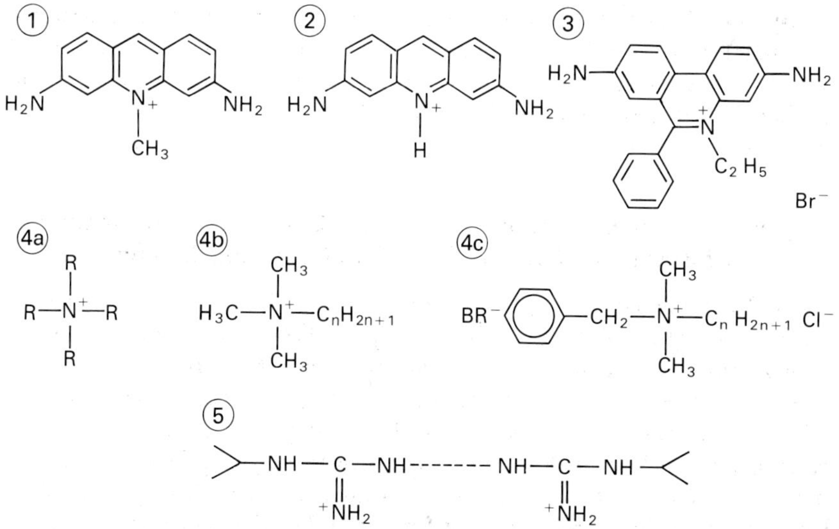

FIG. 7. Structure of various organic cations. 1, Euflavine; 2, proflavine; 3, ethidium bromide; 4a, generic structure for quaternary ammonium salts; 4b, cetrimide (a mixture of dodecyl-, tetradecyl- and hexadecyl-trimethyl ammonium bromide, i.e. n = 12, 14 or 16); 4c, benzalkonium chloride (a mixture of alkyldimethyl ammonium chlorides, n = 8–18); 5, a generalized structure of the amidine-derived antimicrobial agents propamidine and chlorhexidine, both of which are bi-guanides. From Chopra (1988b).

Determinant *qac*A mediates Ac−r, Eb−r, Qa−r, Pi−r, Ch−r and Dd−r (Lyon & Skurray 1987; Chopra 1988b) and encodes a protein of mol. wt 38 000 (Yamamoto *et al.* 1988). Determinant *qac*B, which shows some DNA sequence homology with *qac*A, only mediates Ac−r, Eb−r and Qa−r (Lyon & Skurray 1987). The third determinant, *qac*C, does not share homology with either *qac*A or *qac*B and mediates Qa−r and low-level Eb−r (Lyon & Skurray 1987). The products of *qac*B and *qac*C have not yet been characterized.

Ethidium bromide resistance determined by qacC results from energy-dependent efflux of the organic cation from resistant cells by an antiport reaction probably involving an electroneutral exchange of the ethidium cation for a proton (Jones & Midgley 1985; Midgley 1986). It seems likely that *qac*A-, *qac*B- and *qac*C-mediated resistance to other organic cations has a similar energetic basis although the efflux proteins (antiporters) concerned may not be identical in all cases.

Recently, chromosomal mutation to chlorhexidine resistance in *Providencia stuartii* has been reported (Chopra *et al.* 1987). However, in this case no evidence for a chlorhexidine efflux system responsible for resistance has been obtained (I. Chopra, unpublished data). Osmotic shock procedures (Heppel 1968) temporarily sensitize chlorhexidine-resistant strains to the antiseptic, resistance being restored by incubating shocked cells for a short period in growth medium. Recovery is dependent on protein synthesis, but occurs more rapidly than cell division, suggesting that previously injured cells restore resistance more quickly than they divide (I. Chopra, unpublished data). Since osmotic shock removes periplasmic proteins from *Pv. stuartii* (Chopra & Johnson 1987) the results are consistent with a periplasmic resistance mechanism probably dependent upon the presence of one or more proteins. The exact mechanism of protection against chlorhexidine is presently unclear. In antibiotic resistant bacteria periplasmic enzymes are frequently responsible for drug inactivation (Foster 1983; Chopra 1988a). However, since chlorhexidine-resistant strains of *Pv. stuartii* do not inactivate the antiseptic (Thomas & Stickler 1979), the possibility remains that the periplasmic protective protein(s) binds and traps chlorhexidine thereby preventing it from interacting with its normal target, i.e. the cytoplasmic membrane (Chopra *et al.* 1987).

Silver

Several workers have reported the occurrence of bacterial plasmids that encode resistance to silver ions (see Chopra 1987). Although the mechanism of plasmid-encoded silver ion resistance is not well understood, Misra *et al.* (1984) have suggested that sensitive bacteria bind silver ions so avidly that they extract it from AgCl and other salts, whereas cells with resistance plasmids are prevented from sequestering silver ions.

Acquired resistance to silver by chromosomal mutation has also been reported. For instance, chromosomally encoded silver resistance in *E. coli*, which arises at a fairly high frequency, results from a decrease in silver binding by a major outer membrane protein (Pugsley & Schnaitman 1978). Evidence for chromosomal resistance to silver in other bacterial species has also been obtained (Summers 1984).

Tellurium

Bacterial resistance to tellurium salts is widespread in nature and in many cases is known to be plasmid-determined (Trevors *et al.* 1985). Jobling & Ritchie (1987) have studied the basis of inducible tellurium resistance encoded by a plasmid originally isolated from an *Alcaligenes* strain. The resistance determinant, located in a 3.55-kb region of the plasmid, encodes four polypeptides of molecular weights 15.5, 22, 23 and 41 kDal, but the mechanism by which these products confer resistance is unknown.

Methods for Studying the Molecular and Biochemical Basis of Resistance

The methods used to study the topics presented here virtually encompass the complete range of techniques now available to the molecular biologist. Clearly, a comprehensive practical guide to all these techniques is beyond the scope of this chapter. Accordingly, a few selected techniques are fully described and key references given for other methods which cannot be provided here.

Molecular cloning and DNA sequencing

These techniques have been of major importance in unravelling the detailed molecular basis of resistance to arsenicals, copper, mercurials, organic cations and tellurium. Practical guidance can be found in the texts by Maniatis *et al.* (1982), Davies (1982) and Brown (1984).

Identification of cloned gene products in E. coli *minicells*

The expression of gene products in minicells has contributed greatly to our understanding of resistance to arsenicals, mercurials and tellurium. This author has also used *E. coli* minicells for the detection of cloned or plasmid-encoded gene products (Eccles & Chopra 1984; Davies *et al.* 1988; Shohayeb & Chopra 1988) and the general laboratory protocol is described below. The procedure employs the *E. coli* minicell-producing strain DS410 (*lac* str−r, *min*A, *min*B) carrying an appropriate plasmid of interest.

Preparation of minicells

1 Inoculate 500−1000 ml of Brain Heart Infusion Broth (Difco, Surrey, UK) with a single colony and incubate at 37°C overnight with aeration.

2 Cool culture on ice and subject it to low-speed differential centrifugation (1000−2000 g, 5 min, 4°C) to pellet whole cells and leave the majority of minicells in the supernatant fraction.

3 Decant the supernatant liquid and centrifuge it (12 000−15 000 g, 10 min, 4°C) to collect the minicells.

4 Resuspend the pellet in about 12 ml of M9 salts solution (0.6% (w/v) Na_2HPO_4, 0.3% (w/v) KH_2PO_4, 0.05% (w/v) NaCl, 0.1% (w/v) NH_4Cl) containing cycloserine (100 μg/ml). Carefully layer 3-ml aliquots on to 35-ml sucrose gradients (or pro rata) in tubes suitable for use in a low-speed, swing-out, centrifuge rotor (e.g. a Sorvall HS-4 swinging bucket rotor). Satisfactory gradients can be made by thawing tubes containing frozen 20% (w/v) sucrose (in M9 salts) in a 30°C water bath for 1.5 h. Alternatively, gradients can be made immediately before use with a conventional gradient maker using 5% (w/v) and 20% (w/v) sucrose solutions.

5 Centrifuge for 10−15 min (*c.* 2000 g, 4°C). Under these conditions residual whole cells should be pelleted and minicells contained in an upper band. Remove the upper portion of the minicell band with a Pasteur pipette or syringe.

6 Collect minicells by centrifugation (repeat of step 3).

7 Repeat steps 4−6 a further two times i.e. purify minicells by fractionation on two further sucrose gradients.

8 Repeat step 6 and re-suspend the final minicell pellet in *c.* 5-ml M9 salts containing cycloserine (100 μg/ml).

9 Examine the preparation by phase-contrast microscopy. If no whole cells can be detected in a single field at ×40 magnification, the minicell preparation is satisfactory. The minicell content can be determined approximately by measuring the absorbance of the suspension at 640 nm on the basis that an absorbance value of 1 is equivalent to about 1×10^{10} minicells/ml.

10 Collect minicells by centrifugation (step 3) and resuspend to 2×10^{10} minicells/ml in M9 salts containing cycloserine (100 μg/ml) and glycerol (3% v/v). Store suitable aliquots (e.g. 0.5 ml) at −70°C or in liquid nitrogen.

Labelling of minicells and detection of plasmid-encoded proteins

1 Thaw 0.5 ml of frozen minicells. Wash twice with 1-ml volumes of M9 salts containing cycloserine (100 μg/ml). A bench microfuge (e.g. Eppendorff) is suitable at this stage.

2 Resuspend the minicell pellet in 200 μl M9 medium. M9 medium (sterile) comprises per 10 ml: 9.8 ml M9 salts solution, 1 mg cycloserine, 90 μl 1 mol/l

$MgSO_4$, 5 µl 1 mol/l $CaCl_2$, 5 µl 1 mmol/l $FeCl_3$, 100 µl glucose solution (40% w/v). Add 10 µl Methionine Assay Medium (Difco) and pre-incubate at 37°C for 1 h to allow minicells to reach maximum metabolic activity.

3 Add $3.7-7.4 \times 10^5$ Bq of ^{35}S-labelled methionine and incubate at 37°C for 2 h.

4 Add phenylmethylsulphonyl fluoride (PMSF) to 1 mmol/l, (PMSF stock solutions of 100 mmol/l can be made in ethanol: CAUTION! PMSF is a protease inhibitor) and pellet minicells in a microfuge as in step 1.

5 Resuspend pellet in 200 µl of a suitable sample buffer (see Hames 1968) prior to sodium dodecyl sulphate polyacrylamide gel electrophoresis.

6 Subject the sample to electrophoresis and detect labelled products by auto-radiography or fluorography. Detailed practical guidance on electrophoresis and detection methods is provided by Hames (1981) and William & Gledhill (this book).

Comments

Detection of various plasmid-encoded products using the minicell system is illustrated in Fig. 8. In addition, minicells can be fractionated to produce subcellular fractions. Figure 9 shows enrichment of the pBR322-encoded tetracycline efflux protein in the minicell inner membrane following fraction-ation of whole minicells to produce membrane material. Further details of these and other techniques using minicells can be found in the articles by Stoker *et al.* (1984) and Dougan & Kehoe (1984).

Transport studies

Studies on the movement of inhibitors across cell membranes has led to an improved understanding of resistance mechanisms to some of the inhibitors described earlier. To some extent these advances have depended upon the development of transport assays using *E. coli* membrane vesicles. Techniques are therefore described for the preparation of right-side-out vesicles (for studying solute influx) and everted vesicles (for studying solute efflux).

Preparation of right-side-out vesicles

The technique is based on that of Kaback (1971) and uses the prototrophic *E. coli* strain ML308−225 (*lac*I, *lac*Y, *lac*Z).

1 Grow a 1000−1500-ml culture of strain ML308−225 in a basal salts medium containing 0.5−1.0% glucose, glycerol or succinate as a carbon source to the late exponential phase of growth (absorbance at 675 nm of *c.* 0.8 u).

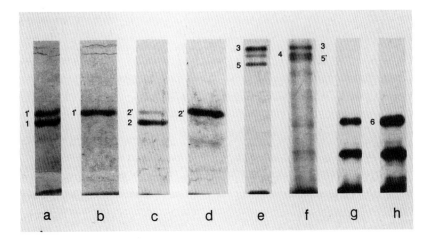

FIG. 8. Detection of plasmid-encoded and cloned gene products in *E. coli* minicells. ^{35}S-methionine-labelled proteins synthesized in minicells were separated by polyacrylamide gel electrophoresis and detected by fluorography. The numbers show the position of the processed and precursor forms of the pUC9 encoded β-lactamase (1, 1' respectively), the processed and precursor forms of the pRW83 encoded β-lactamase (2, 2' respectively), the α and γ forms of penicillin-binding protein 1b (3, 4 respectively), the processed and precursor forms of tonA (5, 5' respectively), and penicillin-binding protein 4 (6). The profiles in tracks b, d, f, h were obtained under conditions where protein processing is inhibited. From Davies *et al.* (1988).

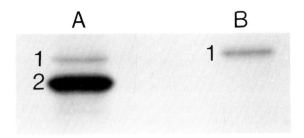

FIG. 9. Fractionation of minicells containing labelled pBR322 encoded proteins. ^{35}S-methionine-labelled proteins synthesized in minicells were separated by polyacrylamide gel electrophoresis and detected by fluorography. A, Profile from whole minicells; B, profile of inner membranes recovered from minicells. Protein 1, the tetracycline efflux protein conferring pBR322 encoded tetracycline resistance, is located in the inner membrane, whereas protein 2, the pBR322 encoded TEM1 β-lactamase, is not found in the inner membrane.

2   Wash the cells twice (12 000–15 000 *g*, 4°C, 15 min) in 10 mmol/l Tris-HCl buffer (pH 8.0).

3   Resuspend 1g (wet weight) of cells, or pro rata, in 80 ml 30 mmol/l Tris-HCl buffer (pH 8.0) containing 20% (w/v) sucrose. Add potassium EDTA

and lysozyme to give final concentrations of 10 mmol/l and 0.5 mg/ml, respectively. The EDTA solution should be added slowly. Incubate with stirring at room temperature for 30 min.

4 Check the efficiency of spheroplasting by examining the preparation with a phase-contrast microscope. Spheroplasts appear as rounded forms that have lost the normal rod-shaped morphology of whole bacteria.

5 Subject the spheroplasts to centrifugation (12 000–15 000 g, 4°C, 15 min).

6 Add 3 ml of 0.1 mol/l potassium phosphate buffer (pH 6.6) containing 20% (w/v) sucrose and 20 mmol/l $MgSO_4$ to the spheroplast pellet. Homogenize the pellet either in a Teflon–Glass homogenizer or using a syringe fitted with a 19 G needle. Add 9 mg each of deoxyribonuclease and ribonuclease.

7 Pour the spheroplast suspension into 400 ml 0.1 mol/l potassium phosphate buffer pH 6.6 and incubate with stirring at 37°C.

8 Add potassium EDTA (10 mmol/l) and incubate for 15 min at 37°C, followed by magnesium sulphate (15 mmol/l) and incubation for another 15 min. At this stage the spheroplasts should have lysed and the absence of major whole cell contamination should be checked by phase-contrast microscopy (see comments under minicell preparation, page 56).

9 Centrifuge the lysate (12 000–15 000 g, 4°C, 30 min).

10 Resuspend the pellet by homogenization in 0.1 mol/l potassium phosphate buffer (pH 6.6) containing 10 mmol/l EDTA.

10 Subject the suspension to low-speed centrifugation (c.800 g, 4°C, 30 min).

12 Discard the pellet (residual intact cells).

13 Repeat steps 11 and 12 then subject the final suspension to high-speed centrifugation (45 000 g, 4°C, 30 min).

14 Repeat step 13 four to six times using the buffer described at step 10.

15 Perform a protein assay on the membranes recovered at step 14 and resuspend them in 0.1 mol/l potassium phosphate buffer pH 6.6 to give a concentration of 1 mg protein/ml. Store small aliquots in liquid nitrogen.

Comments

Various transport assays can be performed with vesicles prepared as described above. These assays can be conducted with a variety of radio-labelled solutes using several types of energy source. Invariably the assays involve collection of vesicles on membrane filters that are washed to remove free (non-transported) solute. Detailed methodology of transport assays can be found in the articles by Kaback (1971), Silver & Bhattacharyya (1974), and Marquis (1981). Consideration has to be given to the type of membrane filters used because this can influence the retention of vesicles (Rosen & Tsuchiya 1979). An

TABLE 2. *Proline transport into* E. coli *membrane vesicles*

	Counts per min/mg vesicle protein	
Conditions	Cellulose nitrate filters	Cellulose acetate filters
Vesicles without added energy source	5775	1915
Vesicles with lithium D-lactate (20 mmol/l)	68 540*	15 220

Uptake of ^{3}H-proline ($10\,\mu M$; 1.85×10^5 Bq ml) by membrane vesicles was determined. Vesicles from glucose-grown cells of *E. coli* ML308−225 were assayed at pH 6.6 for proline transport (30 min) according to the procedure of Kaback (1971) using either Whatman cellulose nitrate filters or Sartorius cellulose acetate filters (each type 25 mm diameter, 0.45-μm pore size). Values shown are the means of duplicate determinations. Radioactivity trapped by the filters in the absence of vesicles has been subtracted.
* Assuming an internal volume of $1\,\mu l$/mg vesicle protein (Hirata *et al.* 1974) this represents an intravesicular concentration of $348\,\mu mol/l$ i.e. establishment of a 35-fold concentration gradient. This value is comparable with that reported by Kaback & Stadtman (1966) for proline transport into *E. coli* membrane vesicles.

example is provided with data obtained in the author's laboratory (Table 2) which indicate that retention of vesicles on cellulose acetate filters is less efficient than retention on nitrocellulose filters. It is also wise to confirm that any particular batch of vesicles will support dehydrogenase-coupled transport, e.g. that of proline (see Table 2 for typical results obtained in the author's laboratory).

Preparation of everted membrane vesicles

Everted membrane vesicles are useful for studying both proton motive force-dependent and ATP-dependent efflux of inhibitors from cells. A comprehensive description of the method for preparing everted vesicles and their use in transport assays is given by Rosen & Tsuchiya (1979) to which the reader is referred for practical guidance. The preparation of everted membrane vesicles usually involves the disintegration of bacteria in a French Pressure Cell. In the UK commercial French Pressure Cells can be purchased from DG Electronics, 16/20 Camp Road, Farnborough, Hampshire GU14 6EW.

Hydropathy analysis

Hydropathy analysis of membrane proteins has proved valuable in predicting the nature of their folding within the bacterial cytoplasmic membrane. In the context of this article hydropathy analysis has been applied to proteins involved in resistance to arsenicals and mercurials. Kyte & Doolittle (1982) presented a useful method which the present author has also used. The original computer program presented by Kyte & Doolittle (1982) was written in the language 'C', but this can relatively easily be rewritten in other languages e.g. the present author has been using hydropathy analysis with a BBC microcomputer having converted the original program to Basic. Other approaches to hydropathy analysis are also available and these have recently been reviewed by Wallace *et al.* (1986).

Conclusions

Studies on the genetic and biochemical basis of bacterial resistance to anti-septics, disinfectants and toxic metal ions are not as advanced as those dealing with antibiotic resistance. However, it is already evident that resistance mechanisms to non-antibiotic inhibitors are, in many cases, similar to those responsible for antibiotic resistance. For instance, energy-dependent efflux of arsenicals, cadmium and organic cations is formally similar to efflux of the antibiotic tetracycline from resistant organisms (Chopra 1988b) and enzymatic reduction of mercuric ions to metallic mercury bears a resemblance to enzymic modification of beta-lactams, aminoglycosides and chloramphenicol (Foster 1983; Chopra, 1988a). It can, therefore, be anticipated that future work will continue to indicate that the mechanisms used to protect bacteria from inhibition by non-antibiotic agents are fundamentally the same as those conferring antibiotic resistance.

Note Added in Proof

Recent observations (P. McNicholas and I. Chopra, manuscript in preparation) indicate that the protein band labelled 1 in Fig. 9 contains two poly-peptides: the tetracycline efflux protein and a precursor form of protein 2 (i.e. the pBR322 encoded β-lactamase). These polypeptides apparently co-migrate in the gel system described and also co-fractionate with the inner membrane.

References

BROWN, N.L. 1984. DNA sequencing. In *Methods in Microbiology*, Vol. 17, ed. Bennett, P.M. & Grinsted, J. pp. 259–313. London: Academic Press.

CHOPRA, I. 1987. Microbial resistance to veterinary disinfectants and antiseptics. In *Disinfection in Veterinary and Farm Animal Practice*, ed. Linton, A.H., Hugo, W.B. & Russell, A.D. pp. 43−65. Oxford: Blackwell Scientific Publications.

CHOPRA, I. 1988a. Mechanisms of resistance to antibiotics and other chemotherapeutic agents. *Journal of Applied Bacteriology Symposium Supplement No. 17* **65**, 149S−166S.

CHOPRA, I. 1988b. Efflux of antibacterial agents from bacteria. In *Homeostatic Mechanisms in Micro-Organisms*, ed. Whittenbury, R., Gould, G.W., Banks, J.G. & Board, R.G. pp. 146−158. FEMS Symposium No. 44, Bath University Press.

CHOPRA, I. & JOHNSON, S.C. 1987. Fractionation of the *Providencia stuartii* cell envelope. *Journal of General Microbiology* **133**, 1767−1773.

CHOPRA, I., JOHNSON, S.C. & BENNETT, P.M. 1987. Inhibition of *Providencia stuartii* cell envelope enzymes by chlorhexidine. *Journal of Antimicrobial Chemotherapy* **19**, 743−752.

COOKSEY, D.A. 1987. Characterization of a copper resistance plasmid conserved in copper-resistant strains of *Pseudomonas syringae* pv. *tomato*. *Applied and Environmental Bacteriology* **53**, 454−456.

COTTER, C.M., TREVORS, J.T. & GADD, G.M. 1987. Decreased cupric ion uptake as the mechanism for cupric ion resistance in *Escherichia coli*. *FEMS Microbiology Letters* **48**, 299−303.

DAVIES, D.B., SHOHAYEB, M. & CHOPRA, I. 1988. Prediction of signal-sequence dependent protein translocation in bacteria: assessment of the *Escherichia coli* minicell system. *Biochemical and Biophysical Research Communications* **150**, 371−375.

DAVIES, R.W. 1982. DNA sequencing. In *Gel Electrophoresis of Nucleic Acids, a Practical Approach*, ed. Rickwood, D. & Hames, B.D. pp. 117−172. Oxford: IRL Press.

DOUGAN, G. & KEHOE, M. 1984. The minicell system as a method for studying expression from plasmid DNA. In *Methods in Microbiology*, Vol. 17, ed. Bennett, P.M. & Grinsted, J. pp. 233−258. London: Academic Press.

ECCLES, S.J. & CHOPRA, I. 1984. Biochemical and genetic characterization of the *tet* determinant of *Bacillus* plasmid pAB124. *Journal of Bacteriology* **158**, 134−140.

ERARDI, F.X., FAILLA, M.L. & FALKINHAM, J.O. 1987. Plasmid-encoded copper resistance and precipitation by *Mycobacterium scrofulaceum*. *Applied and Environmental Microbiology* **53**, 1951−1954.

FOSTER, T.J. 1983. Plasmid-determined resistance to antimicrobial drugs and toxic metal ions in bacteria. *Microbiological Reviews* **47**, 361−409.

FOSTER, T.J. 1987. The genetics and biochemistry of mercury resistance. *CRC Critical Reviews in Microbiology* **15**, 117−140.

GROVES, D.J. & YOUNG, F.E. 1975. Epidemiology of antibiotic and heavy metal resistance in bacteria: resistance patterns in staphylococci isolated from populations not known to be exposed to heavy metals. *Antimicrobial Agents and Chemotherapy* **7**, 614−621.

HAMES, B.D. 1981. An introduction to polyacrylamide gel electrophoresis. In *Gel Electrophoresis of Proteins: a Practical Approach*, ed. Hames, B.D. & Rickwood, D. pp. 1−91. London: IRL Press.

HANCOCK, R.E.W. & NICAS, T.I. 1980. Outer membrane protein H1 of *Pseudomonas aeruginosa*: involvement in adaptive and mutational resistance to ethylenediamine tetraacetate, polymyxin B, and gentamicin. *Journal of Bacteriology* **143**, 872−878.

HANCOCK, R.E.W. & NICAS, T.I. 1984. Resistance to antibacterial agents acting on cell membranes. In *Antimicrobial Drug Resistance*, ed. Bryan, L.E. pp. 147−171. New York & London: Academic Press.

HEPPEL, L.A. 1968. Preparation of cells of *Escherichia coli* with altered permeability. *Methods in Enzymology* **12B**, 841−846.

HIRATA, H., ALTENDORF, K. & HAROLD, F.M. 1974. Energy coupling in membrane vesicles of

Escherichia coli. I. Accumulation of metabolites in response to an electrical potential. *Journal of Biological Chemistry* **249**, 2939–2945.

HUGO, W.B. & RUSSELL, A.D. 1982. Types of antimicrobial agents. In *Principles and Practice of Disinfection, Preservation and Sterilisation*, ed. Russell, A.D., Hugo, W.B. & Ayliffe, G.A.J. pp. 8–106. Oxford: Blackwell Scientific Publications.

ISHIHARA, M., KAMIO, Y. & TERAWAKI, Y. 1978. Cupric ion resistance as a new marker of a temperature sensitive R plasmid, Rts1 in *Escherichia coli*. *Biochemical and Biophysical Research Communications* **82**, 74–80.

JOBLING, M.G. & RITCHIE, D.A. 1987. Genetic and physical analysis of plasmid genes expressing inducible resistance to tellurite in *Escherichia coli*. *Molecular and General Genetics* **208**, 288–293.

JONES, I.G. & MIDGLEY, M. 1985. Expression of a plasmid borne ethidium resistance determinant from *Staphylococcus* in *Escherichia coli*: evidence for an efflux system. *FEMS Microbiology Letters* **28**, 355–358.

KABACK, H.R. 1971. Bacterial membranes. *Methods in Enzymology* **22**, 99–120.

KABACK, H.R. & STADTMAN, E.R. 1966. Proline uptake by an isolated cytoplasmic membrane preparation of *Escherichia coli*. *Proceedings of the National Academy of Sciences, USA* **55**, 920–927.

KYTE, J. & DOOLITTLE, R.F. 1982. A simple method for displaying the hydropathic character of a protein. *Journal of Molecular Biology* **157**, 105–132.

LEIVE, L. 1974. The barrier function of the gram-negative envelope. *Annals of the New York Academy of Sciences* **235**, 109–129.

LYON, B.R. & SKURRAY. R. 1987. Antimicrobial resistance of *Staphylococcus aureus*: genetic basis. *Microbiological Reviews* **51**, 88–134.

MANIATIS, T., ERITSCH, E.E. & SAMBROOK, J. 1982. *Molecular Cloning, a Laboratory Manual*. Cold Spring Harbor, New York: Cold Spring Harbor Laboratory.

MARQUIS, R.E. 1981. Permeability and transport. In *Manual of Methods for General Bacteriology*, ed. Gerhardt, P. *et al*. pp. 393–404. Washington DC: American Society for Microbiology.

MELLANO, M.A. & COOKSEY, D.A. 1988. Nucleotide sequence and organization of copper resistance genes from *Pseudomonas syringae* pv. *tomato*. *Journal of Bacteriology* **170**, 2879–2883.

MIDGLEY M. 1986. The phosphonium ion efflux system of *Escherichia coli*: relationship to the ethidium efflux system and energetic studies. *Journal of General Microbiology* **132**, 3187–3193.

MISRA, T.K., SILVER S., MOBLEY, H.L.T. & ROSEN, B.P. 1984. Molecular genetics and biochemistry of heavy metal resistance in bacteria. In *Molecular and Cellular Approaches to Understanding Mechanisms of Toxicity*, ed. Tashjian, A.H. pp. 63–81. Boston: Harvard School of Public Health.

PUGSLEY, A.P. & SCHNAITMAN, C.A. 1978. Outer membrane proteins of *Escherichia coli*. VII. Evidence that bacteriophage-directed protein 2 functions as a pore. *Journal of Bacteriology* **133**, 1181–1189.

ROSEN, B.P. 1986. Recent advances in bacterial ion transport. *Annual Review of Microbiology* **40**, 263–286.

ROSEN, B.P. & TSUCHIYA, T. 1979. Preparation of everted membrane vesicles from *Escherichia coli* for the measurement of calcium transport. *Methods in Enzymology* **56**, 233–241.

ROSEN, B.P., WEIGEL, U., KARKARIA, C. & GANGOLA, P. 1988. Molecular characterization of an anion pump. *Journal of Biological Chemistry* **263**, 3067–3070.

RUSSELL, A.D. & HUGO, W.B. 1987. Chemical disinfectants. In *Disinfection in Veterinary and Farm Animal Practice*, ed. Linton, A.H., Hugo, W.B. & Russell, A.D. pp. 12–42. Oxford: Blackwell Scientific Publications.

64 I. CHOPRA

SHOHAYEB, M. & CHOPRA, I. 1988. Multiple isoelectric forms of bacterial penicillin-binding proteins: artefacts or genuine cellular components? *Journal of Antimicrobial Chemotherapy* **22**, 113–118.

SILVER, S. & BHATTACHARYYA, P. 1974. Cations, antibiotics and membranes. *Methods in Enzymology* **32**, 881–893.

STOKER, N.G., PRATT, J.M. & HOLLAND, I.B. 1984. *In vivo* gene expression systems in prokaryotes. In *Transcription and Translation, A Practical Approach*, ed. Hames, B.D. & Higgins, S.J. pp. 153–177. Oxford: IRL Press.

SUMMERS, A.O. 1984. Bacterial metal ion resistances. In *Antimicrobial Drug Resistance*, ed. Bryan, L.E. pp. 345–367. New York and London: Academic Press.

SUTTON, L. & JACOBY, G.A. 1978. Plasmid determined resistance to hexachlorophane in *Pseudomonas aeruginosa*. *Antimicrobial Agents and Chemotherapy* **13**, 634–636.

TETAZ, T.J. & LUKE, R.K.J. 1983. Plasmid-controlled resistance to copper in *Escherichia coli*. *Journal of Bacteriology* **154**, 1263–1268.

THOMAS, B. & STICKLER, D.J. 1979. Chlorhexidine resistance and the lipids of *Providencia stuartii*. *Microbios* **24**, 141–150.

TREVORS, J.T., ODDIE, K.M. & BELLIVEAU, B.H. 1985. Metal resistance in bacteria. *FEMS Microbiology Reviews* **32**, 39–54.

WALLACE, B.A., CASICO, M. & MIELKE, D.L. 1986. Evaluation of methods for the prediction of membrane protein secondary structures. *Proceedings of the National Academy of Sciences, USA* **83**, 9423–9427.

WALSH, C.T., DISTEFANO, M.D., MOORE, M.J., SHEWCHUK, L.M. & VERDINE, G.L. 1988. Molecular basis of bacterial resistance to organomercurial and inorganic mercuric salts. *Federation of American Societies for Experimental Biology Journal* **2**, 124–130.

YAMAMOTO, T., TAMURA, Y. & YOKOTA, T. 1988. Antiseptic and antibiotic resistance plasmid in *Staphylococcus aureus* that possesses ability to confer chlorhexidine and acrinol resistance. *Antimicrobial Agents and Chemotherapy* **32**, 932–935.

Biocide Uptake by Bacteria

W.G. SALT[1] AND D. WISEMAN[2]

[1] Microbiology Unit, Department of Chemistry, Loughborough University of Technology, Loughborough, Leicestershire LE11 3TU, UK; and [2] Postgraduate School of Studies in Pharmacy, University of Bradford, Bradford BD7 1DP, UK

Before any antimicrobial agent can exert biocidal effects it must be taken up by its target cells. Despite this primary importance of uptake there have been far fewer published studies of the uptake process than of the subsequent growth inhibitory and killing effects of such compounds.

Uptake of antimicrobial agents can involve one or more of several processes including adsorption, absorption, chemisorption, partition, diffusion both passive and facilitated, and active transport. Experimental studies of uptake and examination of the resulting uptake isotherms may throw light on the processes involved, help in understanding mechanisms of action and assist in the design and formulation of more effective antimicrobial products.

Uptake Studies

The principles underlying uptake experiments are fundamentally simple involving the following steps:

1 preparation of cell suspensions;
2 preparation of solutions of antimicrobial agent;
3 mixing of 1 and 2 to produce reaction mixtures;
4 removal of samples from reaction mixtures after appropriate time intervals and separation of the cells from the suspending fluid;
5 measurement of the amount of agent left in solution and thereby the cellular uptake by difference or more unusually direct measurement of the amount of agent bound to the separated cells.

Although simple in principle, problems arise in practice and each stage of the process will be considered in turn.

Mechanisms of Action of
Chemical Biocides

Preparation of Cell Suspensions

In most studies of the uptake of antimicrobial agents the ultimate intention is to correlate uptake with some measure of biological activity such as cell death, leakage, growth inhibition or enzyme inactivation. If such correlations are to have any meaning it is essential that the condition of the cells and the nature of the suspending medium in the uptake experiments should be as similar as possible to those used in the studies of biological activity.

Growth of cells

No definitive rules for the growth of cultures can be laid down and cells from batch cultures, either from the exponential phase of growth or from the stationary phase, have been used by some workers, whilst others have favoured the use of cells from chemostat cultures. Whatever source of cells is chosen it is important that the conditions of growth are clearly defined and easily reproduced.

The growth requirements of cells may dictate the use of a complex culture medium and in such cases if uptake is to be related to growth inhibition, the nature of the growth medium for inhibition studies will determine the nature of the suspending medium for the uptake studies (see section on suspending media).

Harvesting of cells

In uptake studies the cells usually need to be harvested to allow standardization of cell suspensions and in some cases to produce 'thick cell suspensions' with population densities higher than can be achieved in liquid cultures.

Cells are normally harvested by centrifuging or by membrane filtration, and are then washed with, and finally resuspended in, the appropriate suspending medium. The suspension is then adjusted to the required cell density, usually double that required in the final reaction mixture. Membrane filtration is fast and convenient unless large quantities of cells are being handled.

Suspending media

The composition of the suspending medium can profoundly affect the uptake of antimicrobial agents by changing the surface of the cells, by altering the ionic state of the agent or by competition for binding sites. The presence of magnesium ions, for example, reduces the uptake of cetyltrimethylammonium bromide (CTAB) or chlorhexidine from low concentrations (Salt & Wiseman 1970; Daham & Wiseman 1987), small changes in pH have a large effect on the uptake of chloroquine by *Escherichia coli* (Wiseman 1972), and uptake by active transport will be different in the presence and absence of an energy source.

The nature of the suspending medium may be dictated by the conditions required for any parallel studies of the biological effects of the antimicrobials. Workers studying solely bactericidal activity may be happy to work with water as the suspending medium but studies of growth or enzyme inhibition require the use of more complex media. In the case of simple defined growth media this should cause little difficulty but the use of complex media such as nutrient broth can present problems. Ideally a suspending medium should have a simple, defined, reproducible composition and a buffering capacity.

Buffers

The problems of buffer choice are too complex to be fully covered here but three of the commonest buffers used in uptake studies are Tris (Tris (hydroxy-methylaminomethane)), Mops (3-(N-morpholino) propanesulphonic acid) and phosphate.

Phosphate can give problems of solubility with cationic constituents of suspending media and with the antimicrobial chlorhexidine. Tris has a poor buffering capacity below pH 7.5, can cause changes in cell permeability and has an undesirably high temperature coefficient. Mops has a better pH range than Tris and a better temperature coefficient. Changing buffers can have dramatic effects on both uptake and on biological activity, even when there is no change in pH (Salt & Wiseman 1970).

Reaction Mixtures

Reaction mixtures are prepared by mixing appropriate volumes of cell suspensions and solutions of antimicrobial agent, preferably in the same medium. The mixing of equal volumes of suspension and solution is the preferred practice but when working with compounds near their solubility limit it may be necessary to add small volumes of concentrated cell suspension to large volumes of near-saturated solutions of agent or, if unavoidable, to add small volumes of concentrated solutions of the agent in acid or alkali, or in a solvent such as ethanol, to large volumes of cell suspensions. When using the latter technique, rapid mixing is necessary to prevent localized high concentrations of agent interacting with the cells.

Separation of the cells

Removal of cells from reaction mixtures after the required time can be achieved either by centrifuging or by membrane filtration. Centrifuging at $5000\,g$ for 10 min or some equivalent combination of speed and time will satisfactorily separate most types of cell and allows easy sampling of supernatant fluids; total recovery of the cells free from supernatant is less satisfactory.

Centrifuging of samples takes several minutes even when using high speeds and studies of the early stages of rapid uptake are not possible using this method. Separation of cells by membrane filtration, on the other hand, is fast and can be achieved in a few seconds, allowing rates of uptake to be measured.

Separation of cells by membrane filtration has been successfully used in studies of the uptake of nutrients but presents problems with antimicrobial compounds, mainly because of uptake of the compounds by the membranes and by the filter support. This problem can be overcome to some extent when using radio-labelled compounds by employing a pair of stacked membranes. In this technique the reaction mixture is filtered through two membranes, one on top of the other, and the radioactivity retained by the two membranes measured separately. The difference between the two counts then represents the activity associated with the cells retained on the uppermost membrane.

Most uptake studies, however, continue to use centrifuging as the separation technique.

Measurement of uptake

After the separation of cells from reaction mixtures, uptake can be determined either directly by assay of the agent retained by the cells, or indirectly by assay of the compound in the supernatant fluid. Subtraction of this from the concentration in the original reaction mixture gives the uptake.

Direct measurement of compounds in the presence of separated cells presents technical problems and may require extraction procedures to be used. In addition to this, separated cells retain interstitial fluid which will contain unbound antimicrobial agent which cannot be removed by washing without also removing reversibly bound material.

Because of these problems the indirect method is by far the most commonly used, but this method can also give problems. If uptake represents only a small proportion of the total amount of agent present, it has to be calculated as the difference between two high concentrations, with a resulting inevitably high standard error. Moreover, if there is significant adsorption of the anti-microbial agent on the glass or plastic ware being used in experiments, then the uptakes obtained represent the combined uptake by the cells and the apparatus. This source of error can be particularly important with surface-active compounds.

Both these problems can be reduced by the use of thick cell suspensions and with some compounds cell densities as high as 10^{11}/ml have been used (Bean & Das 1966; Lang & Rye 1972). With such high cell densities, corrections for the volume of cells must be made (Lang & Rye 1972). Where possible, the use of such thick cell suspensions should be avoided.

The problem of adsorption on to glassware can be minimized by using the final centrifuge tubes as the reaction vessels and by preparing the solutions of antimicrobial agent by dilution of a concentrated stock solution directly into these tubes. A correction can also be made by running parallel control experiments, with no cells present in the reaction mixtures, to estimate uptake by the centrifuge tubes alone.

This problem can be avoided entirely when using radio-labelled compounds, by measuring the activity in samples of the reaction mixture, cells and suspending fluid together, immediately before centrifuging, followed by measurement of the activity of the supernatant fluid after centrifuging. The difference between the two activities represents uptake by the cells with no contribution from uptake by the tubes.

Radio-labelled compounds

The direct measurement of cell-bound antimicrobial agents is most easily achieved by the use of radio-labelled compounds. Compounds labelled with ^{14}C or tritium, in cell pellets from centrifuge tubes or on membrane filters, can be assayed using liquid scintillation counting, while ^{14}C compounds in cells held on membranes can be assayed by planchet counting. Iodine-containing compounds can be labelled with the gamma-emitting isotopes of iodine, ^{131}I or ^{125}I, and can most easily be assayed using solid scintillation counting. Radio-labelling can also be used to assay compounds in supernatant fluids.

Although the use of radio-labelled compounds has some advantages, their use is limited by the need for specialized equipment and accommodation for their handling, by the limited number of labelled antimicrobial compounds readily available, and finally, by the high cost of such materials.

Non-radio-labelled compounds

The assay of non-radio-labelled compounds bound to cells normally requires an extraction procedure, although pyrolytic methods may be applicable in some cases.

The method of choice for the assay of non-radio-labelled compounds in supernatant fluids will depend on the particular compound being studied and may involve direct spectrophotometric assays, colorimetric methods, fluorimetry and high pressure liquid chromatography (HPLC). Where appropriate, direct spectrophotometry has been the most commonly used method, but with many compounds, cellular exudate in the supernatant fluids has caused problems. Solvent extraction techniques have been used in attempts to overcome this problem (Bean & Das 1966) but the choice of an appropriate HPLC method should, nowadays, allow clear separation of the antimicrobial from the cellular material.

Presentation of Results

Results from uptake studies are normally presented as isotherms, i.e. as graphs of uptake of antimicrobial agent plotted against concentration remaining in the supernatant solution. The units used for both uptake and supernatant concentration, are often wt (µg or mg)/ml but where possible, it is better to plot uptake as moles per gram of cells (mol/g) and supernatant concentrations as molarities. This mode of presentation makes comparisons between different compounds, particularly compounds within a homologous series, much easier.

Classification and interpretation of uptake isotherms

The most widely used and useful classification system for the uptake isotherms is that described and developed by Giles et al. (1960, 1974a,b). In the latter two papers, there is a theoretical treatment of adsorption with a classification system for isotherms, together with an examination and interpretation of experimentally observed uptake isotherms taken from the published literature including one for the uptake of CTAB by E. coli published by Salt & Wiseman (1968).

Giles et al. divide isotherms into four main classes according to the initial slope. The four main classes (Fig. 1) are named the S,L. (i.e. 'Langmuir' type), H ('high affinity'), and C ('constant partition') isotherms, and variations in each class are divided into subgroups.

The S-curve usually occurs when three conditions are fulfilled:
1   the solute molecule is mono-functional and has a fairly large hydrophobic residue ($>C_5$);
2   the solute molecule has moderate intermolecular attraction, causing it to pack vertically in regular array in the adsorbed layer;
3   the solute molecule meets strong competition, for substrate sites, from molecules of the solvent or of another adsorbed species.

The L-curve occurs when the adsorbed solute molecules are not vertically orientated or where there is no strong competition from the solvent. The types of system which give this curve thus have one of the following characteristics:
1   the adsorbed molecules are most likely to be adsorbed flat; or
2   if adsorbed end-on, they suffer little solvent competition.

The H-curve is a special case of the L-curve, in which the solute has such high affinity for the adsorbent that in dilute solutions it is taken up completely, so that the initial part of the isotherm is vertical.

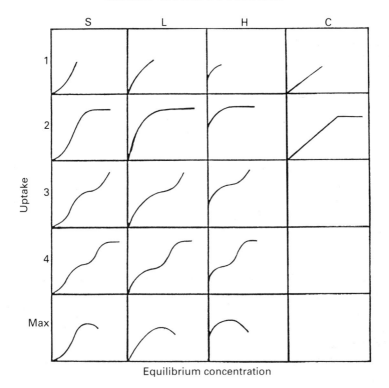

Fɪɢ. 1. Uptake classification scheme. After Giles *et al.* (1974a).

The C-curve is characterized by constant partition of solute between solution and substrate, right up to the maximum adsorption, where an abrupt change to a horizontal plateau occurs. One of the major conditions favouring the C-curve is that the solute has better penetrating power than the solvent and can therefore penetrate porous substrates (Giles *et al.* 1974a).

Diphasic isotherms with both primary and secondary saturation plateaux have been classified for S, L and H isotherms and are designated subgroup 4. In these complex isotherms, a short primary plateau suggests that the adsorbing solute molecules expose a surface which has an affinity similar to that of the original surface; a long plateau suggests that a high-energy barrier has to be overcome before additional adsorption occurs on new sites.

Examples of S, L, H and C isotherms have all been reported for the uptake of antimicrobial compounds. S isotherms have been reported for the uptake by *E. coli* of some phenolic compounds (Bean & Das 1966) and of dodecyl diethanolamine (Lambert & Smith 1976). L isotherms have been widely described for antimicrobial agents including CTAB from water (Salton

1951; Salt & Wiseman 1970) chlorhexidine (Hugo & Longworth 1964) and resorcinol (Bean & Das 1966). True H isotherms are less common but have been reported for the uptake of iodine (Hugo & Newton 1964). Several examples of C isotherms have been reported including ones for aromatic alcohols and for *P*-hydroxybenzoates (Lang & Rye 1972, 1973).

More complex isotherms of the S4 and H4 type have also been observed particularly for the uptake of quaternary ammonium compounds and of chlorhexidine by *E. coli* (Figs 2,3, and 4; Salt & Wiseman 1968; Acheampong & Wiseman 1981; Daham & Wiseman 1987). These biphasic isotherms were all obtained using magnesium-containing defined growth media as suspending agents and their difference from the simple L-type isotherms observed for these compounds from water can be explained by competition for the binding sites by the magnesium ions present.

The S-type primary phase of the biphasic isotherms for the quaternary ammonium compounds is consistent with the mono-functional nature of the adsorbed molecules and their long carbon chains whilst the H-type primary phase of the chlorhexidine isotherm even in the presence of magnesium, results from the bifunctional nature of the molecule.

With all these cationic agents termination of the primary uptake phase approximates to the threshold concentration required for bactericidal activity and cell leakage; secondary uptake almost certainly represents penetration to new uptake sites within the cells.

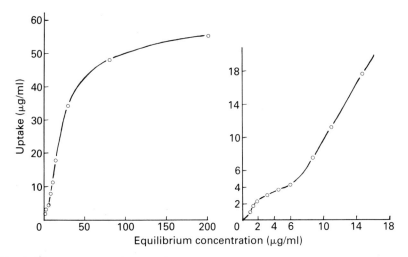

FIG. 2. The uptake of CTAB by *E. coli* suspended in glucose-free Tris mineral salts medium. Temperature 25°C, contact time 15 min, cell concentration 0.125 mg/ml (Salt & Wiseman 1968).

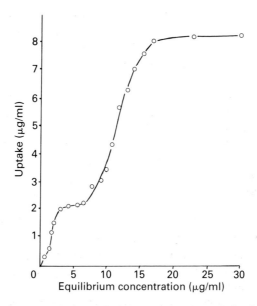

FIG. 3. The uptake of tetradecylbenzyldimethylammonium bromide by *E. coli* suspended in glucose-free Mops mineral salts medium. Temperature 37°C, contact time 15 min, cell concentration 0.08 mg/ml (Acheampong & Wiseman 1981).

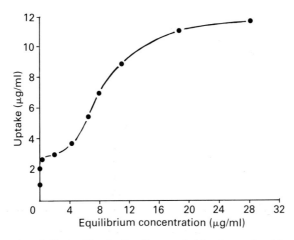

FIG. 4. The uptake of chlorhexidine by *E. coli* suspended in glucose-free Mops mineral salts medium. Temperature 20°C, contact time 15 min, cell concentration 0.04 mg/ml (Daham & Wiseman 1987).

Other complex isotherms have been reported in the literature with perhaps the most notable being Z isotherms for the uptake of 2-phenoxyethanol and 2-phenoxypropanol by *E. coli* (Gilbert *et al.* 1978). With these uptake curves dramatic upward changes in slope again occur at threshold concentrations for leakage with secondary uptake corresponding to penetration into the cell.

In general terms it seems reasonable to assume that any sudden upward change in slope of an uptake isotherm can be taken as prima facie evidence of an increase in cell permeability.

Techniques Supporting Uptake Studies

One of the greatest difficulties in interpreting uptake data is in deciding whether the isotherm produced represents a purely surface phenomenon or whether penetration of the adsorbed solute occurs, through the surface presented for adsorption, into the underlying regions. Additionally, it should not be assumed that, in systems effectively comprising a highly divided surface (cultures of unicellular micro-organisms), that molecules taken up will always be evenly distributed between the individual particles (cells). It is therefore useful to supplement uptake studies with evidence, which need not itself be quantitative, that throws light on the location of the sites of uptake.

Examples of such supplementary techniques include: the measurement of changes in cell-surface charge as shifts in electrophoretic mobility; the assessment of cell size shifts occurring during growth of partially inhibited cultures; the selective use of dyes/stains that are either specific for the components of the subsurface regions or for the molecule the uptake of which is being studied (typically stains with electron microscospy; dyes with optical microscopy); the detection of gross cellular changes that are more likely to occur because of interactions taking place beyond the cell surface, e.g. leakage of cellular constituents or changes in light scatter profile for the treated cellular dispersion.

This section outlines the use of electrophoretic mobility, cell size assessment, optical microscopy and dispersion light scatter (optical density) as supplements to the study of antimicrobial agent uptake.

Electrophoretic Mobility

Generally, microbial cells suspended in an aqueous medium carry a net negative charge due predominantly to the presence at or near the cell surface of ionogenic groups such as phosphate or carboxylate. However, the detection of a net negative charge at a surface in contact with an aqueous medium does not necessarily indicate that the surface is ionogenic in nature. The acquisition of such charges by surfaces known to be non-ionogenic was originally believed to be due to the adsorption of anions from the medium. It is now generally accepted that charges of this type result from the relative distance of the more highly hydrated cations effectively giving rise to an interfacial excess of anions (Briton & Lauffer 1959; Haydon 1961a). Haydon (1961b) suggested that some of the charge carried by *E. coli* might originate by such a mechanism, though the majority of the charge is due to ionogenic groups proximal to the cell surface (Davis *et al.* 1956; James 1957a,b, 1965). For this reason it is often useful to include, for comparative purposes, studies of the behaviour of fine polymer bead suspensions that provide a more predictable surface for drug uptake.

Surface charge may be measured electrophoretically by studying the migration of particles in an applied electric field. A charged particle will be surrounded by a diffuse region of counter ions resulting in the formation of an electric double layer and it is assumed that when the electric field is applied, the migrating particle carries with it a thin layer of the medium, the outside surface of which undergoes continual shear from the bulk medium. The potential at this plane of shear is termed the zeta potential and may be calculated using one of the various forms of the Helmholtz–Smoluchowski equation:

$$\mu = \frac{zD}{4\pi\eta}$$

in which μ is the electrophoretic mobility (velocity per unit field), z is the zeta potential, D is the dielectric constant of the medium, and η is the viscosity of the suspending medium.

Translation of zeta potential to surface charge density (σ) involves use of equations of the type used by Heard & Seaman (1960):

$$\sigma = 3.52 \times 10^4 I^{1/2} \sinh(z/51.3),$$

in which I is the ionic strength of the suspending medium. Both equations, however, make numerous assumptions (e.g. the particle is small with a surface that is non-conducting and does not interfere with the applied electric field; values for dielectric constant, conductivity and viscosity are the same within the double layer and the bulk medium; the film of medium at the particle surface has the velocity of the particle; the viscosity and ionic strength of the medium are low).

Many of these assumptions do not hold for microbial cells suspended in ionically complex growth media, resulting in errors in calculating both zeta potentials and surface charge densities (James 1957b; Wunderlich 1982; Zukoski & Saville 1986). Additionally, the concept of a cell surface as an open matrix penetrable to counter ions with consequent shielding of surface groups may lead to a gross underestimation of true surface charge (Heard & Seaman

1960; Haydon 1961a). This, plus the possibility of changes in the orientation of subsurface components induced by the adsorbed molecular species, makes the quantitative translation of electrophoretic mobility to surface charge density speculative and in the comparative analysis of drug-treated and control suspensions, probably unnecessary.

Despite these limitations micro-electrophoresis is one of the few techniques available for the study of the comparative responses of the individual cells in a suspension to changes in their environment. It has been used most notably in the evaluation of interactions between charged antimicrobial agents such as quaternary ammonium compounds, and microbial cells (Dyar & Ordal 1946; McQuillen 1950; Hugo & Frier 1969; Salt 1970).

The technique is relatively simple and a range of manual and automatic devices are commercially available (e.g. Rank Brothers, Bottisham, Cambridge, UK; Carl Zeiss Jena, GDR). Variations allow for improved optical resolution and in-built television cameras may reduce operator tedium by permitting video recording. Direct assessment of electrophoretic mobility/surface charge density is also possible, within the constraints of the limitations discussed earlier.

A typical, simple, manual system has been described by Bangham *et al.* (1958), the essential features of which are common to all devices. In general, the apparatus comprises a glass, cylindrically capillary or fine flat chamber, with electrodes at each end. The cell suspension under investigation fills the chamber so that the electrodes are immersed, and the chamber is then sealed. The whole unit is immersed in a temperature-controlled water bath and the electrodes connected to a suitable direct current power pack capable of providing a controlled potential gradient of *c.* 5 V/cm (current 1−2 mA to minimize thermal effects) across the chamber.

Under such conditions two electrokinetic effects occur. There is movement of the cells relative to the suspending medium (electrophoretic mobility) and a movement of the suspending medium relative to the wall of the chamber (electro-osmosis) with a consequent return of the medium down the centre of the chamber. This results in a parabolic distribution of cell velocities across the chamber and the formation of a stationary layer of medium in which the mobility of the cells alone (10−20 individual measurements) can be observed using an in-built travelling microscope fitted with water immersion objective lenses. Individual cell movement is timed over a known distance using a precalibrated eyepiece graticule. The direction of current should be reversed half way through each reading to minimize polarization and to average out 'drift'.

Though cylindrical cells may give some image distortion (reduced by water immersion) electro-osmotic flow is less affected by wall effects than in the flat chamber and medium convection is minimized by more even heat exchange.

Cylindrical chambered units have the additional advantage that the location of the stationary layer can be calculated directly from the radius of the bore (Bangham *et al.* 1958). Flat chambers require preliminary experimentation with cell suspensions of known electrophoretic mobility (usually red blood cells) to locate the stationary layer as the area between oppositely moving bands of cells (electrophoretic mobility vs. electro-osmosis) under a constant potential gradient.

The potential gradient is calculated directly from the distance between the electrodes and the appplied potential. Electrophoretic mobility is expressed as microns per second per volt per centimetre and tables of mobilities for some bacteria have been listed by James (1957b). Typical results for both Gram-positive (vegetative *Bacillus megaterium*) and Gram-negative (*E. coli*) bacteria suspended in water and a chemically defined mineral salts medium containing hexadecyltrimethylammonium bromide (HTAB) are shown in Fig. 5. Both types of organism responded to the presence of HTAB in a similar manner, in that increasing the HTAB concentration reduced the cells' electrophoretic mobility, eventually causing charge reversal. Gram-positive cells, however, are apparently unaffected by low HTAB concentrations and a threshold for effect is notable. Similar observations were reported by McQuillen (1950) for HTAB-treated suspensions of *Staphylococcus aureus* and *E. coli*.

Charge reversal is also induced by inorganic cations and, by using various inorganic salts, it is possible to plot charge reversal spectra that relate to the nature of the surface of the dispersed system under investigation. Such a

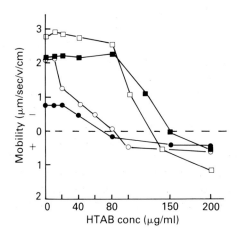

FIG. 5. The effect of HTAB on the electrophoretic mobility of *E. coli* suspended in: (○) water; (●) mineral salts medium; and *Bacillus megaterium* suspended in: (□) water; (■) mineral salts medium. Temperature 25°C.

method, developed by Bungenberg de Jong (1949) for the study of the surfaces of colloidal particles, may be applied to microbial suspensions (James 1957a; Salt 1970). Essentially, the electrophoretic mobility of the particles or cells is assessed in the presence of inorganic cations of various valencies and at different strengths. Graphs of mobility vs. inorganic salt concentration are plotted (Fig. 6) from which the salt concentration neutralizing or just reversing the surface charge can be deduced (if necessary by extrapolation). This information may then be used to construct charge reversal spectra (Fig. 7 a, b, and c). These can then be compared with either standard systems of known surface chemistry and/or with spectra for drug-treated suspensions.

Cell Size Distributions During the Growth of Partially Inhibited Cultures

This approach is applicable to Gram-negative bacteria and uses ampicillin at low levels to inhibit cellular division whilst permitting cellular mass increase to occur at the same rate as untreated controls. It therefore requires preliminary experimentation to establish the required ampicillin concentration (typically $1-3\,\mu g/ml$ for *E. coli* but may be $20-50\,\mu g/ml$ for resistant organisms such as *Klebsiella pneumoniae*). This should be done by constructing growth curves of the appropriate organism in shaken cultures ($2-4$ h) in the desired medium containing a range of ampicillin concentrations. Samples should be subjected to microscopy to confirm the absence of cell wall deformations during experimental times. Additionally there must be no synergism/antagonism etc. be-

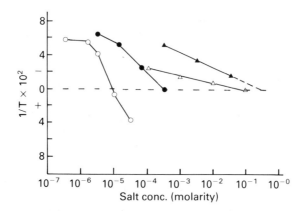

FIG. 6. Effect of electrolytes on the electrophoretic mobility (reciprocal of time, T, to travel a fixed distance under a fixed potential gradient) of cells of *E. coli*. Temperature 25°C. Salts: (○) thorium; (●) uranyl; (△) magnesium; (▲) potassium.

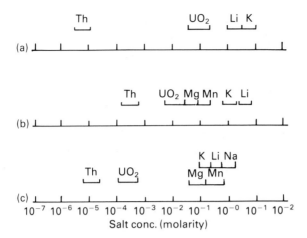

FIG. 7. Charge reversal spectra for: (a) polystyrene beads; (b) *Bacillus megaterium*; (c) *E. coli*.

tween the ampicillin and the test drug. This may be assessed by diffusion tests such as that described by Maccacaro (1961; also Bloomfield (this book)).

The method of assessing the proportion of the population able to grow in the presence of the drug has been described by Rye & Wiseman (1968). Essentially cells are incubated in shaken flasks at the appropriate temperature containing:

1 the chosen medium supplemented with ampicillin at the determined level to inhibit division; and

2 in the same medium as in 1 but containing a range of subinhibitory concentrations of the drug. Samples (1–5 ml) are taken at zero time and at 20–30-min intervals. Ideally, optical density (650 nm: 1-cm path-length) should be assessed to establish a growth profile before cells are isolated (filtration or centrifugation) and resuspended in Isoton (Coulter Electronics, Luton, UK) or electrolyte solution containing 0.2% formaldehyde. Dilution, in the same suspending medium, provides samples suitable for cell size distribution analysis by Coulter counter or other similar analyser. A uniform response following a drug-(pyrithione/*K. pneumoniae*) induced lag phase (Khattar *et al.* 1988, 1990) is shown in Fig. 8 and a non-uniform response (HTAB/*E. coli*) in Fig. 9.

Interactions Between Dyes and Adsorbed Antimicrobial Agents

Many different stains/dyes are available for the selective staining of the cell surface/subsurface regions and the simple displacement of such stains from drug-treated cells or distinct changes in a cell's response to a standard stain

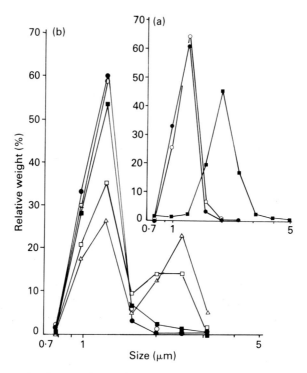

FIG. 8. Cell size distributions of *K. pneumoniae* growing at 37°C: (a) in a chemically defined medium containing no ampicillin (untreated control) at (0) (○) and 120 min (●) or 50 μg/ml ampicillin after 0 (○) and 120 min (■); (b) in the same medium containing 50 μg/ml ampicillin and 2.0 μg/ml pyrithione at 0 min (●), 120 min (○), 240 min (■) 360 min (□) and 480 min (△).

following drug treatment, may be used as an indicator of drug location following uptake. Other stains are not readily taken up by intact cells; their uptake being related to cellular permeability. Though they may be used to detect drug-induced changes in cell permeability (Dyar 1947; Chaplin 1952; Scharff & Maupin 1960) they would not necessarily provide information on the sites of drug uptake.

Ideally, any coloured material used in the location of molecules taken up by microbial cells would combine with the adsorbed species but would have little or no affinity for the cell itself. Since selectivity is the essential feature, a check through the assay procedures available for the antimicrobial agent is often fruitful. For example, complex formation between bromothymol blue (BTB) or bromophenol blue (BPB) and quaternary ammonium compounds (QACs) forms the basis of some methods for QAC analysis (Auerbach 1943) and depends on the availability of the positive charge associated with the QAC

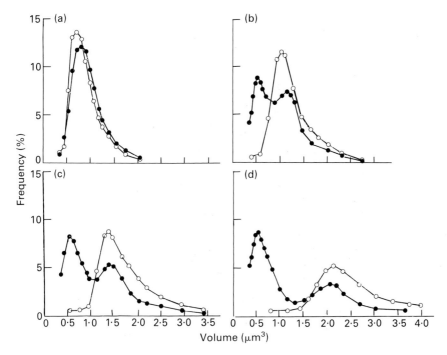

FIG. 9. The size distributions of cells of *E. coli* growing in a chemically defined medium containing ampicillin (2 µg/ml). Incubation times: (a) 0 min, (b) 34 min, (c) 60 min, (d) 95 min. (○) Control cells; (●) cells pretreated with 2 µg/ml HTAB in glucose-free medium for 10 min prior to the addition of glucose and ampicillin.

for combination with up to three sites within the BTB or BPB molecule. The detection of the uptake of stains like BPB by cells treated with charged antimicrobials may thus give evidence as to the orientation and, perhaps, location of the compound in individual cells and may additionally enable comparisons of drug distribution between the numerous members of typical cell suspensions (Salt 1970). BPB uptake following drug treatment may be simply observed using BPB as part of a standard staining routine for optical microscopy and examining the uniformity of the stain distribution. Alternatively, stain uptake may be quantified by resuspending cells, previously subjected to drug treatment under standard conditions, for 1−2 min in a solution of BPB (10 µg/ml) and assessing changes in supernatant BPB levels by colorimetry at 608 nm (Fig. 10).

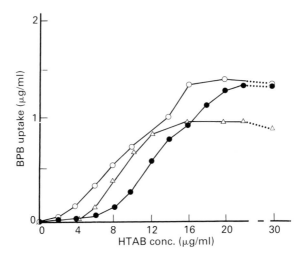

FIG. 10. Uptake of BPB by HTAB-treated suspensions of: (●) *E. coli*; (△), polystyrene beads; (○) *Bacillus megaterium*, plotted as a function of HTAB concentration.

Drug-Induced Turbidity Increases

Non-growing bacterial suspensions have been observed to increase in turbidity as a result of interactions with a variety of different antimicrobial agents. These include phenolic agents (Beckett *et al.* 1959; Lamikanra & Allwood 1977), cationic surfactants (Hugo & Longworth 1964; Hugo & Frier 1969; Salt & Wiseman 1970; Salt 1976), aldehydes (Munton & Russell 1970), local anaesthetics (Salt & Traynor 1979; Fazly Bazaz & Salt 1980, 1983) and β-adrenergic blocking agents (Salt 1982). Though not produced by all anti-microbial agents, when detected, such drug-induced changes occur rapidly and in the presence or absence of a carbon source. Suggestions as to their basis include: changes in cell size, leakage of intracellular contents, shifts in cellular reflectance or refractive index and the precipitation of cellular contents. Whatever the cause, such changes relate to drug uptake and may be used as a rapid preliminary screen of compound−cell interaction (Salt & Wiseman 1970).

Essentially, the procedure entails mixing cell suspensions and drug to give a range of reaction mixtures with constant cell density and various drug concentrations in the desired medium (as for uptake studies). After a fixed contact time (typically 10 min) the optical density of each mixture is assessed (650 nm; 1 cm path-length). Results are typified in Fig. 11 and any apparent shifts in optical density should be compared with the relevant uptake isotherm as appropriate.

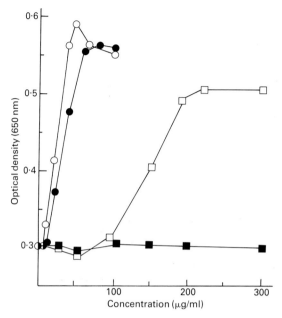

FIG. 11. Induced turbidity increases (optical density; 650 nm) in cells of *E. coli* suspended in a glucose-free, mineral salts medium containing different homologues of HTAB, plotted as a function of the homologue concentration. Temperature 25°C, contact time 15 min. (○) C18; (●) C16; (□) C14; (■) C12.

Summary

Since the primary step in drug action is drug uptake, any study of drug—cell interactions must be considered incomplete if the mode of drug uptake is not understood. Uptake isotherms are simple to construct from easily obtained data. In conjunction with supplementary techniques, such as micro-electrophoresis, and with an understanding of drug-induced cell responses, such isotherms can be interpreted to provide a quantitative picture of both intercellular and intracellular drug distribution.

References

Acheampong, Y.B. & Wiseman, D. 1981. The uptake of nonyl and tetradecylbenzyldimethylammonium compounds by *Escherichia coli*. *Journal of Pharmacy and Pharmacology*, **33**, 30P.

Auerbach, M.E. 1943. Germicidal quaternary ammonium salts in dilute solution. A colorimetric assay method. *Industrial and Engineering Chemistry, Analytical edition*, **15**, 492–493.

BANGHAM, A.D., FLEMANS, R., HEARD, D.H. & SEAMAN, G.V.F. 1958. An apparatus for microelectrophoresis of small particles. *Nature, London*, **182**, 642−644.

BEAN, H.S. & DAS, A. 1966. The absorption by *E. coli* of phenols and their bactericidal activity. *Journal of Pharmacy and Pharmacology*, **18**, 1075−1135.

BECKETT, A.H., PATKI, S.J. & ROBINSON, A.E. 1959. The interaction of phenolic compounds with bacteria. II. The effects of various substances on the interaction of hexylresorcinol with *E. coli*. *Journal of Pharmacy and Pharmacology* **11**, 367−373.

BRINTON, C.C. & LAUFFER, M.A. 1959. The electrophoresis of viruses, bacteria and cells and the microscope method of electrophoresis. In *Electrophoresis*, Vol. 1, ed. Brier, M. pp. 427−492. New York and London: Academic Press.

BUNGENBERG DE JONG, H.G. 1949. Reversal of charge phenomena, equivalent weight and specific properties of the ionised groups. In *Colloid Science*, Vol. 2, ed. Kruyt, H.R. pp. 259−334. Amsterdam: Elsevier.

CHAPLIN, C.E. 1952. Bacterial resistance to quaternary ammonium compounds. *Journal of Bacteriology*, **63**, 453−458.

DAHAM, S.A.M. & WISEMAN, D. 1987. The uptake of chlorhexidine by *Escherichia coli* and its effects on viability in the absence and presence of EDTA. *Journal of Pharmacy and Pharmacology* **39**, 16P.

DAVIS, J.T., HAYDON, D.A. & RIDEAL, E.K. 1956. Surface behaviour of *Bacterium coli*. I. The nature of the surface. *Proceedings of the Royal Society London* **B145**, 375−383.

DYAR, M.T. 1947. A cell wall stain employing a cationic surface active agent as a mordant. *Journal of Bacteriology* **53**, 498.

DYAR, M.T. & ORDAL, E.J. 1946. Electrokinetic studies on bacterial surfaces. I. The effects of surface active agents on the electrophoretic mobility of bacteria. *Journal of Bacteriology* **51**, 149−167.

FAZLY BAZAZ, B.S. & SALT, W.G. 1980. Antimicrobial activity in local anaesthetics: a possible screen for tissue toxicity. *Journal of Pharmacy and Pharmacology* **31** (suppl), 57P.

FAZLY BAZAZ, B.S. & SALT, W.G. 1983. Local anaesthetic induced turbidity increases: implications of interactions with intact bacterial cells and with subcellular fractions. *Microbios* **36**, 135−147.

GILBERT, P., BEVERIDGE, E.G. & SISSONS, I. 1978. The uptake of some membrane-active drugs by bacteria and yeast; possible microbiological examples of "Z" curve adsorption. *Journal of Colloid and Interface Science* **64**, 377−379.

GILES, C.H., MACEWAN, T.H., NAKHWA, S.A. & SMITH, D. 1960. A system of classification of solution adsorption isotherms, and its use in diagnosis of adsorption mechanisms and in measurement of specific surface areas of solids. *Journal of Chemical Society* **III**, 3973−3993.

GILES, C.H., SMITH, D. & HUITSON, A. 1974a. A general treatment and classification of the solute adsorption isotherm. 1. Theoretical. *Journal of Colloid and Interface Science* **47** 755−765.

GILES, C.H., D'SILVA, A.P. & EASTON, I.A. 1974b. A general treatment and classification of the solute adsorption isotherm. Part II. Experimental Interpretation. *Journal of Colloid and Interface Science* **47**, 766−778.

HAYDON, D.A. 1961a. The surface charge of cells and some other small particles as indicated by electrophoresis. I. The zeta potential surface charge relationship. *Biochimica et Biophysica Acta* **50**, 450−456.

HAYDON, D.A. 1961b. The surface charge of cells and some other small particles as indicated by electrophoresis. II. The interpretation of the electrophoretic charge. *Biochimica et Biophysica Acta* **50**, 457−462.

HEARD, D.H. & SEAMAN, G.V.F. 1960. The influence of pH and ionic strength on the electrokinetic stability of the human erythrocyte membrane. *Journal of General Physiology* **43**, 635–654.

HUGO, W.B. & FRIER, M. 1969. Mode of action of the antimicrobial compound dequalinium acetate. *Applied Microbiology* **17**, 118–127.

HUGO, W.B. & LONGWORTH, A.R. 1964. Some aspects of the mode of action of chlorhexidene. *Journal of Pharmacy and Pharmacology* **16**, 655–662.

HUGO, W.B. & NEWTON, J.M. 1964. The adsorption of iodine from solution by micro-organisms and by serum. *Journal of Pharmacy and Pharmacology* **16**, 49–55.

JAMES, A.M. 1957a. Identification of surface components on the bacterial cell wall. *Proceedings of the Second International Congress on Surface Activity*, Vol 4, ed. Schulman, J.H. pp. 254–261.

JAMES, A.M. 1957b. The electrochemistry of the bacterial surface. *Progress in Biophysics and Biophysical Chemistry* **8**, 95–142.

JAMES, A.M. 1965. Surface active agents in microbiology. In *Symposium on Surface Activity and the Microbial Cell*, London, 1964. Society of Chemical Industry Monograph No. 19, pp. 3–24.

KHATTAR, M.M., SALT, W.G. & STRETTON. R.J. 1988. The influence of pyrithione on the growth of micro-organisms. *Journal of Applied Bacteriology* **64**, 264–272.

KHATTAR, M.M., SALT, W.G. & STRETTON, R.J. 1990. Growth and survival of *Klebsiella pneumoniae* in the presence of pyrithion. *Proceedings of the 6th Mediterranean Congress of Chemotherapy, Taormina-Giardini Naxos, Italy, 1988* 224–226.

LAMBERT, P.A. & SMITH, A.R.W. 1976. Antimicrobial action of dodecyldiethanolamine: induced membrane damage in *Escherichia coli*. *Microbios* **15**, 191–202.

LAMIKANRA, A. & ALLWOOD, M.C. 1977. Effect of polyoxyalkylphenols on the optical density of *Staphyloccocus aureus*. *Journal of Applied Bacteriology* **42**, 387–392.

LANG, M. & RYE, R.M. 1972. The uptake by *Escherichia coli* and growth inhibitory properties by benzyl alcohol and phenethyl alcohol. *Journal of Pharmacy and Pharmacology* **24**, 219–226.

LANG, M. & RYE, R.M. 1973. A correlation between the antibacterial activity of some *p*-hydroxy-benzoate esters and their cellular uptake. *Microbios* **7**, 199–207.

MCQUILLEN, K. 1950. The bacterial surface. I. Effect of cetyltrimethylammonium bromide on the electrophoretic mobility of certain Gram positive bacteria. *Biochimica et Biophysica Acta* **5**, 463–471.

MACCACARO, G.A. 1961. The assessment of the interaction between antibacterial drugs. *Progress in Industrial Microbiology* **3**, 173–210.

MUNTON, T.J. & RUSSELL, A.D. 1970. Aspects of the action of glutaraldehyde on *Escherichia coli*. *Journal of Applied Bacteriology* **33**, 410–419.

RYE, R.M. & WISEMAN, D. 1968. The partially inhibited growth of *Escherichia coli* in the presence of some antibacterial agents. *Journal of Pharmacy and Pharmacology* **20**, 697–703.

SALT, W.G. 1970. The uptake of CTAB by bacteria in relation to its antimicrobial action. *PhD thesis*, University of Bradford.

SALT, W.G. 1976 Induced turbidity changes in non-growing cultures of *Escherichia coli*. *Journal of Pharmacy and Pharmacology* **28**, 263.

SALT, W.G. 1982. β-blocker induced turbidity changes in non-growing bacterial cell suspensions. *Microbios Letters* **19**, 125–128.

SALT, W.G. & TRAYNOR, J.R. 1979. Interactions between amethocaine (tetracaine) and non-growing cultures of *Escherichia coli*. *Journal of Pharmacy and Pharmacology* **31**, 41–42.

SALT, W.G. & WISEMAN, D. 1968. The uptake of cetyltrimethylammonium bromide by *Escherichia coli*. *Journal of Pharmacy and Pharmacology* **20** 14–17S.

SALT, W.G. & WISEMAN, D. 1970. The effect of magnesium ions and Tris buffer on the uptake of cetyltrimethylammonium bromide by *Escherichia coli*. *Journal of Pharmacy and Pharmacology* **22**, 767–773.

SALTON, M.R.J. 1951. The adsorption of CTAB by bacteria, its action in releasing cellular contituents and its bactericidal effects. *Journal of General Microbiology* **5**, 391–404.

SCHARFF, T.G. & MAUPIN, W.C. 1960. Correlation of the metabolic effects of benzalkonium chloride with its membrane effects in yeast. *Biochemical Pharmacology* **5**, 79–86.

WISEMAN, D. 1972. The uptake of chloroquine by *Escherichia coli. Journal of Pharmacy and Pharmacology* **24**, 161P.

WUNDERLICH, W. 1982. The effects of surface structure on the electrophoretic mobility of large particles. *Journal of Colloid and Interfacial Science* **88**, 385–397.

ZUKOSKI, C.F. & SAVILLE, D.A. 1986. The interpretation of electrokinetic measurements using a dynamic model of the Stern layer. II. Comparisons between theory and experiment. *Journal of Colloid and Interfacial Science* **114**, 45–53.

Fractionation of Bacterial Cells and Isolation of Membranes and Macromolecules

P. WILLIAMS AND L. GLEDHILL

Department of Pharmaceutical Sciences, University of Nottingham, University Park, Nottingham NG7 2RD, UK

To be effective, an antimicrobial agent must not only gain access to, but also attain an effective concentration and contact time at its site of action. The biochemical target site(s) of antimicrobial agents may be located within the cell envelope, cytoplasmic membrane or cytoplasm. Access to such sites will depend upon the surface architecture and permeability of the bacterial cell. Failure to achieve effective antimicrobial activity at the target site, may occur as a result of more or less harmless interactions between the antimicrobial agent and a variety of cellular components.

The chemical composition, structure and function of Gram-negative and Gram-positive bacterial cell envelopes are very different. The Gram-negative cell envelope is a complex structure consisting of outer and inner or cytoplasmic membranes separated by a thin layer of peptidoglycan and a cellular compartment called the periplasm. This compartment forms a micro-environment between the external medium and the cell cytoplasmic membrane and cytoplasm and contains proteins and some oligo- and polysaccharides. These macromolecules are involved in a variety of cellular functions including cell wall synthesis and maintenance of periplasmic osmolarity (Lugtenberg & van Alphen 1983; Hammond *et al.* 1984). In contrast, the Gram-positive cell wall consists of a thick layer of peptidoglycan through which are interwoven polysaccharides, lipoteichoic acids, teichoic or teichuronic acids and proteins (Hammond *et al.* 1984). Whilst the Gram-negative outer membrane is an effective permeability barrier for molecules greater than about 600 Da (Nikaido & Vaara 1985), the Gram-positive cell wall is essentially an open matrix surrounding the cytoplasmic membrane with an exclusion limit for large molecules of 10 kDa or greater. Nevertheless, charged species within the Gram-positive cell wall may function as ion-exchangers which can remove highly charged molecules from solution (Gilbert & Wright 1987). Thus, in

Mechanisms of Action of
Chemical Biocides

Gram-positive cells, a biocide may still be prevented from reaching the cytoplasmic membrane or cytoplasmic target until all the unoccupied cell wall binding sites are filled. The progress of a charged antimicrobial agent across the cell envelope may also be retarded by highly charged acidic exopolysaccharides which may be present on the surface of either Gram-positive or Gram-negative cells as a discrete capsule or loosely associated slime layer (Sutherland 1977). In addition, it should also be borne in mind that the macromolecular structure and function of the cell envelope is not constant but is largely determined by the prevailing growth environment (Brown & Williams 1985; Williams 1988). Every cell envelope constituent is capable of undergoing structural modification and changes in distribution and quantity. Such plasticity considerably influences susceptibility to antimicrobial agents.

The purpose of this paper is to review selectively methods for disrupting and fractionating bacterial cells and the subsequent isolation of their macromolecular constituents. These approaches may be employed in the study of interactions between antimicrobial agents and bacterial cells thereby facilitating determination of the molecular basis of the action of, and resistance to, antimicrobial agents. Methods for quantitating the changes occurring in bacterial cell envelopes following exposure to biocides are described by Lambert (this book). An extensive review of the current techniques available for the detailed study of bacterial cell envelopes has been compiled by Hancock & Poxton (1988).

Disruption of Bacterial Cells

Gram-negative bacteria are intrinsically more resistant to many biocides than are Gram-positive bacteria, a phenomenon which is largely due to the function of the outer membrane as a permeability barrier. At minimal growth inhibitory concentrations (MIC), many biocides exert their bacteriostatic effects at the cytoplasmic membrane. Resistance to such agents may be due to the nature and composition of the cell envelope. For example, the sensitivity of intact cells of *Escherichia coli* and *Staphylococcus aureus* to the membrane-active agent tetrachlorosalicylanilide differs by a factor of 200 whereas sphaeroplasts prepared from both organisms are equally sensitive (Gilbert & Wright 1987). Growth rate and nutrient limitation both influence the sensitivity of *Bacillus megaterium* to lysozyme and to the membrane active agents 2-phenoxyethanol and chlorhexidine. However, protoplasts from these cells grown under different conditions showed similar sensitivities and the differences were interpreted in terms of altered cell wall permeability (Gilbert & Brown 1979).

Thus, comparison of the susceptibility of whole cells and sphaeroplasts or protoplasts to biocides may provide a useful indication of failure to permeate through the cell wall and therefore identify a possible factor in resistance. The susceptibility of protoplasts or sphaeroplasts to an antimicrobial agent can be assessed simply by measuring lysis rates in isotonic media as determined by monitoring changes in the optical density (absorbance) of a sphaeroplast/ protoplast suspension. In addition, the preparation of these osmotically fragile forms is frequently the first stage in the disruption of bacterial cells prior to the isolation of membranes or cytoplasmic constituents. Methods for preparing these wall-deficient forms will be outlined prior to describing the mechanical techniques available for the disruption of bacterial cells.

Preparation of protoplasts and sphaeroplasts

The term protoplast describes that part of a bacterial cell which consists of the cytoplasmic membrane and the cell material enclosed within it. Protoplasts can be prepared from Gram-positive bacteria by incubating the cells in the presence of a peptidoglycan-degrading enzyme such as lysozyme. Protoplasts are spherical regardless of the original shape of the cell and since they are osmotically fragile, must be maintained in an isotonic or a hypertonic medium. The peptidoglycan of certain Gram-positive bacteria, notably the staphylococci and streptococci, is resistant to digestion by lysozyme. Streptococcal lysozyme sensitivity can be increased by prior culture in media containing high levels of threonine or glycine (Scholler et al. 1983). Alternatively, the enzymes lysostaphin and mutanolysin, which are commercially available, can be used instead of lysozyme for the preparation of protoplasts from staphylococci (Cheung & Fischetti 1988) and streptococci (Siegel et al. 1981), respectively.

Similar procedures can be used to prepare round, osmotically fragile forms from Gram-negative bacteria. They will, however, differ from the protoplasts of Gram-positive bacteria in that the enzyme-treated cells will retain parts of their outer membranes and are called sphaeroplasts rather than protoplasts. If sphaeroplasts are to be prepared from Gram-negative bacteria using lysozyme, some disruption of the outer membrane is first required using an agent such as ethylene diamine tetraacetic acid (EDTA) which enables the enzyme to gain access to the underlying peptidoglycan (Lugtenberg & van Alphen 1983).

Methods

Gram-positive protoplasts

1 Resuspend a washed cell suspension to an absorbance at 650 nm (A_{650}) of c. 1.0 in 10 mmol/l Tris-HCl buffer (pH 7.4) containing 0.01 mol/l $MgCl_2$, 0.5 mol/l sucrose and 50 µg lysozyme/ml. To control proteolytic activity which may be released by the cell during digestion, protease inhibitors such as

benzamidine (1 mg/ml) and phenylmethylsulphonyl fluoride (PMSF, 2 mg/ml) can be added. For staphylococci and streptococci, lysozyme should be replaced by lysostaphin (100 μg/ml) or mutanolysin (50 μg/ml), respectively. The stability of the protoplasts obtained may be increased by replacing the sucrose with 30 or 40% (w/v) raffinose (Siegel *et al.* 1981).

2   Incubate the cell suspension at 37°C without shaking for 15−30 min. Protoplast formation can be assessed either by phase contrast microscopy or by measuring the decrease in A_{650} after diluting an aliquot of the suspension in distilled water. Alternatively, a lytic control of cells suspended in digestion buffer without sucrose can be included to follow the time course of enzyme activity.

3   Protoplasts can be harvested by centrifugation at room temperature (6000 *g*, 15 min), washed in the stabilization buffer (without lysozyme), and resuspended in isotonic or hypertonic test media.

Gram-negative sphaeroplasts

1   Resuspend a washed cell suspension to an A_{650} of 1.0 in 10 mmol/l Tris-HCl buffer (pH 7.4) containing 0.5 mol/l sucrose, 1.0 mmol/l EDTA and 50 μg lysozyme/ml.

2   Incubate the suspension at 37°C without shaking for 15−30 min or until sphaeroplast formation is complete, determined as described above for Gram-positive bacteria.

3   Sphaeroplasts can be harvested by centrifugation at room temperature (6000 *g*, 15 min), washed in the stabilization buffer (without lysozyme and EDTA), and resuspended in isotonic or hypertonic test media.

Mechanical bacterial cell disruption methods

The preliminary purification of bacterial cell envelopes, membranes and cytoplasmic constituents generally requires efficient disruption of bacterial cells (Hancock & Poxton 1988). This can be achieved using enzymes to obtain protoplasts or sphaeroplasts as described above, which are subsequently lysed by resuspension in distilled water. Alternatively, mechanical methods which employ ultrasonic radiation (sonic probe), explosive decompression (e.g. French Press) or rapid agitation in the presence of small (0.1−0.2 mm diameter) glass beads (e.g. in a Mickle tissue disintegrator or Braun homogenizer) can be employed. Such methods are often limited in their range of applications through poor temperature control, incomplete cell disruption or the extended processing time required. Recently, we have successfully employed a laboratory microfluidizer to disrupt both bacterial and fungal cells prior to the purification of cell membranes, surface proteins and intracellular enzymes (Figgitt *et al.* 1988). This instrument is essentially a high-pressure homogenizer in which two similar liquid streams travelling at high velocities interact in precisely defined microchannels.

The final choice of disruption method will depend on the organism under investigation and the purpose of the preparation. Examples of the use of enzymatic degradation, sonication and the French press will be found in the following sections.

Isolation of Gram-Positive Cytoplasmic Membranes and Extraction of Cell Wall Macromolecules

Preparation of cell wall and membrane proteins

Enzymatic digestion of the cell wall peptidoglycan in a hypertonic medium to prepare protoplasts can be used to release cell wall proteins, and teichoic acids. Removal of the protoplasts by centrifugation yields a supernatant containing cell wall macromolecules. Following lysis of the protoplast pellet in a hypotonic medium, the cytoplasmic membrane can be separated from the cytoplasmic contents by high-speed centrifugation. This technique has been used to prepare streptococcal M proteins (Fischetti *et al.* 1984) staphylococcal protein A (Sjoquist *et al.* 1972) and teichoic acids (Kaya *et al.* 1985). An example of the method used for the preparation of staphylococcal cell wall and membrane proteins is outlined below:

Method

1   Collect the bacterial cells obtained by centrifugation of a washed 25-ml suspension (A_{650} 1.0) in 0.6 ml of digestion buffer containing 100 µg of lysostaphin, 10 µg of deoxyribonuclease I, 0.6 mg PMSF and 0.6 mg benzamidine. The digestion buffer consists of 30% (w/v) raffinose with 0.145 mol/l NaCl in 50 mmol/l Tris-HCl (pH 7.5). For other Gram-positive bacteria except for the streptococci, lysozyme should be used instead of lysostaphin. For the streptococci, efficient digestion can be achieved with mutanolysin.
2   Incubate the cell mixture with gentle agitation for 1 h at 37°C.
3   Remove protoplasts by centrifugation at 6000 *g* for 10 min and recentrifuge the supernatant liquid (6000 *g* for 10 min). The supernatant obtained, which contains cell wall components, can be frozen in aliquots or used for the further purification of specific macromolecules.
4   Cytoplasmic membranes and cytoplasmic constituents can be prepared by resuspending the protoplast pellet in water and/or by sonicating the suspension in an ice bath. Membranes can be collected by centrifugation at 4°C at

40 000 g for 60 min or 100 000 g for 15 min, resuspended in water and the centrifugation step repeated.

The proteins released from each fraction can be analysed by sodium dodecyl sulphate polyacrylamide gel electrophoresis (SDS-PAGE, see Appendix 1) prior to further purification. An SDS-polyacrylamide gel of the cell wall and cytoplasmic membrane proteins obtained from *Staphylococcus epidermidis* using this technique is shown in Fig. 1. As can be seen from this figure, a proportion of the wall-degrading enzyme used remained associated with both the cell wall and cytoplasmic membrane fractions. These enzymes may be removed from the cell membrane preparation by washing with 0.2 mol/l KCl.

Extraction of lipoteichoic acids

Lipoteichoic acids (LTAs) are amphiphilic polymers which are found in most Gram-positive bacteria. They are generally glycerol teichoic acids with terminal glycolipid or diglyceride moeities. LTAs are located mainly on the outer surface of the cytoplasmic membrane with their glycerolphosphate polymeric chains enmeshed within the cell wall peptidoglycan (Hammond *et al.* 1984). They can be conveniently extracted from whole or disrupted cell suspensions

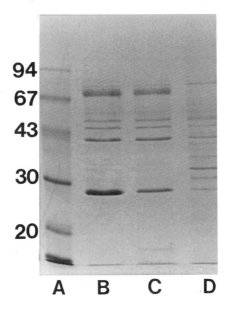

FIG. 1. SDS-PAGE showing the wall (lanes B and C) and cytoplasmic membrane (lane D) proteins of *Staphylococcus epidermidis* grown in human peritoneal dialysate. Lane A shows the molecular weight marker proteins (kDa). The major protein migrating just below 30 kDa in lanes B, C and D is the enzyme lysostaphin.

with hot aqueous phenol. As this procedure will also extract nucleic acids, lipids and glycolipids, the cells may require an initial defatting step (Heckels & Virji 1988).

Method

1 800 mg wet wt/ml of freshly harvested bacteria are resuspended in 0.1 mol/l sodium acetate buffer (pH 4.5, adjusted with acetic acid) and defatted by shaking for 16−18 h at room temperature with 2 vol. of methanol and 1 vol. of chloroform. Bacteria are harvested and resuspended in 0.1 mol/l sodium acetate buffer (pH 5.0).

2 LTAs are extracted from the defatted cells by mixing an equal volume of the cell suspension with 80% (w/v) aqueous phenol at 65°C. The mixture, maintained at 65°C in a water bath, is stirred continuously for 45 min and then cooled to 4°C in an ice bath. GREAT CARE MUST BE TAKEN WHEN HANDLING PHENOL. IT IS CAUSTIC AND EXTREMELY TOXIC WHEN ABSORBED THROUGH THE SKIN.

3 The emulsion formed on cooling can be separated by centrifugation at 5000 g for 30 min at 4°C. The upper aqueous phase which contains the LTAs is collected and dialysed extensively against distilled water to remove the phenol.

Contaminating nucleic acids can be degraded and removed by incubation with ribo- and deoxyribo-nucleases followed by a second extraction with hot phenol. The resulting material can be lyophilized and if necessary, further purification can be achieved by chromatography on Sepharose 6B as described by Coley et al. (1975).

Isolation of Gram-Negative Cell Membranes, Lipopolysaccharides and Exopolysaccharides

The Gram-negative cell envelope consists of an outer and an inner membrane separated by a layer of peptidoglycan (Lugtenberg & van Alphen 1983; Nikaido & Vaara 1985). Whilst the inner cytoplasmic membrane resembles that of Gram-positive bacteria, the outer membrane is unusual. The distribution of phospholipids within the outer membrane is asymmetric (they are present on the inner but not the outer face), it contains a unique macromolecule, lipopolysaccharide, and relatively few dominant proteins which are present at high copy number. Following disruption and digestion of the peptidoglycan layer, Gram-negative cell membranes can be separated using isopycnic sucrose density gradient ultracentrifugation (Schnaitmann 1970). The method can be used to yield qualitative and quantitative data on both gross and specific changes occurring in cells exposed to antimicrobial agents. Changes in the buoyant density and composition of *E. coli* outer membranes after exposure to sub-growth inhibitory concentrations of antibacterial agents have been reported (Leying *et al.* 1986; Suerbaum *et al.* 1987).

An alternative and more rapid method of isolating outer membranes from disrupted cells employs detergents such as sodium N-lauroyl sarcosinate (sarkosyl) (Filip *et al.* 1973) or Triton X-100 (Schnaitmann 1971). These detergents selectively solubilize the cytoplasmic membrane and the outer membrane−peptidoglycan complex can be recovered by high-speed centrifugation. This technique is useful for the rapid preparation of outer membrane proteins. However, it results in the loss of some lipid and lipopolysaccharide and so cannot be used to prepare intact outer membranes for quantitative analysis.

Isolation of outer membranes

Separation of outer and inner membranes by sucrose density ultracentrifugation

The method described is based on that of Hancock & Carey (1979):

1   8 l of cells, grown overnight to stationary phase, are harvested by centrifugation, washed in 30 mmol/l Tris-HCl (pH 8.0) and resuspended in 20 ml of 30 mmol/l Tris-HCl (pH 8.0) at 4°C containing 20% (w/v) sucrose, 2 mg/ml PMSF, 0.1 mg/ml deoxyribonuclease, 0.1 mg/ml ribonuclease.

2   The cell suspension is passed through a French Press at 103 500 kPa (15 000 p.s.i.) or microfluidizer at 69 000 kPa (10 000 p.s.i.). The procedure should be repeated at least once to ensure adequate disruption of the cells.

3   4 mg of lysozyme is added to the lysate and incubated at room temperature for 30 min.

4   The lysate is diluted with 40 ml of 30 mmol/l Tris-buffer (pH 8.0) and centrifuged twice at 5000 g for 10 min to remove unbroken cells. The supernatant fraction obtained is centrifuged at 40 000 g for 60 min and the resulting pellet resuspended in 20 ml of 20% (w/v) sucrose in 30 mmol/l Tris-HCl (pH 8.0).

5   2-ml samples are layered on to a two-step sucrose gradient containing 9.0 ml each of 70% and 60% (w/v) sucrose in 30 mmol/l Tris-HCl (pH 8.0).

6   The gradient is centrifuged at 100 000 g at 4°C for 18 h.

7   The membrane bands obtained at different buoyant densities can be removed with a syringe, diluted in 30 mmol/l Tris-HCl (pH 8.0) and centrifuged at 40 000 g for 60 min. The membrane pellet obtained should be washed in buffer and recentrifuged to remove the sucrose.

The outer membrane usually has the highest buoyant density i.e. it is the lowest band observed. Apart from the lighter cytoplasmic membrane band, several intermediate bands may be seen. These may represent different functional regions of the cell envelope or outer membrane−cytoplasmic membrane hybridizations. The identity of each band should be confirmed by assaying for cytoplasmic membrane marker enzymes such as succinate dehydrogenase and NADH oxidase (Osborn *et al.* 1972). For certain bacteria, successful separation of the outer and inner membranes may be achieved without prior digestion of the peptidoglycan with lysozyme. The presence of peptidoglycan may aid separation of the two membranes by increasing the buoyant density of the outer membrane.

Isolation of the outer membrane using sodium N-lauroyl sarcosinate (sarkosyl)

1   100 ml of bacteria (A_{650} 1.0) are resuspended in 10 ml of distilled water and broken by sonication (3×60 s with a 30-s cooling period between each burst) at 4°C. Any intact cells remaining can be removed by centrifugation at $5000\,g$ for 10 min.

2   1 ml of 20% (w/v) sodium N-lauroyl sarcosinate is added and the mixture incubated at room temperature for 30 min. A visible clearing of the envelope suspension indicates solubilization of the cytoplasmic membrane.

3   The outer membrane−peptidoglycan complex is recovered by centrifugation at $40\,000\,g$ for 60 min, washed twice in distilled water containing 1 mg/ml benzamidine and/or 2 mg/ml PMSF, resuspended in 0.5 ml of the same solution and stored frozen at -20°C.

Examples of the outer membrane protein profiles of several different Gram-negative bacteria prepared using the sarkosyl method are shown in Fig. 2 (lanes B−E).

Extraction of lipopolysaccharide

Lipopolysaccharide (LPS) plays an essential role in the assembly and maintenance of the outer membrane as a permeability barrier (Hancock 1984; Nikaido & Vaara 1985) and makes an important contribution to the pathogenicity and antigenicity of Gram-negative bacteria (Jann & Jann 1985). As LPS carries a net negative charge it is generally responsible for conferring a strong negative surface charge on Gram-negative bacteria. Structurally, LPS is usually composed of three covalently linked regions: the inner lipid A, the central core polysaccharide and the outer O-antigen polysaccharide side chain. This type of LPS is called 'smooth' LPS to distinguish it from the 'rough' LPS of certain genera (e.g. *Neisseria* and *Haemophilus*) which does not contain an O-antigen. O-antigens consist of a variable number of repeating tri- to penta-saccharides which can range from 1 to as many as 40 units, giving rise to the characteristic ladder-like pattern observed on SDS-PAGE gels (Fig. 2, lane G). LPS appears to be anchored in the outer membrane by binding to outer membrane proteins, possibly through hydrophobic interactions via its

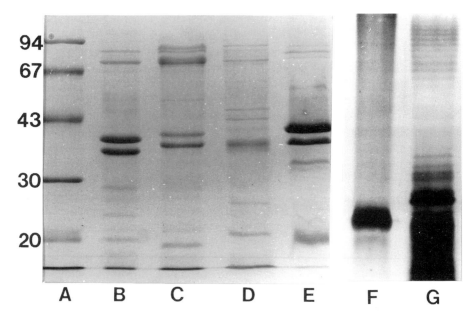

FIG. 2. SDS-PAGE showing the outer membrane proteins (lanes B–E) and lipopolysaccharides of Gram-negative bacteria (lanes F and G). Lane A, molecular weight marker proteins (kDa); lane B, *Escherichia coli*; lane C, *Klebsiella pneumoniae*; lane D, *Pseudomonas aeruginosa*; lane E, *Haemophilus influenzae* type b. Outer membranes were prepared, using the sarkosyl method, from bacteria grown under conditions of iron-deprivation and show the presence of iron-regulated proteins in the 67–94 kDa range. Lanes F and G show the lipopolysaccharides of *Bordetella pertussis* (rough LPS) and *E. coli* 0111 (smooth LPS), respectively.

lipid component and by the formation of non-covalent metal-cation (e.g. Mg^{2+}) cross-bridges between adjacent LPS molecules. Polycationic compounds including several biocides, are capable of destabilizing and making permeable the outer membrane by interacting at these cationic bridges (Hancock 1984). LPS can be isolated from whole cells and outer membranes either by extraction with phenol (Westphal & Jann 1965) or by digestion with proteinase K (Hitchcock & Brown 1983). The latter method can be carried out on very small samples. Methods for quantitating LPS based on the analysis of hydroxy fatty acids or 2-keto-3-deoxy-*manno*-octulosonic acid (KDO) are described by Lambert (this book).

Methods

Phenol extraction

1   Resuspend a bacterial wet weight of *c.* 10 g in 175 ml of distilled water and warm to 65°C in a water bath.

2 Add an equal volume of 90% (w/v) aqueous phenol at the same temperature and stir vigorously for 5 min. Cool rapidly in an ice bath and centrifuge at 5000 g for 30 min to permit phase separation.

3 Carefully remove the upper aqueous phase and dialyse against running tap water for at least 24 h to remove the phenol.

4 Centrifuge the dialysate at 10 000 g for 10 min to remove any insoluble debris. The LPS can then be collected as a clear viscous gel after a further centrifugation stage at 100 000 g for 4 h and subsequently lyophilized, if required.

The method described above is suitable for the extraction of smooth LPS but extracts rough LPS inefficiently. An alternative method using aqueous phenol, chloroform and low-boiling petroleum ether (40−60°C) has been described for this purpose (Galanos *et al.* 1969).

Isolation of lipopolysaccharide using proteinase K

1 Take 0.1 ml of an overnight suspension of bacteria containing *c.* 10^9 cells/ml. Add 0.05 ml of SDS-PAGE sample buffer (see Appendix 1) and boil at 100°C for 10 min.

2 After cooling to room temperature, add 0.05 ml of a solution of proteinase K (1 mg/ml) in 10 mmol/l Tris-HCl containing 5 mmol/1 $MgCl_2$ (pH 7.3).

3 Incubate the mixture at 60° for 60 min and then boil again at 100°C for 5 min to inactivate the proteinase K.

4 5−10-μl samples are taken for electrophoretic analysis on SDS-PAGE gels as described in Appendix 1. LPS can be revealed by staining with silver (see Appendix 1, page 103).

Using the proteinase K technique, cleaner preparations of LPS may be obtained from cell envelopes or isolated outer membranes instead of whole cells.

Examples of patterns observed on SDS-PAGE gels for smooth (*E. coli* 0111) and rough (*Bordetella pertussis*) LPS are shown in Fig. 2 (lanes F and G).

Extraction of exopolysaccharides

The surface of many Gram-positive and Gram-negative bacteria is covered extensively by an exopolysaccharide layer either as a discrete capsule or a loosely attached slime layer (Sutherland 1977). These surface polymers, which are composed of repeating units of one or more monosaccharides, are usually acidic polysaccharides. Whilst they are not essential for cell viability, they are important virulence determinants and may present a barrier to the penetration of antimicrobial agents (Sutherland 1977; Brown & Williams 1985; Williams

1988). Their production is considerably influenced by the growth environment and by the presence of antimicrobial compounds (Brown & Williams 1985; Williams 1988). Exopolysaccharides can be conveniently isolated from cell supernatants by precipitation with organic solvents such as acetone or ethanol. For bacteria which produce copious amounts of loosely associated material, the polysaccharides are precipitated from the spent growth medium after removal of the cells. Alternatively, bacteria grown on solid media (which often increases exopolysaccharide production) may require gentle blending or homogenizing. Once isolated, exopolysaccharides can be assayed by chemical or immunochemical methods (see Lambert, this book) and a polyacrylamide gel electrophoretic method for their analysis has also been described (Pelkonen *et al.* 1988).

Method

1   Ice-cold acetone or ethanol (4 vol.) is added to either (a) spent cell-free growth medium or (b) the supernatant fraction obtained after centrifuging a gently blended or homogenized cell suspension in phosphate-buffered saline (pH 7.4) at room temperature. Prior to the addition of solvent, high-speed centrifugation (40 000 g) may be required to removed whole cells because of the viscous nature of the exopolysaccharide solution

2   The precipitate, which may take up to 24 h to form at 4°C is recovered by centrifugation at 10 000 g. It should be washed at least twice in acetone and can be freeze-dried at this stage if required.

The precipitate obtained will consist of a crude mixture of exopolysaccharide, RNA, LPS and some protein. The exopolysaccharide can be further purified by fractional precipitation using cetyltrimethylammonium bromide (CTAB) (Jann 1985) as follows:

3   The precipitate is centrifuged at 100 000 g for 4 h to remove LPS and is subsequently lyophilized.

4   To a solution of 500 mg of the lyophilized material in 50 ml of 0.25 mmol/l NaCl, 1.0 g of CTAB in 25 mol of 0.25 mol/l NaCl is added with stirring to precipitate insoluble CTAB-RNA salts. After incubating the mixture with stirring for 15 min at room temperature, the precipitated CTAB−RNA salts can be removed by centrifugation at 10 000 g for 60 min.

5   3 vol. of water are slowly added to the clear supernatant liquid, the mixture is allowed to stand in an ice bath for at least 2 h and the resulting precipitate collected by centrifugation for 60 min at 10 000 g.

6   The precipitate thus obtained is dissolved in 5−8 ml of 1 mol/l NaCl (the smallest volume possible should be used) and reprecipitated by adding 8−10 vol. of ethanol. The mixture should be incubated for 2 h in an ice bath and the precipitate collected by centrifugation.

7   The procedure in 6 should be repeated and the resulting precipitate dissolved in water and dialysed against distilled water. If opalescent, the solution should be recentrifuged at 100 000 g at 4°C for 2 h prior to freeze-drying.

Purification of Soluble and Membrane-Bound Enzymes

In vitro studies of the molecular basis of antimicrobial action may require the isolation and extensive purification of the target enzyme(s). Such investigations depend on the availability of a sensitive detection system for the enzyme and/or its enzymatic activity. Preliminary purification procedures generally involve disruption of the bacterial cells and separation of soluble and membrane fractions. Further purification steps will depend upon the physico-chemical properties of the protein and the need to retain its enzymic activity (Scopes 1987). For many proteins, an initial concentration step employing fractional precipitation with salts (e.g. ammonium sulphate) or neutral organic solvents (e.g. acetone) acts as a useful preliminary purification stage. After crude fractionation, low-resolution column chromatographic systems such as molecular size exclusion and/or ion-exchange chromatography are used (Scopes 1987). These systems may be replaced by affinity chromatography (Dean *et al.* 1985). Both the resolution and speed of such techniques is increased by the availability of medium- and high-performance liquid chromatography (HPLC) (Fallon *et al.* 1987). The purity of the fractions obtained can be conveniently assessed by SDS-PAGE, particularly using minigel systems (see Appendix 1)

Whilst an extensive review of such methodology is beyond the scope of this paper, the purification of an extracellular enzyme, β-lactamase I, is given as an example. This enzyme, which is produced by *Bacillus cereus*, is secreted into the medium during growth. Its purification is complicated by the production, in similar concentrations, of a second enzyme, β-lactamase II. This enzyme shares similar physico-chemical properties with β-lactamase I. Following fractional precipitation from spent growth medium, the fraction containing β-lactamase activity is dialysed and loaded on to a cation-exchange column. The results are shown in Fig. 3, in which the presence of protein in the eluted fractions was determined by measurement of absorbance at 280 nm. β-lactamase activity was detected by using the chromogenic cephalosporin nitrocefin (O'Callaghan *et al.* 1972) and purity confirmed by SDS-PAGE.

Electrophoretic and HPLC Methods for Studying the Interaction of an Inhibitor with its Target Enzyme

The interaction of a biocide with an enzyme system is generally examined by determining the loss of specific enzyme activity (see Fuller, this book).

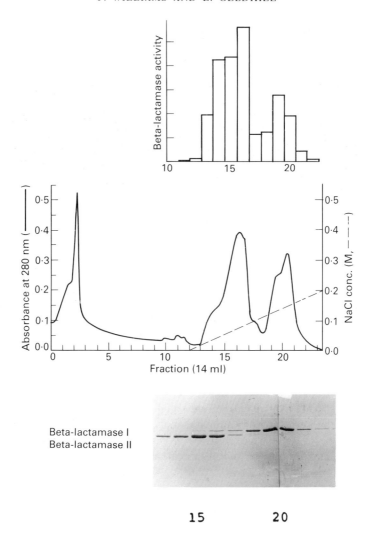

FIG. 3. Purification of β-lactamase I by cation exchange column chromatography on CM-Trisacryl-M and eluting with increasing concentrations of sodium chloride. The central panel shows the absorbance of each eluted fraction at 280 nm, the upper and lower panels denote the β-lactamase activity (as determined by the chromogenic cephalosporin nitrocefin) and purity (as determined by SDS-PAGE), respectively.

Another approach which has proved useful is isoelectric focusing, which can be used to study the effect of a biocide on the physico-chemical properties of the enzyme. Information on the antimicrobial agent's target site/enzyme active site can also be obtained by comparison of the peptide fragmentation

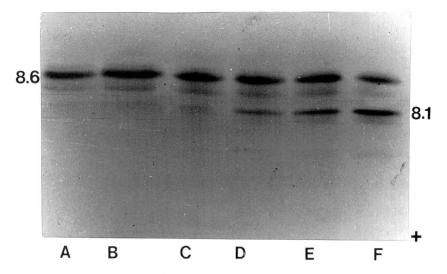

FIG. 4. The effect of irreversible inhibition on the isoelectric point of β-lactamase I isoenzymes inactivated by the β-lactamase inhibitor RES462A. After incubation in the presence or absence of RES462A, isoenzymes were focused on ampholine−polyacrylamide gels with a pH range of 3.5−9.5. Lanes A and B, native isoenzymes; lanes C−F, RES462A inhibited β-lactamase I isoenzymes with a percentage inhibition of 6% (C), 40% (D), 58% (E) and 65% (F), respectively. The pI values of the major isoenzymes are noted on both sides of the gel.

patterns derived from native and inhibited enzymes following enzymatic digestion. The two examples given below are based on studies of the interaction of a β-lactamase inhibitor and β-lactamase I purified as described above (Gledhill 1988).

Isoelectric focusing of an inhibited enzyme

The interaction of an antimicrobial agent with its target may alter physicochemical properties of the protein such as its isoelectric point. This can be evaluated by isoelectric focusing of the native and inhibited enzymes in polyacrylamide gels containing carrier ampholines (Dunbar 1987). Figure 4 shows the effect of the β-lactamase inhibitor RES462A on the isoelectric point of β-lactamase I, in which the isoelectric point of the major isoenzyme is reduced from pI 8.6 to pI 8.1. Both the isoelectric focusing apparatus and precast gels are commercially available.

Analysis of peptide fragmentation patterns of inhibited enzyme systems using HPLC

The covalent labelling of specific sites within an enzyme can be investigated by comparing the peptide fragmentation patterns of native and inhibited enzymes. These patterns are generated by HPLC (Fallon *et al.* 1987) of the peptide fragments obtained following the digestion of the enzyme with a pro-

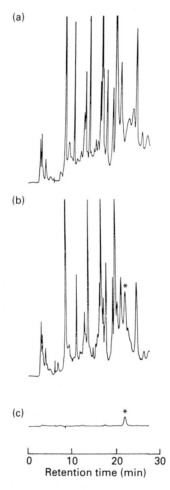

FIG. 5. Peptide fragmentation patterns of native β-lactamase I (a) and β-lactamase I inhibited by 6-β bromopenicillanic acid (b and c). The fragmentation patterns obtained by HPLC of tryptic digests were monitored simultaneously at absorbances of 230 nm (a and b) and 320 nm (c). A new peak* observed in the inhibited enzyme pattern (b) has a chromophore derived from the inhibitor which absorbs at 320 nm (c).

tease such as trypsin. The changes occurring in the peptide fragmentation pattern of β-lactamase I following inhibition with 6-β bromopenicillanic acid are shown in Fig. 5. The patterns were generated by HPLC performed on a C_{18} reverse-phase silica column. By simultaneously monitoring at two wavelengths (i.e. one wavelength to detect the peptides, the other to detect inhibitor-derived chromophores), the existence of peptide-inhibitor fragments can be observed. Such fragments can be collected and the inhibitor target site(s) identified by determination of the amino acid sequence of the purified peptide(s).

Appendix I
Sodium dodecyl sulphate polyacrylamide gel electrophoresis (SDS-PAGE)

Polyacrylamide gel electrophoresis is a versatile technique which can be used for both qualitative and quantitative analysis of soluble and membrane-bound proteins under denaturing (i.e. in the presence of SDS (SDS-PAGE)) or under non-denaturing (i.e. in the absence of SDS) conditions (Dunbar 1987). Proteins electrophoresed on sodium dodecyl sulphate polyacrylamide gels are separated according to molecular weight. The technique can be used to resolve complex mixtures of proteins and can be further enhanced by using two-dimensional systems. In these systems, the samples are separated according to charge on isoelectric focusing gels in the first dimension prior to electrophoresis on SDS-polyacrylamide gels in the second (Dunbar 1987). SDS-PAGE can also be used in the analysis of LPS and exopolysaccharides. A variety of different polyacrylamide slab gel systems are available commercially. These include minigel systems in which fast separations (less than 60 min) can be achieved with very small sample volumes.

The buffer system described below is based on that given by Lugtenberg et al. (1975) and is suitable for separating proteins and in particular the outer membrane proteins of Gram-negative bacteria. Lipopolysaccharides can also be electrophoresed using this buffer system although a number of modified systems have been suggested to improve the resolution of the O-antigen ladder patterns (Hancock & Poxton 1988). For exopolysaccharides, the buffer system described by Pelkonen et al. (1988) should be used.

Gels consisting of a separating gel containing 15, 12.5 or 10% acrylamide are cast, overlaid with SDS-PAGE electrode buffer containing 20% (v/v) methanol and are allowed to polymerize. After setting, the buffer is replaced with the stacking gel solution. The reagents are mixed as described in Table 1.

Following electrophoresis, proteins are stained with Coomassie Brilliant Blue R250 as described below. Alternatively, they can be stained with silver, a procedure that is approximately 100-fold more sensitive. Commercial kits for silver staining polyacrylamide gels are available although the reagents can be prepared from laboratory materials (Hancock & Poxton 1988). LPS and exopolysaccharides are also conveniently stained with silver.

TABLE 1. *Preparation of SDS-polyacrylamide gels*

Reagent	Separating gel: volume (ml) to give acrylamide concentration of			Stacking gel (ml)
	15%	12.5%	10%	
Stock I	6.17	5.17	4.17	—
Stock II	—	—	—	2.5
SDS 10% (w/v)	0.5	0.5	0.5	0.15
Tris-HCl 1.5 mol/l (pH 8.8)	6.17	6.17	6.17	—
Tris-HCl 0.5 mol/l (pH 6.8)	—	—	—	3.75
Distilled water	6.67	7.67	8.67	8.0
APS 10% (w/v)	0.07	0.07	0.07	0.07
TEMED	0.05	0.05	0.05	0.05

Where Stock I consists of 44% (w/v) acrylamide and 0.8% (w/v) N, N'-methylene-bis-acrylamide (BIS) and Stock II consists of 30% (w/v) acrylamide and 0.8% (w/v) BIS (ACRYLAMIDE IS NEUROTOXIC AND SHOULD BE HANDLED WITH CARE). TEMED is NNN'N' tetramethy-lethylene diamine and APS is ammonium persulphate. APS should be made fresh each day. Polymerization is initiated by the addition of TEMED.

Method

Protein samples are prepared for electrophoresis by mixing in a 1:1 ratio with sample buffer (see below) and are then heated at 100°C for 5–10 min. Gels are electrophoresed, according to the manufacturer's instructions, in an electrode buffer consisting of 0.025 mol/l Tris, 0.192 mol/l glycine and 0.1% (w/v) SDS. The pH of this buffer is 8.3 and should not be adjusted with acid or base.

Sample buffer pH 6.8

Tris-HCl 0.5 mol/l (pH 6.8)	5.0 ml
SDS 10% (w/v)	10.0 ml
2-mercaptoethanol	0.5 ml
Glycerol	5.0 ml
Distilled water	10.0 ml
Bromophenol blue 0.1% (w/v)	0.1 ml

After electrophoresis, gels are fixed and stained in 0.1% Coomassie Brilliant Blue R250 in 50% (v/v) methanol and 10% (v/v) glacial acetic acid in distilled water. Gels are destained in 40% (v/v) methanol with 10% (v/v) glacial acetic acid in distilled water and stored in a 10% (v/v) methanol/5% (v/v) glacial acetic acid mix.

Appendix II
Equipment and biochemicals suppliers

Chemical and biochemical compounds

Sigma Chemical Company, Fancy Road, Poole, Dorset BH17 7TH, UK.
BDH Ltd, Broom Road, Poole BH12 4NN, UK.

Electrophoresis equipment, chromatography columns and supports

Bio-Rad Laboratories Ltd, Caxton Way, Watford Business Park, Watford, Hertfordshire WD1 8RP, UK.
Pharmacia-LKB, Pharmacia House, Midsummer Boulevard, Milton Keynes MK9 3HP, UK.

Cell disruption equipment

French Press: Aminco, Silver Springs, Maryland, USA.
Sonicator: MSE Scientific Instruments, Manor Royal, Crawley, West Sussex RH10 2QQ, UK.
Microfluidizer: Microfluidics, Newton, Massachusetts USA.
Braun Homogenizer: Braun Melsungen International GMBH, Schwartzerbergerweg 23, D-3508, Federal Republic of West Germany.
Mickle Disintegrator: Mickle Laboratory Engineering Co., Ltd, Mill Works, Gomshall, Surrey GU5 9LJ, UK.

HPLC equipment

Anachem Ltd, 20 Charles St, Luton, Bedfordshire LU2 OEB, UK.
Beckman Instruments, Sands Industrial Estate, Lane End Road, High Wycombe, Buckinghamshire HP12 4JL, UK.

References

BROWN, M.R.W. & WILLIAMS, P. 1985. The influence of environment on envelope properties affecting survival of bacteria in infections. *Annual Review of Microbiology* **39**, 527–556.
CHEUNG, A.L. & FISCHETTI V.A. 1988. Variation in the expression of cell wall proteins of *Staphylococcus aureus* grown on solid and liquid media. *Infection and Immunity* **56**, 1061–1065.
COLEY, J., DUCKWORTH, M. & BADDILEY, J. 1975. Extraction and purification of lipoteichoic acids from Gram-positive bacteria. *Carbohydrate Research* **41**, 41–52.
DEAN, P.D.G., JOHNSON, W.S. & MIDDLE, F.A. 1985. *Affinity Chromatography: a Practical Approach*. Oxford: IRL Press.
DUNBAR, B.S. 1987. *Two-Dimensional Electrophoresis and Immunological Techniques*. New York: Plenum Press.

FALLON, A., BOOTH, R.F.G. & BELL, L.D. 1987. *Applications of HPLC in Biochemistry, Laboratory Techniques in Biochemistry and Molecular Biology*, Vol. 17, ed. Burdon, R.H. & Van Knippenberg, P.H. Amsterdam: Elsevier.

FIGGITT, D., CASTON, A., DENYER, S.P., WILLIAMS, P., JACKSON, D.E., WASHINGTON, C. & STEVENSON, N. 1988. Disruption of microbial cells using a laboratory microfluidiser. *Journal of Pharmacy and Pharmacology*, 40(S), 138P.

FILIP, C., FLETCHER, G., WULFF, J.L. & EARHART, C.F. 1973. Solubilisation of the cytoplasmic membrane of *Escherichia coli* by the ionic detergent sodium lauryl sarcosinate. *Journal of Bacteriology* 115, 717–722.

FISCHETTI, V.A., JONES, K.F., MANJULA, B.N. & SCOTT, J.R. 1984. Streptococcal M6 protein expressed in *Escherichia coli*. Localisation, purification and comparison with streptococcal-derived M-protein. *Journal of Experimental Medicine* 159, 1083–1085.

GALANOS, C., LUDERITZ, O. & WESTPHAL, O. 1969. A new method for the extraction of R lipopolysaccharides. *European Journal of Biochemistry* 9, 245–249.

GILBERT, P. & BROWN, M.R.W. 1980. Cell wall-mediated changes in sensitivity of *Bacillus megaterium* to chlorhexidine and 2-phenoxyethanol, associated with growth rate and nutrient limitation. *Journal of Applied Bacteriology* 48, 223–230.

GILBERT, P. & WRIGHT, N. 1987. Non-plasmidic resistance towards preservatives of pharmaceutical products. In *Preservatives in the Food, Pharmaceutical and Environmental Industries*, ed. Board, R.G., Allwood, M.C. & Banks, J.G. pp. 255–279. Society for Applied Bacteriology Technical Series No. 22. Oxford: Blackwell Scientific Publications.

GLEDHILL, L. 1988. The antimicrobial and β-lactamase inhibitory properties of chlorinated 6-spiroepoxy penicillins. *PhD thesis*, Nottingham University.

HAMMOND, S.M., LAMBERT, P.A. & RYCROFT, A.N. 1984. *The Bacterial Cell Surface*. London: Croom Helm.

HANCOCK, I.C. & POXTON, I.R. 1988. *Bacterial Cell Surface Techniques*. Chichester: John Wiley & Sons.

HANCOCK, R.E.W. 1984. Alterations in outer membrane permeability. *Annual Reviews in Microbiology* 38, 237–264.

HANCOCK, R.E.W. & CAREY, A.M. 1979. Outer membrane of *Pseudomonas aeruginosa*: heat modifiable and 2-mercaptoethanol modifiable proteins. *Journal of Bacteriology* 140, 902–910.

HECKELS, J.E. & VIRJI, M. 1988. Separation and purification of surface components. In *Bacterial Surface Techniques*, ed. Hancock I.C. & Poxton I.R. Chichester: John Wiley & Sons.

HITCHCOCK, P.J. & BROWN T.M. 1983. Morphological heterogeneity among *Salmonella* lipopolysaccharide chemotypes in silver-stained polyacrylamide gels. *Journal of Bacteriology* 154, 269–277

JANN, K. 1985. Isolation and characterization of capsular polysaccharides (K antigens) from *Escherichia coli*. In *The Virulence of* Escherichia coli; *Reviews and Methods*, ed. Sussman, M. pp. 375–379. London: Academic Press.

JANN, K. & JANN, B. 1985. Cell surface components and virulence: *Escherichia coli* O and K antigens in relation to virulence and pathogenicity. In *The Virulence of* Escherichia coli; *Reviews and Methods*, ed. Sussman, M. pp. 157–176. London: Academic Press.

KAYA, S., ARAKI, Y. & ITO, E. 1985. Characterisation of a novel linkage unit between ribitol teichoic acid and peptidoglycan in *Listeria monocytogenes* cell walls. *European Journal of Biochemistry* 146, 517–522.

LEYING, H., SUERBAUM, S., KROLL, H-P., KARCH, H. & OPERKUCH, W. 1986. Influence of beta-lactam antibiotics and ciprofloxacin on composition and immunogenicity of *Escherichia coli* outer membrane. *Antimicrobial Agents and Chemotherapy* 30, 475–480.

LUGTENBERG, B., MEIJERS, J., PETERS, R., VAN DER HOEK, P. & VAN ALPHEN, L. 1975. Electrophoretic resolution of the 'major outer membrane protein' of *Escherichia coli* K-12 into four bands. *FEBS Letters* **58**, 254–258.

LUGTENBERG, B. & VAN ALPHEN, L. 1983. Molecular architecture and functioning of the outer membrane of *Escherichia coli* and other Gram-negative bacteria. *Biochimica et Biophysica Acta* **737**, 51–115.

NIKAIDO, H. & VAARA, M. 1985. Molecular basis of bacterial outer membrane permeability. *Microbiological Reviews* **49**, 1–32.

O'CALLAGHAN, C.M., MORRIS, A., KIRKBY, S.M. & SHINGLER, A.H. 1972. Novel method for detection of β-lactamase by using a chromogenic cephalosporin substrate. *Antimicrobial Agents and Chemotherapy* **1**, 283–288.

OSBORN, M.J., GANDER, J.E. & PARISI, E. 1972. Mechanism of assembly of the outer membrane of *Salmonella typhimurium*. Isolation and characterisation of the cytoplasmic and outer membranes. *Journal of Biological Chemistry* **247**, 3962–3972.

PELKONEN, S., HAYRINEN, J. & FINNE, J. 1988. Polyacrylamide gel electrophoresis of the capsular polysaccharides of *Escherichia coli* K1 and other bacteria. *Journal of Bacteriology* **170**, 2646–2653.

SCHNAITMANN, C.A. 1970. Examination of the protein composition of the cell envelope of *Escherichia coli* by polyacrylamide gel electrophoresis. *Journal of Bacteriology* **104**, 882–889.

SCHNAITMANN, C.A. 1971. Solubilisation of the cytoplasmic membrane of *Escherichia coli* by Triton X-100. *Journal of Bacteriology* **108**, 545–552.

SCHOLLER, M., KLEIN, J.P., SOMMER, P. & FRANK, R. 1983. Protoplast and cytoplasmic membrane preparations from *Streptococcus sanguis* and *Streptococcus mutans*. *Journal of General Microbiology* **129**, 3271–3279.

SCOPES, R.K. 1987. *Protein-Purification: Principles and Practice*. New York: Springer Verlag.

SIEGEL, J.L., HURST, S.F., LIBERMAN, E.S., COLEMAN, S.E. & BLEIWEISS, A.S. 1981. Mutanolysin-induced spheroplasts of *Streptococcus mutans* are true protoplasts. *Infection and Immunity* **31**, 808–815.

SJOQUIST, J., MELHOUN, B. & HJELM, H. 1972. Protein A isolated from *Staphylococcus aureus* after digestion with lysostaphin. *European Journal of Biochemistry* **29**, 572–578.

SUERBAUM, S., LEYING, H., KROLL, H-P., GMEINER, J. & OPFERKUCH, W. 1987. Influence of β-lactam antibiotics and ciprofloxacin on cell envelope of *Escherichia coli*. *Antimicrobial Agents and Chemotherapy* **31**, 1106–1110.

SUTHERLAND, L.W. 1977. *Surface Carbohydrates of the Prokaryotic Cell*. London: Academic Press.

WESTPHAL, O. & JANN, K. 1965. Bacterial lipopolysaccharides: extraction with phenol/water and further applications of the procedure. In *Methods in Carbohydrate Chemistry*, Vol. 5, ed. Whistler, R.L. pp. 83–89. New York: Academic Press.

WILLIAMS, P. 1988. Role of the bacterial cell envelope in adaptation to growth *in vivo* in infections. *Biochimie* **70**, 987–1011.

Studies Involving Anaerobic Organisms

P.N. Levett

*Department of Biological and Biochemical Sciences, University of Ulster, Coleraine
BT52 1SA, UK*

Over 100 years have passed since the first methods for culture of anaerobic bacteria were described. The ubiquitous nature of anaerobes has led to the recognition of their importance in disease, food manufacture and spoilage, as contaminants in industrial processes and in environmental microbiology.

Determination of the susceptibility of anaerobes to antibacterial agents still presents problems to microbiologists. Since most sensitivity testing of anaerobes is done on clinical isolates this chapter will concentrate on methods used in clinical microbiology, with examples drawn from other areas wherever possible. However, the methods described using antibiotics are equally applicable to biocides. One of the most extensive studies of the mode of action of a biocide (chlorhexidine) on an anaerobe (*Clostridium perfringens*) was carried out by Hugo & Daltrey (1974) and Daltrey & Hugo (1974). In these papers many of the techniques described elsewhere in this volume were adapted to anaerobic conditions. Further details will be found in Daltrey (1973).

Preparation of Cells

For routine sensitivity testing, the inoculum should be prepared from a young culture, preferably in late log phase growth. In practice this may best be achieved by incubating a broth (e.g. Brain Heart Infusion supplemented with 0.5% yeast extract) culture for 4−5 h, or for more slowly growing anaerobes for 18 h, in an anaerobic cabinet. Alternatively, a suspension may be prepared from a fresh culture on an appropriate solid medium such as blood agar. The culture is diluted or suspended in saline or broth to a density of approximately 1×10^8 c.f.u./ml. Incubation is most conveniently carried out within anaerobic cabinets, thus providing optimum growth conditions throughout the experiments. However, acceptable results may be obtained using anaerobic jars

* Present Address: University of the West Indies, Faculty of Medical Sciences, Queen Elizabeth Hospital, St Michael, Barbados.

Mechanisms of Action of
Chemical Biocides

(Ralph & Kirby 1975; Stratton *et al.* 1987). If anaerobe jars are used a longer initial lag phase will be observed.

For biochemical studies, Hugo & Daltrey (1974) used a strain of *Cl. perfringens* (NCTC 8247), selected for its inability to spore readily in artificial media and for its aerotolerant nature, which permits harvesting under aerobic conditions. The culture was routinely maintained in cooked meat medium. For experimentation, cells were grown in the medium of Mossell *et al.* (1965) without agar. The medium was steamed and cooked before inoculation. After growth, the cells were harvested by centrifugation, washed twice with quarter-strength Ringer solution and finally suspended in 0.026 mol/l phosphate buffer (pH 7.0), or an alternative medium, to a density of *c.* 3.5×10^8 cells/ml. The cells were used immediately as they tended to form sphaeroplasts if stored. A summary of the subsequent anaerobic impositions on mode of action experiments is made in Table 1.

Assessment of Antimicrobial Activity against Anaerobes

A prelude to mechanism of action studies is the determination and quantification of antimicrobial effect. This section will consider methods appropriate to sensitivity testing and antibacterial assessment in anaerobes.

Disc diffusion assays

A suitable qualitative method is that based on the method of Stokes (1968) using antimicrobial-impregnated filter paper discs. A control organism of known sensitivity is inoculated on to the same plate as the test organism, providing both an indication of sensitivity or resistance of the test isolate and a check on the activity of the antimicrobial-impregnated discs. A suitable medium is Iso-Sensitest agar (Oxoid, Basingstoke, UK) with the addition of 5% (v/v) lysed horse blood. Other suitable basal media include DST agar (Oxoid) and Wilkins–Chalgren agar. Some media may require the addition of haemin and menadione in order to support the growth of some non-intestinal *Bacteroides* spp. It should be realized that added reducing agents such as L-cysteine and thioglycollate may inhibit the action of some antimicrobial substances. Plates should be freshly poured and dried at 37°C to prevent swarming of motile organisms (such as some clostridia). If necessary they can be prereduced in an anaerobic cabinet prior to use.

The test isolate is inoculated in the centre of the plate while the sensitive control strain is inoculated around the edge of the agar surface. Up to six discs may be applied to the interface between the two inocula, and the zones of inhibition may readily be compared after a suitable period of incubation (usually 48 h at 37°C).

TABLE 1. *Summary of mechanism of action techniques when using an anaerobe. Based on Daltrey (1973), Daltrey & Hugo (1974) and Hugo & Daltrey (1974)*

Mechanism of action parameter	Method and mode of anaerobiosis
MIC	Broth dilution in anaerobic jar (10% CO_2: 90% H_2)
Bactericidal activity	Biocide–cell interaction studied under 95% N_2: 5% CO_2 gas mixture. Survivors plated by the method of Miles *et al.* (1938) and incubated in an anaerobic jar
Adsorption of antimicrobial agent to cells	Pregassing with N_2: CO_2 atmosphere
Leakage (pentoses and 260-nm absorbing material)	Action of biocide on cells studied under N_2: CO_2 gas mix
Precipitation of nucleic acid and protein	Action of biocide on cell extract studied under N_2: CO_2 mix
Formation of sphaeroplasts	Treatment with lysozyme, lysozyme and EDTA, or left to autolyse. All carried out in N_2: CO_2 atmosphere
Sphaeroplast permeability	Permeability in presence of salt solutions which had been pregassed for 15 min with N_2
Cell metabolism: 1 Dehydrogenase activity	1 Thunberg technique, an anaerobic method, with N_2: CO_2 mix
2 Macromolecular synthesis	2 ^{14}C-glutamic acid, uracil and thymidine incorporation studied in cells growing under N_2: CO_2 mix
Transmembrane proton flux	Studies made in a vessel containing electrodes to monitor pH. The vessel was continuously gassed with N_2
Amino acid uptake	Use of ^{14}C-labelled amino acids in a system under H_2
ATP-ase activity	Crude cell extract was incubated with ATP in an anaerobic jar under H_2. Inorganic phosphorus production was followed.

The problems associated with disc diffusion include those common to sensitivity testing of aerobic organisms, namely relating to the depth of medium in the Petri dish, disc content and the relative rate of diffusion of different antimicrobial agents. However, most of these difficulties are largely overcome by the use of Stokes' method since the sensitive control strain is included on each plate. Ideally, an isolate with similar characteristics to that under test (of the same genus, for instance) should be selected for the control strain.

Minimum growth inhibitory concentration (MIC) determination

MICs may be determined either by broth dilution or by agar dilution. Broth dilution methods may be conducted in conventional test tubes or bottles (macrodilution) or in microtitre trays (microdilution). Macrodilution techniques are laborious and costly, while the advantages of microdilution methods may sometimes be offset by failure of organisms to grow in the wells close to the edge of the tray.

Broth dilution is used to determine the efficiency of biocides against sulphate-reducing bacteria (*Desulfovibrio* spp). The method used was described in detail by Sharma *et al.* (1987). The tests are performed in prereduced anaerobically sterilized media; growth is measured by absorbance at 580 nm and bactericidal activity by performing viable counts after 9 h incubation. Metabolic activity and biocide-induced inhibition is determined by following the reduction in sulphate concentration in the medium during the incubation period. A comprehensive listing of useful inhibitors active against sulphate-reducing bacteria was given by Postgate (1984). Microbiological problems, including those caused by sulphate-reducing anaerobes, in the offshore oil and gas industries are discussed by Battersby *et al.* (1985).

Agar dilution is the most widely accepted method of MIC determination for antibiotics against anaerobes and a reference method has been developed (NCCLS 1985). The inoculum is prepared in the manner described for routine sensitivity testing. Twofold dilutions of antimicrobial agents are prepared and plates are poured containing the appropriate dilutions in 20-ml portions of Wilkins–Chalgren agar. Two antimicrobial-free plates serve as controls. All plates should be dried to prevent swarming.

The plates are inoculated with up to 20 isolates using either a Steers replicator or a Denley multi-point inoculator. Both types of inoculator deliver a final inoculum of 1 µl, equivalent to 10^5 c.f.u. Inoculum size can significantly affect MIC (Brown 1988). The use of control strains of known MIC is essential.

One control plate may be incubated aerobically to check for aerobic contamination, while the other plate is incubated anaerobically to check growth on the basal medium. After incubation in an anaerobic atmosphere for 48 h, the plates are examined. If growth on the anaerobic medium control is adequate the MIC for each test isolate is determined as the lowest concentration showing no growth, a single discrete colony, or a fine, barely visible haze.

Organisms that do not grow sufficiently well on Wilkins—Chalgren agar may necessitate the use of other basal media, such as those used for disc-diffusion testing.

Kinetics studies

While the disc diffusion and MIC methods are of value in determining anaerobe sensitivity they provide little information about the way in which antibacterial agents inhibit anaerobic bacteria. Kinetics studies (or killing curves) yield data on the rate at which antimicrobial agents kill or otherwise inhibit the growth of bacteria, yet they have been relatively little used in studies of antibacterial action against anaerobes (Ralph & Kirby 1975; Crouch 1983; Ronning & Frank 1987; Stevens *et al.* 1987; Stratton *et al.* 1987).

The following method has been found reliable. All media are prereduced in an anaerobic cabinet for 24 h. Killing curve determinations are performed in 50-ml volumes of Brain Heart Infusion in 100-ml Duran bottles (these bottles have a neck sufficiently wide to allow the insertion of a micropipette). Strains to be tested are inoculated into 10-ml volumes of brain—heart infusion and incubated at 35°C for 13–14 h. Immediately before use sterile solutions of the antibacterial agents are prepared so that less than 1 ml of the antibacterial-containing solution is added to 50 ml of Brain Heart Infusion, in order to minimize dilution errors. After thorough mixing, 0.5 ml of the culture is inoculated into a control bottle and each of the test bottles containing the desired concentrations of the antibacterial agents under study. After inoculation cultures are incubated for 24 h. Samples are removed for viable counts immediately after inoculation and then at regular intervals (usually 4 h, but for some rapidly bactericidal agents more frequent sampling is necessary).

This method has been used to study the action of metronidazole and vancomycin upon *Cl.difficile* (Levett, unpublished results). Subinhibitory concentrations of either agent have little, if any, effect upon the growth curve of *Cl.difficile* (Fig. 1). However, at concentrations greater than the MICs for the two antibiotics, marked inhibition occurs with a significant bactericidal effect from metronidazole (Fig. 2), whereas vancomycin at high concentrations is bacteriostatic.

Performance of viable counts at frequent intervals over 24-h periods becomes exceedingly tedious. Growth or inhibition may be followed by indicators other than total viable count. Examples include continuous opacity measurement (Eley & Greenwood 1984), toxin production (Stevens *et al.* 1987), evolution of $^{14}CO_2$ using the Bactec system (Collins & Levett 1989),

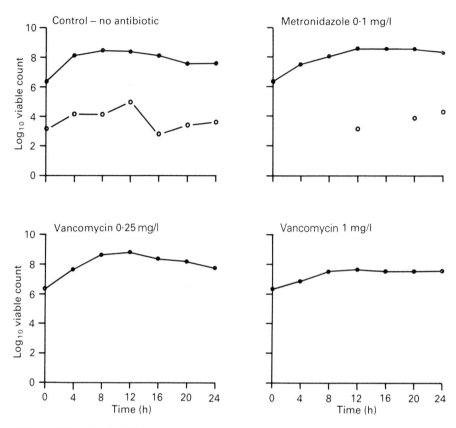

FIG. 1. Effect of subinhibitory concentrations of metronidazole and vancomycin on growth of *Cl. difficile*. Total viable count (●); spore count, (○).

changes in cellular morphology detected by microscopy (Eley & Greenwood 1984), inhibition of amino acid uptake and protein synthesis (Ronning & Frank 1987), reduction of sulphate by sulphate-reducing bacteria (Sharma *et al*. 1987) and changes in the phosphorylated nucleotide pool (Ronning & Frank 1987). Automated growth detection systems such as Bactec or the Abbott MS-2 may remove a considerable amount of the tedium from studies of time-dependent killing of anaerobes (Yourassowsky *et al*. 1981; Murray & Niles 1982).

It must be recognized that kinetics studies performed in batch cultures under optimum conditions, with a constant antibacterial concentration, yield highly artificial results, extrapolation to the practical situation may thus prove

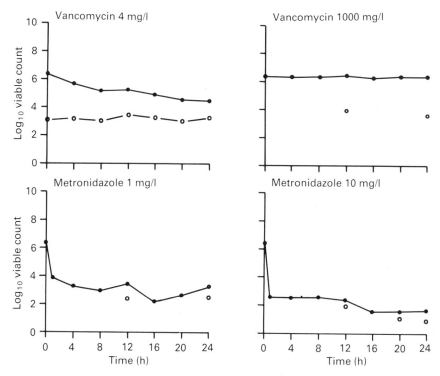

FIG. 2. Effect of supraMICs of metronidazole and vancomycin on growth of *Cl. difficile*. Total viable count (●); spore count (○).

difficult. One way in which these studies may be made more closely to resemble the *in vivo* environment would be by the use of continuous culture. Several such models of intestinal and ruminal bacteriology have been described (Slyter & Putnam 1967; Onderdonk *et al.* 1976; Freter *et al.* 1983; Edwards *et al.* 1985), some of which have been used to study the inhibitory effects of intestinal bacteria on anaerobes (Ushijima & Ozaki 1986; Wilson & Freter 1986). Models which mimic the hydrokinetics of urinary tract infection and treatment have been evolved (Greenwood & O'Grady 1978) and it may prove possible to develop models of this nature applicable to obligate anaerobes in other environmental situations.

Most probable number methods

The probability of growth of *Cl. botulinum* under a variety of conditions has been studied in a series of elegant experiments (Lund & Wyatt 1984; Graham

& Lund 1987; Lund *et al.* 1987), using either vegetative cells or spores of *Cl. botulinum.*

Peptone—yeast—glucose—starch medium is dispensed in 9-ml aliqouts in glass vials under a headspace of 85% N_2, 10% H_2 and 5% CO_2 (Lund & Wyatt 1984). The desired concentration of the inhibitor being studied is included in the medium and a standard inoculum of spores or vegetative cells is added. The most probable number of bacteria capable of growth in the test conditions after the appropriate incubation time is determined (Hurley & Roscoe 1983). The probability of growth from a single spore or vegetative cell is then calculated using formulae described by Hauschild (1982).

Using this approach, the inhibitory effects of temperature, pH, redox level, and preservatives such as sodium chloride, citric acid and sorbic acid have been investigated, individually and in combination.

Inhibition of spore germination

Inhibitors of spore germination and outgrowth are used in the food industry to prevent the growth of, and production of, toxin by several pathogenic organisms, amongst them *Cl. botulinum* (Sofos *et al.* 1986).

The effect of such inhibitors may be quantified by measuring the optical density at 600 nm of a spore suspension in an appropriate buffer. As spores germinate the OD_{600} decreases. Smoot & Pierson (1981) demonstrated reversible inhibition of germination of *Cl. botulinum* spores by potassium sorbate. Other methods of germination inhibition were reviewed by Cook & Pierson (1983).

Co-culture

A novel approach to the simulation of *in vivo* conditions during the study of antibacterial activity against anaerobes utilizes co-culture of an obligate anaerobe with a facultative anaerobe (usually *Escherichia coli*). Using such a model Ingham *et al.* (1981) demonstrated that the rate of killing of *B. fragilis* by metronidazole was proportional to the degree of oxygen scavenging by *E. coli.*

Variables affecting susceptibility

A number of factors may influence the *in vitro* action of antibacterial agents against obligate anaerobes. Many of these variables affect action against aerobes also, such as medium composition, pH and inoculum size. However several factors relate specifically to anaerobes.

The addition of CO_2 to the anaerobic atmosphere to stimulate growth lowers the pH and may reduce the activity of antibiotics (Ingham *et al.* 1970;

Rosenblatt & Schoenknecht 1972) and biocides such as cationic quaternary ammonium disinfectants. Tetracycline however, is more active when the pH is lowered (Rosenblatt & Schoenknecht 1972) as are phenols and organic acid preservatives. Failure to achieve adequate anaerobiosis may cause the action of some agents to be misrepresented.

References

BATTERSBY, S., STEWART, D.J. & SHARMA, A.P. 1985. Microbiological problems in the offshore oil and gas industries. *Journal of Applied Bacteriology Symposium Supplement* **59**, 227S–235S.

BROWN, W.J. 1988. National Committee for Clinical Laboratory Standards agar dilution susceptibility testing of anaerobic Gram-negative bacteria. *Antimicrobial Agents and Chemotherapy* **32**, 385–390.

COLLINS, T. & LEVETT, P.N. 1989. Radiometric studies on the use of selective inhibitors in the identification of *Mycobacterium* spp. *Journal of Medical Microbiology* **30**, 175–181.

COOK, F.K. & PIERSON, M.D. 1983. Inhibition of bacterial spores by antimicrobials. *Food Technology* **37**, 115–126.

CROUCH, B.A. 1983. Evaluation of biocides for use in North Sea oil operations. In *Biodeterioration*, Vol. 5, ed. Oxley, T.A. & Barry, S. pp. 725–730. Chichester: John Wiley.

DALTREY, D.C. 1973. Studies in the mode of action of chlorhexidine on *Clostridium perfringens*. *PhD thesis*, University of Nottingham.

DALTREY, D.C. & HUGO, W.B. 1974. Studies on the mode of action of the antibacterial agent chlorhexidine on *Clostridium perfringens* 2. Effect of chlorhexidine on metabolism and the cell membrane. *Microbios* **11**, 131–146.

EDWARDS, C.A., DUERDEN, B.I. & READ, N.W. 1985. Metabolism of mixed human colonic bacteria in a continuous culture mimicking the human cecal contents. *Gastroenterology* **88**, 1903–1909.

ELEY, A. & GREENWOOD, D. 1984. Variations in susceptibility to latamoxef (moxalactam) and cefoxitin within the *Bacteroides fragilis* group. *Journal of Antimicrobial Chemotherapy* **13**, 245–255.

FRETER, R., STAUFFER, E., CLEVEN, D., HOLDEMAN, L.V. & MOORE, W.E.C. 1983. Continuous-flow cultures as *in vitro* models of the ecology of large intestinal flora. *Infection and Immunity* **39**, 666–675.

GRAHAM, F.G. & LUND, B.M. 1987. The combined effect of sub-optimal temperature and sub-optimal pH on growth and toxin formation from spores of *Clostridium botulinum*. *Journal of Applied Bacteriology* **63**, 387–393.

GREENWOOD, D. & O'GRADY, F. 1978. An *in vitro* model of the urinary bladder. *Journal of Antimicrobial Chemotherapy* **4**, 113–120.

HAUSCHILD, A.H.W. 1982. Assessment of botulism hazards from cured meat products. *Food Technology* **36**, 95–104.

HUGO, W.B. & DALTREY, D.C. 1974. Studies on the mode of action of the antibacterial agent chlorhexidine on *Clostridium perfringens*. Adsorption of chlorhexidine on the cell, its antibacterial activity and physical effects. *Microbios* **11**, 119–129.

HURLEY, M.A. & ROSCOE, M.E. 1983. Automated statistical analysis of microbial enumeration by dilution series. *Journal of Applied Bacteriology* **55**, 159–164.

INGHAM, H.R., SELKON, J.B., CODD, A.A. & HALE, J.H. 1970. The effect of carbon dioxide on the sensitivity of *Bacteroides fragilis* to certain antibiotics *in vitro*. *Journal of Clinical Pathology* **23**, 254–258.

INGHAM, H.R., SISSON, P.P., EISENSTADT, R.L., SPROTT, M.S., BYRNE, P.O. & SELKON, J.B. 1981. Enhancement of activity of metronidazole by *Escherichia coli* under sub-optimal anaerobic conditions. *Journal of Antimicrobial Chemotherapy* 8, 475−479.

LUND, B.M., GEORGE, S.M. & FRANKLIN, J.G. 1987. Inhibition of type A and type B (proteolytic) *Clostridium botulinum* by sorbic acid. *Applied and Environmental Microbiology* 53, 935−941.

LUND, B.M. & WYATT, G.M. 1984. The effect of redox potential, and its interaction with sodium chloride concentration, on the probability of growth of *Clostridium botulinum* type E from spore inocula. *Food Microbiology* 1, 49−65.

MILES, A.A., MISRA, S.S. & IRWIN, J.O. 1938. The estimation of the bactericidal power of the blood. *Journal of Hygiene, Cambridge* 38, 732−749.

MOSSELL, D.A.A., BEERENS, H., TAHON-CASTEL, N.M., BARON, G. & POLSPEL, B. 1965. Etude des millieux utilsés pour le dénombrement des spores des bactéries anaérobies en microbiologie alimentaire. *Annales de l'Institut Pasteur, Lille* 16, 147−156.

MURRAY, P.R. & NILES, A.C. 1982. Adaptation of an automated microbiology system for the growth of anaerobes and performance of antimicrobial susceptibility tests. *American Journal of Clinical Pathology* 78, 457−561.

NATIONAL COMMITTEE FOR CLINICAL LABORATORY STANDARDS 1985. *Reference agar dilution procedure for antimicrobial susceptibility of anaerobic bacteria.* Approved standard Mll-A. Villanova, Pennsylvania: NCCLS.

ONDERDONK, A.B., JOHNSTON, J., MAYHEW, J.W. & GORBACH, S.L. 1976. Effect of dissolved oxygen and E_h on *Bacteroides fragilis* during continuous culture. *Applied and Environmental Microbiology* 31, 168−172.

POSTGATE, J.R. 1984. *The Sulphate-Reducing Bacteria*, 2nd edn. Cambridge: Cambridge University Press.

RALPH, E.D. & KIRBY, W.M.M. 1975. Unique bactericidal action of metronidazole against *Bacteroides fragilis* and *Clostridium difficile. Antimicrobial Agents and Chemotherapy* 8, 409−414.

RONNING, I.E. & FRANK, H.A. 1987. Growth inhibition of putrefactive anaerobe 3679 caused by stringent-type response induced by protonophoric activity of sorbic acid. *Applied and Environmental Microbiology* 53, 1020−1027.

ROSENBLATT, J.E. & SCHOENKNECHT, F. 1972. Effect of several components of anaerobic incubation on antibiotic susceptibility test results. *Antimicrobial Agents and Chemotherapy* 1, 433−440.

SHARMA, A.P., BATTERSBY, N.S. & STEWART, D.J. 1987. Techniques for the evaluation of biocide activity against sulphate-reducing bacteria. In *Preservatives in the Food, Pharmaceutical and Environmental Industries*, ed. Board, R.G., Allwood, M.C. & Banks, J.G. pp. 165−175. Society for Applied Bacteriology Technical Series No. 22. Oxford: Blackwell Scientific Publications.

SLYTER, L.L. & PUTNAM, P.A. 1967. *In vivo* vs *in vitro* continuous culture of ruminal microbial populations. *Journal of Animal Science* 26, 1421−1427.

SMOOT, L.A. & PIERSON, M.D. 1981. Mechanisms of sorbate inhibition of *Bacillus cereus* T and *Clostridium botulinum* spore germination. *Applied and Environmental Microbiology* 42, 477−483.

SOFOS, J.N., PIERSON, M.D., BLOCHER, J.C. & BUSTA, F.F. 1986. Mode of action of sorbic acid on bacterial cells and spores. *International Journal of Food Microbiology* 3, 1−17.

STEVENS, D.L., MAIER, K.A. & MITTEN, J.E. 1987. Effect of antibiotics on toxin production and viability of *Clostridium perfringens. Antimicrobial Agents and Chemotherapy* 31, 213−218.

STOKES, E.J. 1968. *Clinical Bacteriology*, 3rd edn. London: Edward Arnold.

STRATTON, C.W., WEEKS, L.S. & ALDRIDGE, K.E. 1987. Comparison of kill-kinetic studies with agar and broth microdilution methods for determination of antimicrobial activity of selected agents against members of the *Bacteroides fragilis* group. *Journal of Clinical Microbiology* **25**, 645–649.

USHIJIMA, T. & OZAKI, Y. 1986. Potent antagonism of *Escherichia coli*, *Bacteroides vulgatus*, *Fusobacterium varium* and *Enterococcus faecalis*, alone or in combination, for enteropathogens in anaerobic continuous flow cultures. *Journal of Medical Microbiology* **22**, 157–163.

WILSON, K.H. & FRETER, R. 1986. Interaction of *Clostridium difficile* and *Escherichia coli* with microfloras in continuous-flow cultures and gnotobiotic mice. *Infection and Immunity* **54**, 354–358.

YOURASSOWSKY, E., VAN DER LINDEN, M.P., LISMOUNT, M.J., LABBE, M. & CROKAERT, E. 1981. The effect of β-lactam antibiotics on the growth curves of *Bacteroides fragilis*, obtained with the MS-2 system. *Journal of Antimicrobial Chemotherapy* **8**, 219–224.

Action on Cell Walls and Outer Layers

P.A. LAMBERT

*Pharmaceutical Sciences Institute, Department of
Pharmaceutical Sciences, Aston University, Aston Triangle,
Birmingham B4 7ET, UK*

Some biocides have dramatic effects upon the integrity of bacterial envelopes, causing lysis or massive leakage of cellular constituents. These effects can be detected by a decrease in turbidity of the cell suspension or the appearance of cytoplasmic constituents in the surrounding medium, and are described by Denyer & Hugo (this book). However, some agents cause subtle changes in cell envelope structure which require more sensitive techniques for detection. The purpose of this contribution is to outline methods for the quantitative assessment of changes in bacterial envelopes induced by the action of biocides.

Detection of Envelope Damage by
Changes in Permeability

The outer membrane (OM) of Gram-negative bacteria acts as a permeability barrier (Nikaido & Vaara 1985). The restrictive size of the porin channels in the OM effectively excludes hydrophilic molecules with masses in excess of *c.* 600 Da. In some smooth strains, the polysaccharide chains of the lipopolysaccharide (LPS) O-antigen present a barrier to the penetration of hydrophobic molecules. A hydrophobic uptake pathway is recognized in strains which lack O-antigen (e.g. *Neisseria gonorrhoeae*) whilst some compounds (e.g. the aminoglycoside antibiotics) can penetrate cells by a self-promoted uptake pathway by partially disrupting the permeability barrier. Damage to the OM resulting in release of LPS and associated OM components can be detected by changes in the ability of molecules to penetrate the envelope (Hancock 1984). Two kinds of marker molecules are useful in this respect: substrates for periplasmic enzymes and hydrophobic fluorescent probes. The following are examples of how such probes can be used.

Mechanisms of Action of
Chemical Biocides

Nitrocefin hydrolysis by whole cells

Nitrocefin is a chromogenic cephalosporin which changes colour from yellow to red when hydrolysed by β-lactamases (O'Callaghan *et al.* 1972). Biocide-induced OM damage is indicated by an increase in hydrolysis rate of nitrocefin by whole cells (Hancock & Wong 1984). This could be due either to increased penetration of the OM by nitrocefin, or to release of β-lactamase from the periplasm. The activity of β-lactamase is retained in the presence of many biocides. To obtain sufficient activity a cell density of 10^9 cells/ml is normally required using sodium phosphate buffer at pH 7. As this density is markedly turbid, it is desirable to use a 1-mm path-length microcuvette to minimize light scattering. The absorbance of the suspension at 482 nm is monitored after addition of the biocide. If possible, the cuvette should be maintained at a constant temperature of 25°C in the spectrophotometer. Higher rates of hydrolysis are obtained by working at 37°C but storage of the test cell suspension at this temperature can lead to gradual lysis and release of β-lactamase. As a control, sonically disrupted cells can be used to measure the maximum hydrolysis rate in the absence of a permeability barrier. The effect of the biocide on this control rate should be investigated to establish any effect upon the enzyme. The rate of hydrolysis of nitrocefin by intact cells depends upon the permeability characteristics of the organism and the amount of β-lactamase present. If the control rates are too low then it can be advantageous to induce the enzyme level in the cells by use of an agent such as 6-aminopenicillanic acid (6-APA, 50 μg/ml). In principle, any Gram-negative organism can be used, since most express some β-lactamase activity in the periplasm. For organisms with low activity which cannot be induced with 6-APA, a plasmid-mediated β-lactamase can be introduced.

The kinetics of this system are obviously complex; some of the cells might become completely permeabilized, giving the substrate free access to the enzyme, and others only partially damaged by the biocide. Additionally, the biocide might partly inhibit (or stimulate) the β-lactamase. For these reasons it is advisable not to interpret the data in terms of rigorous enzyme kinetics. Any β-lactam can be used, adjusting the wavelength accordingly to detect the hydrolysis products (Nikaido *et al.* 1983). For cephaloridine the reduction in absorbance at 255 nm gives a measure of hydrolysis of the cephalosporin (Holt *et al.* 1983). However, nitrocefin is the most convenient agent, the red colour gives a clear indication of hydrolysis and release of cytoplasmic constituents does not interfere with the detection at 482 nm.

Method

1   Prepare cell suspension of test organism (any Gram-negative organism producing moderate levels of β-lactamase can be used) in 10 mmol/l sodium

phosphate buffer (pH 7.0) containing 10^9 cells/ml and place in a water bath at 25°C.

2 Prepare nitrocefin solution by dissolving 1 mg (available as 1-mg amounts of lyophilized powder in vials, Oxoid SR112, Oxoid Ltd, Basingstoke UK) in 2 ml of sodium phosphate buffer and place in a water bath at 25°C. It may help to dissolve the solid nitrocefin in 20 µl of dimethyl sulphoxide before adding the buffer; if this is done, a control experiment must be carried out to ensure that the solvent does not permeabilize the cells. This can be checked by pretreating the cell suspension with the final concentration of solvent in the absence of nitrocefin for 30 min, then adding nitrocefin solution. If any permeabilization has occurred, the initial rate should be increased.

3 Place 0.1 ml of cell suspension in a glass microcuvette (1 mm path-length, 0.3 ml vol.) with 0.1 ml of phosphate buffer. Add 0.1 ml of nitrocefin solution, mix rapidly and monitor absorbance at 482 nm over 10–20 min. As the nitrocefin penetrates the cells and is hydrolysed by the periplasmic β-lactamase, the absorbance at 482 nm increases. The rate of increase is controlled by the amount of β-lactamase in the cells and the permeability of the outer membrane.

4 Repeat experiment with cells pretreated with biocide or add biocide to the cell suspension in the cuvette in place of the 0.1 ml of phosphate buffer. An example of the use of this assay is shown in Fig. 1. Hancock & Wong (1984) have used a similar method to study compounds which increase the permeability of the *Pseudomonas aeruginosa* OM.

Use of the fluorescent probes, ANS and NPN

ANS (6-anilino-1-naphthalenesulphonic acid) and NPN (1-*N*-phenylnaphthylamine) are large hydrophobic fluorescent molecules which cannot normally enter intact Gram-negative bacteria. When the envelope is damaged, they can gain access to the cytoplasmic membrane, to which they bind and fluoresce strongly. The assay is carried out in a quartz fluorimeter cuvette and the fluorescence of a cell suspension is monitored in the presence of the probe before and after addition of the biocide. The method requires relatively low cell densities (10^8 cells/ml) for detection of envelope damage. Control experiments should be done to check that the biocide does not cause the probes to fluoresce. This can occur with detergent biocides where the probes enter the hydrophobic core of micellar aggregates. ANS and NPN are useful probes for monitoring damage in pseudomonads (Anwar *et al.* 1983; Loh *et al.* 1984); NPN has been used extensively to study the effects of a range of 'permeabilizers' on *Pseudomonas aeruginosa* (Hancock & Wong 1984; Hancock 1985; Moore *et al.* 1987). Historically the approach was pioneered by Newton (1955) who used the fluorescent properties of dansyl-polymyxin to monitor the action upon Gram-negative envelopes.

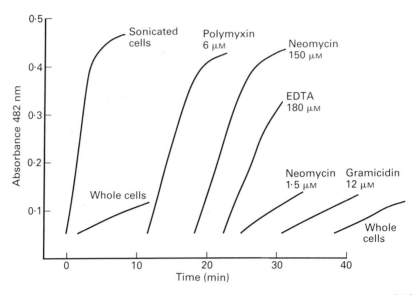

Fig. 1. Time course for hydrolysis of nitrocefin by intact cells of *Pseudomonas aeruginosa* PAO1 containing the R plasmid RP1. A 0.1-ml sample of a washed cell suspension (10^9 cells/ml) in 10 mmol/l sodium phosphate buffer (pH 7.0) was placed in a 1-mm path-length microcuvette with 0.1 ml of phosphate buffer; 0.1 ml of nitrocefin (0.5 mg/ml in similar buffer) was then added and the absorbance at 482 nm monitored over 10 min at 25°C (traces labelled 'whole cells'). The other traces show the effects of the addition of various agents (added in place of the 0.1 ml of phosphate buffer) at the final concentrations shown. One sample of untreated whole cell suspension was subjected to sonic disruption (MSE Soniprep, MSE, Crowley, UK, maximum power, 2×30 s) and nitrocefin then added ('sonicated cells').

Method

1 Prepare a cell suspension (10^8 cells/ml) in phosphate buffer, 0.1 mol/l (pH 7.0) and place in a water bath at 25°C.

2 Prepare stock solution of ANS in ethanol (0.5 mmol/l) and place in a water bath at 25°C.

3 Incubate 4.9 ml of cell suspension with 0.1 ml of ANS solution in a test tube at 25°C for 15 min then measure fluorescence spectrum in a fluorimeter over the wavelength range 380−550 nm with an excitation wavelength of 355 nm. Undamaged intact cells show little fluorescence whereas biocide-damaged cells show a strong fluorescence maximum at 440 nm. When Tris buffer is substituted for phosphate the cells show a marked fluorescence due to the damaging effects of Tris upon the outer membrane.

Where NPN is used in place of ANS the stock solution (0.5 mmol/l) is prepared in acetone, the excitation wavelength is 350 nm and the emission spectrum maximum is 420 nm. For both probes, control experiments must be made to check that the solvents have no effect upon the cell permeability. This is best done by measuring the effect of the solvents upon the rate of nitrocefin hydrolysis in intact cells as described above.

Biocide can be added directly to the test system with ANS or NPN, or the cells can be pretreated with biocide separately and removed before addition of the probes. If the former method is employed, care must be taken to ensure that the biocide does not interact with the probe. By continuous monitoring of fluorescence at the maximum emission wavelengths the time course of damage induced by the biocide can be followed. In either method some caution must be applied to quantitative assessment of damage from the fluorescence intensity produced; quenching effects can reduce the fluorescence considerably. As the method is extremely sensitive, it is advisable to start with low concentrations of biocides which have no effect upon fluorescence and increase the concentration until an increase is detected. An example of the method is given in Fig. 2.

Damage Measured by Changes in Envelope Composition

An excellent source of information on techniques for the isolation, analysis and estimation of bacterial surface components has been compiled by Hancock & Poxton (1988). This should be consulted for methods not covered in this chapter.

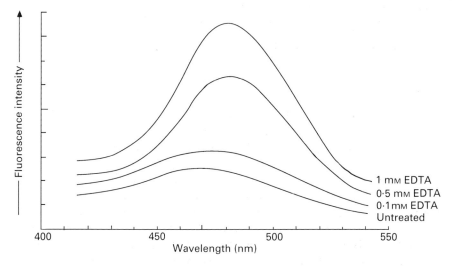

FIG. 2. Effect of EDTA upon the fluorescence of whole cells of *Pseudomonas aeruginosa* PAO1 in the presence of 6-anilino-1-naphthalenesulphonic acid (ANS). Washed cell suspensions (10^8 cells/ml) in 0.1 mol/l sodium phosphate buffer (pH 7.0) were treated with EDTA for 10 min at 25°C. ANS was added to a final concentration of 10 µmol/l and the fluorescence spectrum measured immediately with an excitation wavelength of 355 nm.

Outer membrane components

Measurement of LPS by analysis of hydroxy fatty acids in whole cells

Damage to the envelope of Gram-negative bacteria usually results in release of vesicles containing protein, LPS and phospholipid from the outer membrane. Measurement of an OM marker, such as the 2-keto-3-deoxy-*manno*-octulosonic acid (KDO) component of LPS, before and after exposure of the cells to the biocide should give a measure of the loss of LPS. The thiobarbituric acid method is not reliable when applied to whole cells due to interference by cellular deoxyribonucleotides. A better approach is to use the hydroxy fatty acid substituents of LPS as markers. These are characteristic of particular species, are found only in the LPS (apart from polyhydroxybutyrate which can occur in cytoplasmic storage granules) and can be measured in whole cells by the sensitive technique of gas–liquid chromatography (GLC). The method employs acid hydrolysis to ensure release of amide-linked fatty acids from lipid A and derivatization to fatty acid methyl esters with boron trifluoride/ methanol reagent. In this and all subsequent methods it is assumed that cell suspensions are treated with biocide under desired conditions, then centrifuged, washed once in saline to remove residual biocide, and resuspended to the original volume in water prior to analysis.

Method

The assay is carried out in 15-ml Pyrex hydrolysis tubes fitted with Teflon-lined screw caps.

1   To each of a series of hydrolysis tubes add a measured amount of a fatty acid to act as an internal standard (50 µl of a 0.1 mg/ml solution in hexane). A fatty acid that does not occur in the test organism must be used as the internal standard. Tridecanoic acid is suitable for many Gram-negative organisms. The solvent is allowed to evaporate at room temperature.

2   To each tube is then added 1 ml of cell suspension containing 10^9 cells/ml.

3   4 ml of 6N HCl is added to each tube, the caps are sealed and the tubes heated at 100°C for 4 h.

4   After cooling, methyl esters of the fatty acids released from the cells are formed by addition of 4 ml of boron trifluoride/methanol complex (14% w/v) and heating to 80°C for 5 min.

5   The fatty acid methyl esters are extracted by shaking vigorously with 4 ml of chloroform:hexane (1:4) in the hydrolysis tubes. The upper phase is placed in a glass round-bottom flask and reduced to dryness on a rotary evaporator.

6   The residue in each flask is redissolved in 40 µl hexane and transferred to a small glass vial for storage at −20°C.

7   Before applying to the gas chromatograph the contents of each vial are allowed to evaporate at room temperature to c. 10 μl; a sample of 2 μl is then applied to the column.

8   GLC conditions for packed columns are as described by Lambert & Moss (1983):

Column	3 m × 2 mm internal diameter glass packed with 3% SP-2100 DOH on 100/200 Supelcoport (Supelchem, Saffron Walden, UK).
Conditions	150°C 1 min, increase at 2°C/min to 225°C, hold for 5 min.
Carrier gas	20 ml/min nitrogen.
Detection	Flame ionization, hydrogen/air.
Standards	Reference preparation of 23 bacterial fatty acid methyl esters, 10 mg/ml (Supelchem, Saffron Walden, UK).

The internal standard and fatty acids present in each sample are identified by reference to the retention times of fatty acid methyl esters in a standard mixture (run separately) and quantitated by peak area measurement. Some variation in the amount of internal standard used will be required to ensure that the peak area is similar to those of the cellular fatty acids. Capillary columns offer improved resolution one-packed columns; a 30 m × 0.25 mm ID fused silica column of SPB^{TM}−1 (Supelchem, Saffron Walden, UK) gives excellent results.

Direct measurement of cellular LPS by SDS-PAGE

A direct assessment of LPS content can be made by examination of silver-stained gel patterns following SDS-PAGE of protease K digests of whole cells (see Williams & Gledhill, this book). The method requires small cell samples (1 ml of 10^8 cells/ml) and can give a semi-quantitative evaluation of changes in LPS content, especially when linked to densitometric scanning of the stained patterns (Tilling et al. 1986).

Extraction of LPS and capsular polysaccharide from whole cells for quantitative analysis

A useful micromethod involves phenol extraction of cells and can be carried out in plastic microcentrifuge tubes (e.g. Eppendorf tubes).

1   Cell suspensions are prepared in 3 ml of phosphate buffered saline containing 0.15 mmol/l $CaCl_2$ and 0.5 mmol/l $MgCl_2$, to a density of 10^9 cells/ml.

2 Cells are then pelleted by centrifugation and resuspended in 0.3 ml water in microcentrifuge tubes and transferred to a water bath at 65−70°C.

3 0.5 ml of hot phenol (80% w/w at 65−70°C) is carefully added, the tubes are shaken vigorously and then maintained at this temperature for 15 min. (GREAT CARE MUST BE TAKEN WHEN HANDLING PHENOL, IT IS BOTH CAUSTIC AND EXTREMELY TOXIC WHEN ABSORBED THROUGH THE SKIN.)

4 The suspension is cooled on ice for 30 min and centrifuged at 2400 g for 25 min.

5 The upper aqueous phase is transferred to a 50-ml polypropylene centrifuge tube and the lower phenol phase re-extracted with 0.3 ml of water in the microcentrifuge tube.

6 To the pooled aqueous phases is added 40 μl of 5 mmol/l NaCl followed by 40 ml of 95% ethanol. The suspension is left overnight at −20°C to precipitate the polysaccharide (LPS and capsule, if present).

7 The polysaccharide precipitate is pelleted by centrifugation at 2400 g for 15 min, resuspended in 0.2 ml water and transferred to a microcentrifuge tube. The inner walls of the 50-ml centrifuge tube are rinsed with 1 ml of 95% ethanol to suspend residual precipitate which is then added to the dissolved pellet in the microcentrifuge tube.

8 After centrifugation at 5000 g for 10 min the pellet is resuspended in 50 μl of water and stored at −20°C until required for analysis.

Yields are too small for accurate measurement by weight, but are excellent for SDS-PAGE analysis of LPS profiles or quantitation by chemical analysis or immunoassay as described below.

Estimation of polysaccharide in the phenol extracts by measurement of hexose content

The phenol-sulphuric acid assay can be used to measure the total hexose in the extract (i.e. hexose content of capsular polysaccharide and LPS combined).

Method

1 Two-millilitre samples of glucose standard solutions in water (containing 10−80 μg glucose) are placed in glass test tubes; 10- or 20-μl samples of the extracts are then placed in separate tubes and the volume in each is made up to 2.0 ml with water.

2 To each tube is added 1.0 ml of 5% (w/v) aqueous phenol followed by 5.0 ml of 95% (w/v) H_2SO_4. Both solutions must be added rapidly to ensure thorough mixing and to avoid local overheating. (GREAT CARE MUST BE TAKEN WHEN HANDLING THESE REAGENTS.)

3 After cooling to room temperature the absorbance at 490 nm is measured. (TAKING CARE WHEN FILLING AND EMPTYING THE CUVETTES.)

LPS in the extracts can be estimated by measuring the KDO content with thiobarbituric acid.

Method

1 Samples of KDO standard (10−100 μg, Sigma Chemicals Company Ltd, Poole, UK) or 10−20 μl of the extract solutions prepared as described above are placed in 15-ml pyrex glass hydrolysis tubes; 0.25 ml of 0.05 mol/l H_2SO_4 is added, the tubes are sealed with Teflon-lined caps and heated at 100°C for 30 min.
2 On cooling, 0.25-ml periodic acid (0.025 mol/l in 0.0625 mol/l) H_2SO_4 is added and the tubes are heated to 55°C for 20 min.
3 0.5 ml of 2% (w/v) sodium arsenite in 0.5 mol/l HCl is added and the contents mixed thoroughly.
4 2.0 ml of 0.3% (w/v) thiobarbituric acid in water is added; the tubes are sealed and heated to 100°C for 20 min.
5 After cooling to room temperature the absorbance is measured at 550 nm. The KDO content of the extract is determined from the standard curve. The LPS content can be estimated either by assuming that the KDO content of LPS is 5% (w/w), or by analysis of a purified sample of LPS from the test organism. KDO contents of LPS usually range from 2 to 10% (w/w). An estimate of the capsular polysaccharide in the extract can be obtained from the difference between the LPS and total hexose assays.

For a completely independent measurement of capsular polysaccharide, an immunological assay such as rocket immunoelectrophoresis should be considered. This requires specific antibody to the capsular polysaccharide.

Method

1 Prepare a 1% (w/v) solution of agarose (medium electroendosmosis, LKB) in Tris-barbiturate buffer (pH 8.6) (a stock buffer solution containing 22.4 g diethylbarbituric acid, 44.3 g Tris, 0.533 g calcium lactate and 0.65 g sodium azide is diluted 1:5 before dissolving the agarose by boiling for 5 min).
2 Calculate the volume of molten agarose for each gel from length of gel (cm) × width of gel (cm) × 0.132 ml. Cool to 55°C in a water bath, add antiserum to desired dilution (1/10 to 1/100). Pour on to a glass plate or on to the hydrophilic side of Gelbond (Pharmacia LKB Biotechnology, Milton Keynes, UK) plastic sheet on a level surface.
3 When the gel has set, cut a row of wells at 10-mm intervals, 15 mm from one edge of the plate with a 4- or 5-mm diameter cork borer to give 15- or 25-μl capacity wells.
4 Fill the wells with phenol-extracted polysaccharide solution prepared as described above.

5 Place the gel on the cooling plate of a flat-bed electrophoresis apparatus (e.g. LKB Multiphor or Pharmacia flat-bed apparatus Pharmacia LKB Biotechnology, Milton Keynes, UK). Apply thick paper wicks soaked in Tris-barbiturate buffer to either edge of the plate (sample wells nearest the negative electrode) and electrophorese at 500 V overnight at 10°C.

6 Press the gel dry by covering it with a moist filter paper, several dry paper towels and a glass plate held in place with a heavy weight for 10 min.

7 Rehydrate the gel in water and dry again by pressing. Repeat the pressing and rehydration steps three times. Finally dry to a thin film with a hair drier, stain with coomassie blue (1 g Coomassie Brilliant Blue/90 ml ethanol/20 ml acetic acid/90 ml water) for 10 min and wash with destain solution (90 ml ethanol/20 ml acetic acid/90 ml water) until the background is clear.

The sensitivity of the method and the optimum loadings of sample and antisera will depend upon the particular polysaccharide and the antibody used. Figure 3 shows a typical pattern obtained for *Klebsiella pneumoniae* K1 capsular polysaccharide and antiserum raised in a rabbit. Commercial K-specific typing serum can also be used if available for the organism under study.

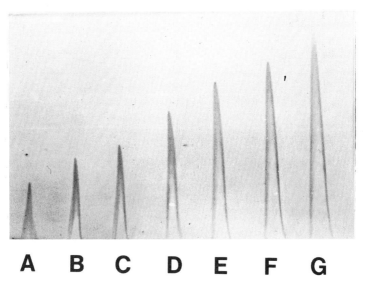

A B C D E F G

FIG. 3. Assay of capsular polysaccharide from *Klebsiella pneumoniae* K1 by rocket immunoelectrophoresis. Phenol-extracted capsular polysaccharide solution (10 µl) was placed in wells A–G and electrophoresed at 500 V overnight at 10°C into agarose containing antiserum to the K1 polysaccharide raised in a rabbit. Wells contained (µg polysaccharide): A, 0.5; B, 1; C, 1.5; D, 2; E, 3; F, 4; G, 5. The agarose (1% w/v in Tris-barbiturate buffer, pH 8.6) contained 0.1 ml of antiserum in 10 ml and was cast on a 10 × 8 cm^2 gelbond sheet. This figure was kindly provided by Dr Julia Lodge.

Peptidoglycan

This method uses boiling sodium dodecyl sulphate (SDS) to remove all non-covalently attached material from the peptidoglycan. It can be applied to Gram-positive and Gram-negative bacteria.

Method

1 Wet bacterial paste (equivalent to 2—4 mg dry wt/ml) is added dropwise to an equal volume of boiling 8% (w/v) SDS. The mixture is boiled for 30 min with continuous stirring, then cooled and left at room temperature overnight.
2 The mixture is centrifuged at 30 000 g for 15 min (for Gram-positives) or 1 h (for Gram-negatives) at 20°C to avoid precipitation of SDS.
3 The pellet is collected and the SDS extraction repeated twice. The final pellet is washed four times with water, twice with 2 mol/l NaCl and finally four times with water.

For Gram-positive bacteria the resulting pellet contains peptidoglycan sacculi and any covalently linked accessory polymers (e.g. teichoic acid or teichuronic acids). For Gram-negative bacteria the pellet comprises peptidoglycan sacculi with covalently linked lipoprotein. Pure peptidoglycan is prepared from the sacculi preparations as follows.

Method for Gram-positive bacteria

1 Suspend sacculi (10 mg/ml) in 0.1 mol/l HCl and heat to 100°C for 1 h.
2 Centrifuge at 30 000 g for 30 min and wash pellet of crude peptidoglycan twice with water.
3 Resuspend pellet (5 mg/ml) in 0.1 mol/l ammonium carbonate and incubate with calf intestinal alkaline phosphatase (200 U/ml, Sigma) at 37°C for 20 h under toluene.
4 Centrifuge at 75 000 g for 30 min to deposit pellet of pure peptidoglycan, wash twice in water and freeze-dry.

Method for Gram-negative bacteria

1 Suspend sacculi from 1 litre of mid-log-phase culture in 2.5 ml of 10 mmol/l Tris-HCl (pH 7.0) and incubate with pronase (200 µg/ml, Sigma) at 60°C for 1 h (a stock solution of 10 mg/ml of the pronase must be pretreated in the same buffer by heating to 60°C for 2 h to inactivate contaminating peptidoglycan-hydrolysing activity).
2 Add an equal volume of 8% (w/v) SDS and boil for 15 min.

3   Dilute the suspension with 3 vol. water, centrifuge at 130 000 g for 1 h at 20°C, wash pellet of pure peptidoglycan three times in water. The total yield of peptidoglycan can be measured as dry weight after freeze-drying, or by measuring the amino acid or hexosamine content after acid hydrolysis (6 mol/l HCl, 100°C, 6 h). Alternatively, the samples can be digested with *Chalaropsis* muramidase (Sigma) and the mucopeptide fragments analysed by HPLC (Glauner & Schwartz 1988).

Phospholipids

Measurement of phospholipids cannot be achieved successfully with small cell samples. Cells from at least 1 litre of culture are required to give sufficient lipid for separation and analysis by thin-layer chromatography.

Method

1   Resuspend cells from 1 to 2 l of culture (equivalent to at least 500 ml of 10^9 cells/ml) in 8 ml water and place in a glass separating funnel.
2   Add 30 ml methanol:chloroform (2:1 v/v) and shake. Add 20 ml of water: chloroform (1:1 v/v) and shake thoroughly. Leave to stand at room temperature for 2 h or until the phases separate.
3   Carefully remove the lower phase which contains the lipid. Filter it through silicone-treated filter paper (Whatman 1PS, Whatman LabSales Ltd, Maidstone, UK) to remove any residual aqueous phase and particulate material.
4   Transfer filtrate to a weighed round-bottom flask and remove solvent on a rotary evaporator at reduced pressure. Store in a vacuum desiccator overnight to remove residual solvent and weigh accurately.

   This gives the total 'readily extractable lipid'. Further fractionation can be carried out as follows.

Method

1   Dissolve extracted lipid in 1 ml chloroform:methanol (2:1 v/v), add 20 ml diethyl ether and leave overnight at −10°C.
2   Remove any precipitate of polyhydroxybutyrate by centrifugation. Evaporate the supernatant to dryness and dissolve the lipid residue in 1 ml chloroform: methanol (2:1 v/v). Add 20 ml acetone and store overnight at −10°C.
3   Deposit the precipitated phospholipids by centrifugation, dry and weigh. Evaporate the remaining acetone supernatant to dryness and weigh. This fraction contains chiefly neutral lipids (e.g. diglycerides and glycolipids).
Individual lipids in the readily extractable lipid fraction or the purified fractions can be examined by thin-layer chromathography on silica gel using chloro-

form:methanol:water (65:25:4 v/v/v) or chloroform:acetic acid:methanol:water (80:18:12:5 v/v/v/v). Two-dimensional separation using each solvent system in turn gives an excellent resolution of the major phospholipids. Suitable detection sprays are: ninhydrin for amino-containing phospholipids; phosphate stain for phospholipids (Vaskovsky & Kostetsky 1968); charring with 5% ethanolic molybdophosphoric acid for glycolipids.

Acknowledgement

I would like to thank Dorothy Townley and Roy Tilling for their help with the development of the assays described in this chapter.

References

ANWAR, H., BROWN, M.R.W., BRITTEN, A.Z. & LAMBERT, P.A. 1983. Disruptive effects of Tris and sodium lauroyl sarcosinate on the outer membrane of *Pseudomonas cepacia* shown by fluorescent probes. *Journal of General Microbiology* **129**, 2017–2020.

GLAUNER, B. & SCHWARTZ, U. 1988. Investigation of murein structure and metabolism by high pressure liquid chromatography. In *Bacterial Cell Surface Techniques*, ed. Hancock, I.C. & Poxton, I.R. pp. 158–171. Chichester: John Wiley & Sons.

HANCOCK, I.C. & POXTON, I.R. 1988. *Bacterial Cell Surface Techniques*. Chichester: John Wiley & Sons.

HANCOCK, R.E.W. 1984. Alterations in outer membrane permeability. *Annual Review of Microbiology* **38**, 237–264.

HANCOCK, R.E.W. 1985. The *Pseudomonas aeruginosa* outer membrane permeability barrier and how to overcome it. *Antibiotics and Chemotherapy* **36**, 95–102.

HANCOCK, R.E.W. & WONG, P.G.W. 1984. Compounds which increase the permeability of the *Pseudomonas aeruginosa* outer membrane. *Antimicrobial Agents and Chemotherapy* **26**, 48–52.

HOLT, J., SIMPSON, I.N. & HARPER, P.B. 1983. Quantitative methods for assessing stability of β-lactam antibiotics to cell-free β-lactamase extracts. In *Antibiotics: Assessment of Antimicrobial Activity and Resistance*, ed. Russell, A.D. & Quesnel, L.B. pp. 127–139. London & New York: Academic Press.

LAMBERT, M.A. & MOSS, C.W. 1983. Comparison of the effects of acid and base hydrolysis on hydroxy and cyclopropane fatty acids in bacteria. *Journal of Clinical Microbiology* **18**, 1370–1377.

LOH, B., GRANT, C. & HANCOCK, R.E.W. 1984. Use of the fluorescent probe 1-*N*-phenylnaphthylamine to study the interactions of aminoglycoside antibiotics with the outer membrane of *Pseudomonas aeruginosa*. *Antimicrobial Agents and Chemotherapy* **26**, 546–551.

MOORE, R.A., WOODRUFF, W.A. & HANCOCK, R.E.W. 1987. Antibiotic uptake pathways across the outer membrane of *Pseudomonas aeruginosa*. *Antibiotics and Chemotherapy* **39**, 172–181.

NEWTON, B.A. 1955. A fluorescent derivative of polymyxin: its preparation and use in studying the site of action of the antibiotic. *Journal of General Microbiology* **12**, 226–236.

NIKAIDO, H., ROSENBERG, E.Y. & FOULDS, J. 1983. Porin channels in *Escherichia coli*: studies with β-lactams in intact cells. *Journal of Bacteriology* **153**, 232–240.

NIKAIDO, H. & VAARA, M. 1985. Molecular basis of bacterial outer membrane permeability. *Microbiological Reviews* **49**, 1–32.

O'CALLAGHAN, C.H., MORRIS, A., KIRBY, S.M. & SHINGLER, A.H. 1972. Novel method for detection of β-lactamases by using a chromogenic cephalosporin substrate. *Antimicrobial Agents and Chemotherapy* **1**, 283−288.

TILLING, R.K., JESSOP, H.I. & LAMBERT, P.A. 1986. A note on the use of a scanning laser densitometer to analyse silver-stained lipopolysaccharide patterns on polyacrylamide gels and antigenic profiles on nitrocellulose sheets produced by immunoblotting. *Letters in Applied Microbiology* **2**, 43−46.

VASKOVSKY, V.E. & KOSTETSKY, E.Y. 1968. Modified spray for detection of phospholipids on thin-layer chromatograms. *Journal of Lipid Research* **9**, 396.

Electron and Light Microscopy of Damaged Bacteria

E.G. BEVERIDGE,[1] I. BOYD,[1] I. DEW,[1] M. HASWELL[2] AND C.W.G. LOWE[1]

[1]Department of Pharmaceutics; and [2]Electron Microscopy Unit, Sunderland Polytechnic, Sunderland SR2 7EE, UK

The Microbe is so very small
You cannot make him out at all,
But many sanguine people hope
To see him through a microscope

Hilaire Belloc (1964)
Selected Cautionary Verses.
Revised Puffin Edition.

Microscope Techniques

Success involving optical or electron microscopic techniques depends upon an understanding of the factors which influence image quality, particularly when working with the subcellular bacterial structures. Quesnel (1971), Lickfeld (1976) and Bulla *et al.* (1973) provide readable explanations of these techniques and their practical application.

Since individual bacteria are virtually transparent to transmitted light it is necessary to work with specimens which have been stained, or to use an optical system that renders transparent objects opaque. Stains may be non-selective, such as crystal violet, or may be chosen to selectively stain nuclear material, capsules, lipid granules or cell wall components, and have been used to determine, for example, the degree of subdivision of the nuclear material in 5-fluorouracil-induced filaments of *Bacillus cereus* (Doolittle *et al.* 1973). We have found that some biocide-induced filaments and sphaeroplasts were particularly unstable to solvent or heat fixation but would withstand gentle air drying, prior to examination.

Phase-contrast or interference-contrast techniques which allow direct examination of unfixed and unstained bacteria permit the direct viewing of

Mechanisms of Action of
Chemical Biocides

135

biocide action upon bacteria in simple agar slide cultures or even as biofilms on test materials. For electron microscopy, with its harsh conditions of high vacuum and low water activity, possible deleterious effects of sample preparation, fixing, staining and sectioning, need to be controlled and distinguishable from any biocide-induced effects (see Glauert 1974; Lewis & Knight 1977). The greater availability of epifluorescence attachments for general use enables the utilization of a wide range of fluorescent reagents to investigate biocidal activity. Fluoresecent-tagged antibodies (Grange *et al.* 1987) and ultraviolet-fluorescing optical brighteners (Paton & Jones 1971) could prove useful in monitoring the disappearance of or unmasking of cell surface groupings by biocides. Some biocides are fluorescent themselves, and we, for example, have investigated the selective accumulation of anthracycline drugs into the kineto-plast of trypanosomes (unpublished, with W.B. Mitchell and J.R. Brown) monitoring its red fluorescence under short-wave ultraviolet-irradiation. Fluorescence-inducing probes such as 8-anilinonaphthalenesulphonic acid (Newton 1956) may give an indication of selective changes in membrane permeability.

Interpretation of data

Biocide-induced structural changes, although interesting *per se*, are usually more valuable as clues to overall modes of action. There is, therefore, a need to appreciate normal bacterial ultrastructure and the various modifications possible under normal (biocide-free) environmental fluctuations, such as the extensive filamentation induced in *Pseudomonas putida* by oxygen-limitation (Jensen & Woolfolk 1985).

Debate still occurs as to whether structures such as mesosomes are real or artefacts of processing, whilst biocide-induced changes can be difficult to interpret as modifications of normal behaviour in the absence of 'normal' counterparts. A useful anthology of relevant literature has been prepared by van Iterson (1984a). In addition to the variable biochemical changes observed with differing biocide levels a variety of structural changes are often seen, also indicating a progressive level of interference; these range from perturbation of growth to extensive cellular disorganization in highly biocidal systems. Observed effects may reflect the direct inhibition of a site such as destruction of the outer membrane or an indirect action such as filamentation by inactivation of DNA synthesis and its subsequent effect on the sequences of the cell growth cycle. Whether structural changes represent the cause(s) or the consequence(s) of death or damage is often difficult to decide and, generally, microscopic evidence will only provide one facet of the solution to be considered in the overall context of studies which should include biochemical and physical studies, and an assessment of quantitative biocide measurements.

Observable effects

Routine examination of cultures and suspensions can provide a pattern of information on size, shape and degree of aggregation, enabling rapid identification of contaminants, unusual changes in cell condition or signs of instability (lysis, plasmolysis), and suitable controlled total cell counts provide a primary standardization for secondary calibration purposes (spectrophotometry etc.). With other techniques, microscopy will assist in assessing formation or degradation of biofilms or confirm the behaviour of cells in hydrophobicity measurements like the bacterial adsorption to hydrocarbons (BATH) technique (see Gorman, this book). Various biocides are reported to induce morphological changes in growing bacteria, possibly the most widely studied class having been the β-lactam antibiotic where the effects include filamentation, and the formation of sphaeroplast, and other variants caused by the selective inactivation of different proteins of the peptidoglycan-synthesizing system (PBPs) (see Reynolds 1985). Fosfomycin (Carlone *et al.* 1982) and possibly glycerol and sucrose esters of fatty acids (Tsuchido *et al.* 1987) induce filamentation in a broadly analogous manner, whilst the mechanisms of others such as phenols (Spray & Lodge 1943), triethylene-melamine (Grant 1968),

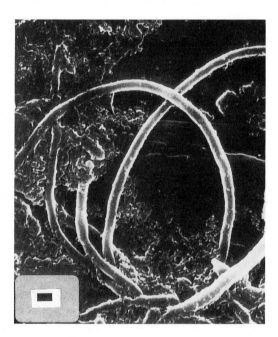

FIG. 1. Filament formation in *E. coli* by subMIC (0.5%) levels of 2-chloroacetamide; bar = 400 nm; scanning electron microscopy. (With permission of S.P. Denyer.)

and 2-chloroacetamide (Fig. 1; Serry *et al.* 1986) are less clear. Direct inhibitory action upon DNA synthesis can, secondarily, disrupt cell division and induce filamentation as reported for 5-fluorouracil (Doolittle *et al.* 1973), and nalidixic acid (Mirelman *et al.* 1977). Often the filaments contain discrete nuclear bodies along their length and are free from internal septa (Katchman *et al.* 1955; Serry *et al.* 1986) and in some cases such as phenylethanol (Silva *et al.* 1976) mesosome-like structures are observed. Quaternary ammonium antimicrobial agents and chlorhexidine induce outer membrane damage, disorganization of cytoplasm and the appearance of membranous and vesicular structures in growing bacteria. At moderately bactericidal levels cytoplasmic membrane damage is evident with loss of cell contents and the formation of 'ghosts'. At highly bactericidal levels, however, cell contents appear to be precipitated within the cell, confirming the biphasic leakage patterns found with these agents (Hugo & Longworth 1965; Hoffman *et al.* 1973; Richards & Cavill 1976).

There is a long ongoing microbiological interest in a 'vital' stain, distinguishing 'live' bacteria from 'dead', although there are varying levels of acceptance of such stains as are in use. We have determined, in part, the degree of 'viability' of *M. leprae* bacilli treated with potential antileprotic agents in a macrophage slide culture system. After treatment, the bacilli are stained with fluorescein diacetate (non-fluorescent) and ethidium bromide. Fluorescein diacetate is considered to penetrate healthy membranes to be hydrolysed to fluorescein by non-specific esterases (green fluorescence, 'viable') whilst ethidium bromide only penetrates markedly damaged membranes and reacts with DNA (red fluorescence, 'dead'). Some correlation is observed with antileprotic activity in this test and in the mouse foot pad technique (Hooper *et al.* 1988).

Results with specific biocide

We wish to illustrate our experience of microscopy as an aid to the study of antimicrobial action by reference to our work on two groups of biocides:
1 2-phenoxyethanol and its analogues are used as preservatives in pharmaceutical, cosmetic and perfumery formulations, and we have identified a variety of interconnected inhibiting mechanisms which include progressive perturbation of membrane function and stability, interference with ATP synthesis and direct interference with DNA biosynthesis (Gilbert *et al.* 1980);
2 Betane (Agma plc, Haltwhistle, Northumberland, UK) is an ampholytic biocide for use in the food, brewing and related industries; it is a complex mixture of alkylaminoalkylglycines and is related to, but different from, the Tego (Th. Goldschmidt Ltd, London, UK) range of ampholytic agents.

Materials and Methods

Preparation and examination of specimens

Optical microscopy involved staining techniques as detailed fully by Norris & Swain (1971) for study of general characteristics such as nuclear bodies, lipid inclusions etc. For phase-contrast examination, bacteria were allowed to settle on a thin tryptone-soy agar film (1 drop, hot slide, 60°, dehydrate for 30 min at room temperature) to minimize movement. Examination of growing cells involved thicker agar films (5 drops) inoculated and incubated in airtight boxes lined with moist filter paper. Periodic viewing provided a review of the sequence of events. Fluorescent antibody staining required conventional methods (Walker *et al.* 1971), our own prepared species-specific antisera (rabbit) and commercially available fluorescent-tagged antirabbit antisera. Electron microscopic procedures closely followed those of Lewis & Knight (1977) and Glauert (1974). Negative staining used carbon-stabilized, Formvar-coated grids, and, generally, silicotungstic acid (1% for 30s) revealed surface detail well. For ultrastructural details, bacteria test suspensions (100 ml) were treated for 5 min at room temperature with 20 ml glutaraldehyde-paraformaldehyde fixative containing calcium chloride in cacodylate buffer (glutaraldehyde, 4%; formaldehyde, 4%; calcium chloride, 0.5%; cacodylate buffer, 0.08 mol/l, pH 7.2) followed by fresh fixative for 6−12 h after which they were washed four times and stored in cacodylate buffer (0.2 mol/l, pH 7.2). The collected pellet was stained with osmium tetroxide (2% for 2 h) and then uranyl acetate (2% for 1 h). Bacteria were then dehydrated with ethanol and embedded in Spurr's resin (Agar Aids, Stanstead, Essex, UK). Ultra-thin sections (50−60 nm) prepared with a diamond knife were further stained with lead citrate solution and examined by transmission electron microscopy (Model 801, AEI Ltd, Manchester, UK; 60 kV accelerating voltage).

Recording of data

Kodak Technical Pan Film (TP 2514) gives good results for phase-contrast work, when rated at 75 ASA, used with a green filter (Wratten No. 58) and developed for high contrast. Kodacolour 400 (Gold) negative film provided good records of epifluorescence data but exposures may need to be long. A particularly useful book dealing with practical aspects of optical photomicrography is that produced by Kodak (Anon 1980). Electron micrographs were made on Ilford Technical Film (EM) and printed on Ilford Multigrade paper for high contrast.

Results and Comments

At concentrations approaching the MIC (*c.* 35−45 μg/ml) 2-phenoxyethanol inhibited bacterial motility and induced filament formation with *E. coli* in broth cultures, the proportion of conversion from normal rods being highest when nearest to the MIC but the largest filaments being induced at slightly lower antimicrobial levels. In slide cultures very long filaments, up to 1000 μm in length, were formed in 16 h (Fig. 2); these were fairly stable to centrifugation and washing, and showed evidence of plasmolysis in hypertonic sodium chloride solution (Fig. 3) indicating a reasonable degree of homeostatic control. Staining with anti-*E. coli* rabbit antiserum followed by fluorescent-tagged antirabbit antiserum (Fig. 4), and negative-staining electron microscopy revealed surface characteristics similar to those of untreated bacteria. Nuclei were evenly distributed along the length of the filaments (Robinow's method). In thin section the filaments were seen to be non-septate with DNA somewhat more diffusely distributed than suggested by the optical nuclear stain. Other structures were similar to those of untreated bacteria with the exception of large lightly stained lamellar inclusions appearing as irregular flattish sheets or concentric tubes (Fig. 5). These were reminiscent of, but different in appearance from, membrane accumulation in *E. coli* grown at 40°C (van Iterson 1984b). When washed and placed in 2-phenoxyethanol-free media filaments

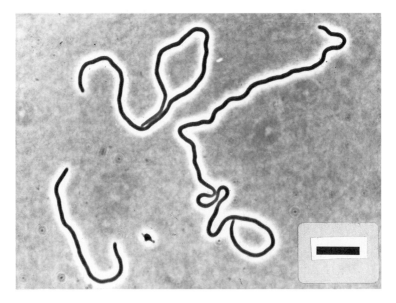

FIG. 2. Filament formation in *E. coli* by 2-phenoxyethanol in slide culture at subMIC concentration (25 μmol/ml); bar = 10 μm; phase-contrast microscopy (PC).

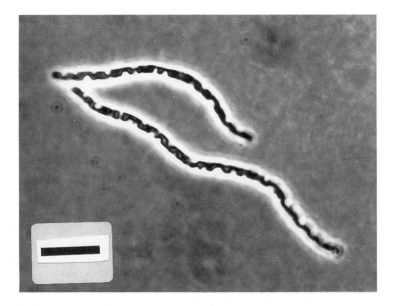

FIG. 3. Filaments of *E. coli* induced by 2-phenoxyethanol (27 μmol/ml) and suspended in hypertonic saline solution (5% NaCl) showing plasmolysis; bar = 10 μm; PC.

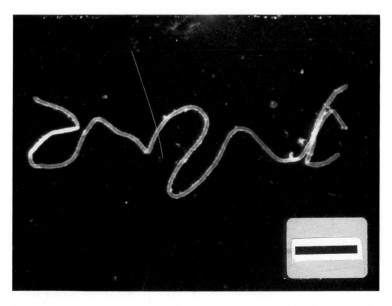

FIG. 4. *E. coli* filament(s) induced by 2-phenoxyethanol (25 μmol/ml) showing staining with species-specific fluorescent antibodies; bar = 10 μm; epifluorescence microscopy.

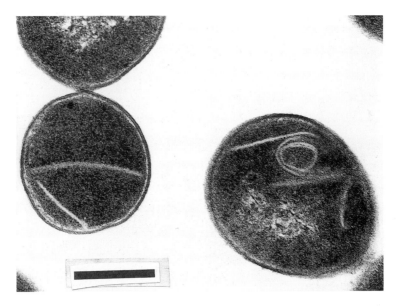

FIG. 5. Lamellar inclusions induced in *E. coli* by subMIC levels of 2-phenoxyethanol (25 μmol/ ml); bar = 400 nm; transmission electron microscopy (TEM).

reverted progressively to rods by initiation of division both at their poles and across their length (Fig. 6), the lamellar inclusions disappearing at an early stage in this process. At concentrations just above the MIC, cells remained static but viable for some considerable time. Sections revealed blebbing of the outer membrane as small attached globules, and signs of plasmolysis indicated reasonable membrane control.

In moderately biocidal levels of 2-phenoxyethanol (1%, LT 90% $\cong$ 10 min)* progressive damage was observed to the outer and cytoplasmic membranes together with the appearance of densely staining 'blisters' on the outer membrane similar to those observed by Hugo & Longworth (1965) for chlorhexidine, with the loss of some cell contents. More biocidal levels (2% 2-phenoxyethanol, LT 90% < 0.5 min) created 'ghosts' comprising surprisingly intact (physically) envelope fractions but almost totally devoid of cell contents. Treatment of *E. coli* with 2-phenoxyethanol levels of *c.* 0.7% rendered them penetrable by 8-anilinonaphthalenesulphonic acid and thus fluorescent under ultraviolet light, suggesting the beginning of significant cytoplasmic membrane damage.

A weakly biocidal analogue of 2-phenoxyethanol, 4-(2-hydroxyethoxy)

* T90%; time taken to kill 90% of bacterial population at a defined biocide concentration.

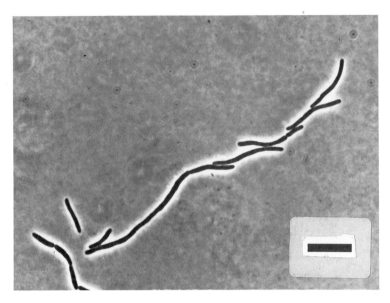

FIG. 6. Resumption of division of 2-phenoxyethanol-induced (25 μmol/ml) *E. coli* filament on drug-free slide culture (35°C, 1.5 h); bar = 10 μm; PC.

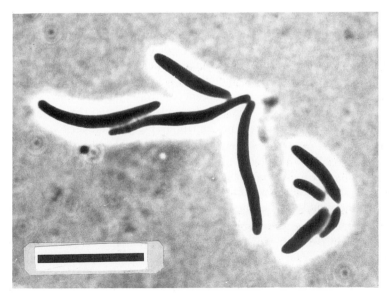

FIG. 7. Fusiform filaments of *E. coli* induced by subMIC levels of 4-(2-hydroxyethoxy) acetanilide (35 μmol/ml); bar = 10 μm; PC.

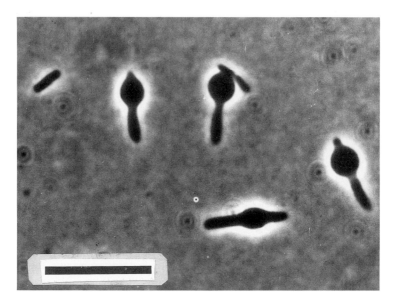

FIG. 8. Sphaeroplast formation by *E. coli* induced with subMIC levels of 4-(2-hydroxyethoxy) acetanilide (35 µmol/ml) in slide culture; bar = 10 µm; PC.

acetanilide, induced shorter (up to 15 µm) fragile swollen fusiform filaments (Fig. 7) and bulbous sphaeroplast-like cells (Fig. 8) near its MIC (*c.* 80 µg/ml). Both only withstood mild handling and the filaments, but not the sphaeroplasts, reverted to normal *E. coli* rods on biocide-free agar. Sections revealed a granular cytoplasm containing membrane-enclosed vacuoles, large amorphous densely stained granules and the absence of distinct nuclei. Evidence of plasmolysis indicated some membrane control. The outer and cytoplasmic membranes were clearly visible but the collapsed peptidoglycan gel usually seen in untreated bacteria was not apparent (Fig. 9 and Fig. 17, inset).

In *Staphylococcus aureus* 2-phenoxyethanol induced cell growth of one and a half to three times the normal diameter, and sections revealed gross interference with cell wall formation, with thickened, distorted walls, incomplete septa and fused undivided cells of various sizes (Fig. 10). These resembled the distortions induced in staphylococci by β-lactam antibiotics (Lorian & Atkinson 1976).

Bacillus subtilis underwent filamentation with 2-phenoxyethanol and the filaments were characterized by irregular, incomplete septa, and nuclei at intervals along their length with mesosome-like inclusions and infoldings of wall material associated with the septa. We have been unable so far to induce filament formation in *Pseudomonas aeruginosa* with 2-phenoxyethanol or its analogues.

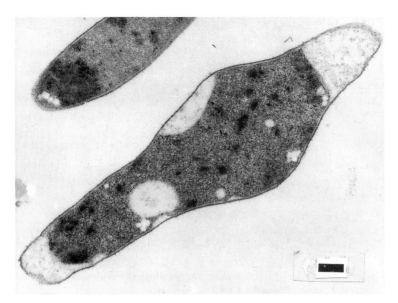

FIG. 9. Fusiform filaments induced in *E. coli* by 4-(2-hydroxyethoxy) acetanilide (35 μmol/ml) in slide culture; bar = 400 nm; TEM.

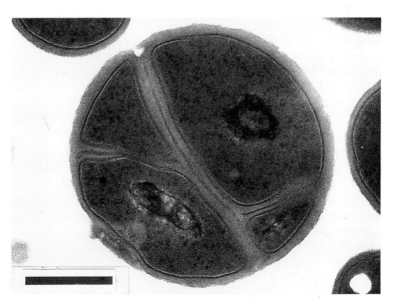

FIG. 10. Large, irregular, fused *Staph. aureus* cell(s) induced by subMIC concentrations of 2-phenoxyethanol (25 μmol/ml) in slide culture; bar = 400 nm; TEM.

These observations are consistent with, and support, the biochemical data available for 2-phenoxyethanol and its analogues which indicate membrane-damaging activities, interference with ATP generation, and a possible direct inhibitory action on DNA synthesis (Gilbert *et al.* 1980). Direct action(s) upon wall synthesis is a possibility from the microscopic findings but needs other supportive data before it can be regarded as likely.

Betane at concentrations close to its MIC (*c.* $1.3 \times 10^{-3}\%$ total solids) induced a variety of morphological changes in growing *E. coli* cultures of increasing instability as the MIC was approached. Initially, in broth, shortish filaments (up to 10 μm, larger on solid media, up to 35 μm) were formed by about 20% of the cells present, which contained nuclei along their length and had a solid appearance under phase-contrast illumination. They withstood centrifugal collection and washing, and plasmolysed in hypertonic sodium chloride solution indicating fairly healthy membrane function. Slightly higher Betane levels yielded higher levels of conversion, with more transparent filaments having a beaded appearance (Fig. 11), a variety of sphaeroplasts and club-shaped cells, similarly transparent, and there were signs of extensive cell lysis with the accumulation of cell debris in the medium. In Betane-free media only the solid-looking filaments reverted to normal bacterial rods with divisions usually starting at their poles and occasionally across their length but

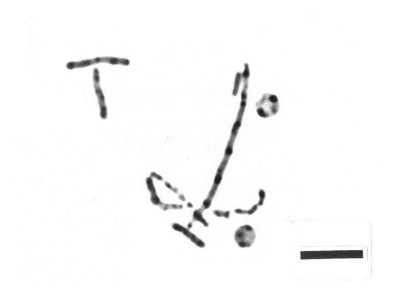

FIG. 11. Beaded, semi-transparent, filaments of *E. coli* and sphaeroplasts induced in broth by subMIC levels of Betane ($0.75 \times 10^{-3}\%$); bar = 10 μm; PC.

generally only after an extended period of further filament extension. On Betane-free media containing chloramphenicol at three times the MIC for normal cells, this further filament growth did not occur but several rounds of division were observed before more activity ceased. This suggested that sufficient previously synthesized protein remained in an active state after treatment to enable some division following biocide removal before becoming inadequate for more division. In section the solid filaments showed globular blebbing of the outer membrane, no internal septa, diffusely distributed DNA and signs of plasmolysis (Fig. 12). The semi-transparent filaments had apparently intact outer and cytoplasmic membranes, a weakly stained cytoplasm with membrane-enclosed vacuoles and densely stained amorphous granules, but there was still evidence of plasmolysis (Fig. 13). Some sphaeroplasts showed marked loss of cytoplasmic contents and the remains (probably) of internal cytoplasmic membranes (Figs 14 and 15). In many cases, however, complex multi-lamellar membranous structures were seen within cells; clearly biocide-induced 'membranes' (Fig. 16).

Bacterial suspensions treated with biocidal (killing) levels of Betane (LT 99% $\cong$ 1 min) (see footnote, p. 142) became very dark under phase-contrast illumination and had a 'warty' appearance although at markedly biocidal concentrations (LT 99% < 0.05 min) (see footnote, p. 142) no 'wartiness'

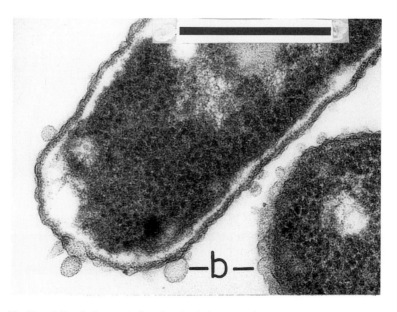

FIG. 12. Tip of *E. coli* filament induced in broth by subMIC concentration of Betane (0.7 × 10^{-3}%); b, outer membrane blebbing; bar = 400 nm; TEM.

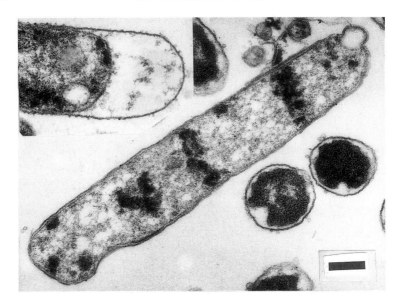

FIG. 13. Semi-transparent *E. coli* filaments similar to those in Fig. 11, (Betane 0.75 $\times$ 10^{-3}%) revealing granular cytoplasm and dense bodies; inset showing plasmolysis, intact cytoplasmic membrane and membrane-enclosed vacuole; bar = 400 nm (inset, bar = 330 nm); TEM.

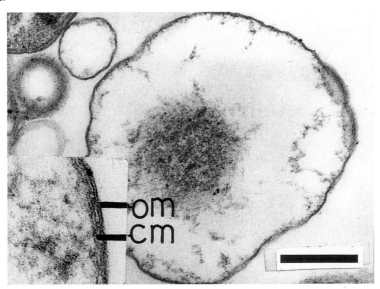

FIG. 14. *E. coli* sphaeroplast with subsequent loss of cell contents ('ghost') induced by subMIC level of Betane (0.72 $\times$ 10^{-3}%); bar = 400 nm; inset, slightly healthier sphaeroplast section with outer (om) and cytoplasmic (cm) membranes; bar = 140 nm; TEM.

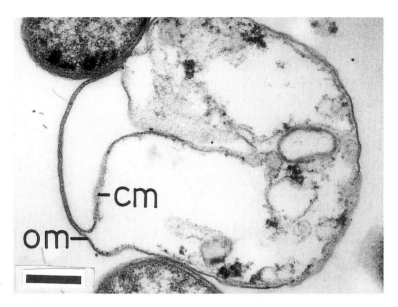

FIG. 15. *E. coli* sphaeroplast formed at subMIC Betane concentration ($0.72 \times 10^{-3}\%$) showing outer (om), cytoplasmic, and internal membranes (cm); bar = 400 nm; TEM.

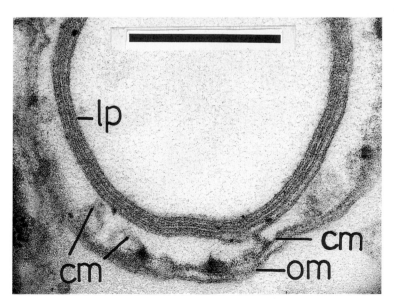

FIG. 16. *E. coli* sphaeroplast from subMIC levels of Betane ($0.72 \times 10^{-3}\%$) showing formation of an internal polyliposome-like structure (lp), cytoplasmic (cm) and outer membranes (om); bar = 400 nm; TEM.

occurred and cells became very refractile. In the BATH test they were so hydrophobic as to form a sticky precipitate with the *n*-octane hydrophobic phase. Additionally, examination of the surface of these bacteria with the fluorescent-tagged double antibody technique resulted in brightly fluorescent cells which might indicate either the uncovering of more antigenic sites in the cell wall or that biocide-induced changes to the surface had influenced the intensity of fluorescence. In section the 'warty' cells showed extensive damage to the outer membrane. Internally signs of the cytoplasmic membrane were very limited and cytoplasm was intensely stained with large irregular vacuoles (Fig. 17). Cytoplasmic material was extensively re-organized into minute lamellae (Fig. 18). The more rapidly killed cells (LT 99% < 0.5 min) however, showed far less outer membrane and cytoplasmic damage, with a densely stained cytoplasm having a mottled and speckled appearance. Nuclear material was visible but more constricted than in untreated cells. This apparent retention of cytoplasmic contents is correlated with our findings of only limited leakage of intracellular components into suspending fluids when cells are treated with Betane. The ampholytic components of Betane are highly surface-active and have been shown to solubilize lipidic material extensively. The cytoplasmic re-organization observed was not therefore totally unexpected.

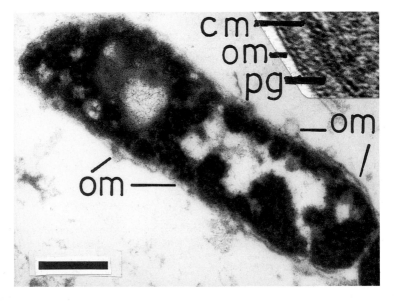

FIG. 17. *E. coli* cell treated with a killing level of Betane (0.005%) showing destruction of outer membrane (om), densely stained cytoplasm and irregular vacuole(s); bar = 400 nm; inset, outer layers of untreated cell including outer (om) and cytoplasmic (cm) membranes and collapsed peptidoglycan layer (pg); bar = 55 nm; TEM.

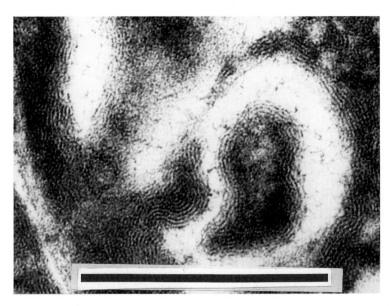

FIG. 18. Multi-lamellar changes induced in *E. coli* cytoplasm by a killing level of Betane (0.005%), bar = 400 nm; TEM.

References

ANON. 1980. *Photography Through the Microscope.* Kodak Publication No. P-2. Rochester: Eastman Kodak Company.

BULLA, L.A., JULIAN, G.ST., HESSELTINE, C.W. & BAKER, F.L. 1973. Scanning electron microscopy. In *Methods in Microbiology,* Vol. 8, ed. Norris, J.R. & Ribbons, D.W. pp. 1–33. London: Academic Press.

CARLONE, N.A., CUFFINI, A.M. & CATTANEO, O. 1982. Structural changes induced by subinhibitory concentrations of fosfomycin on *Staphylococcus aureus* and *Bacillus cereus. Microbios* 33, 119–128.

DOOLITTLE, C.H., MANDEL, H.G. & HAHN, G.A. 1973. Use of fluorouraciluracil combinations to study growth accompanied by insufficient deoxyribonucleic acid synthesis in *Bacillus cereus. Journal of Bacteriology* 113, 1311–1319.

GILBERT, P., BEVERIDGE, E.G. & CRONE, P.B. 1980. Effect of 2-phenoxyethanol upon RNA, DNA and protein biosynthesis in *Escherichia coli* NCTC 5933. *Microbios* 111, 7–17.

GLAUERT, A.M. 1974. *Fixation, Dehydration and Embedding of Biological Specimens,* Vol. 3, Part I, *Practical Methods in Electron Microscopy,* ed. Glauert, A.M. Oxford: North Holland Publishing Company.

GRANGE, J.M., FOX, A. & MORGAN, N.L. (eds) 1987. *Immunological Techniques In Microbiology.* Society for Applied Bacteriology Technical Series No. 24. Oxford: Blackwell Scientific Publications.

GRANT, D.J.W. 1968. The adaptation of *Klebsiella aerogenes* to the inhibitory action of triethylene-melamine on growth and division. *Journal of General Microbiology* 50, 23–35.

HOFFMAN, H.P., GEFTIC, S.G., GELZER, J., HEYMAN, H. & ADIAR, F.W. 1973. Ultrastructural alterations associated with the growth of resistant *Pseudomonas aeruginosa* in the presence of benzalkonium chloride. *Journal of Bacteriology* **113**, 409−416.

HOOPER, M., BHAGRIA, A., BEVERIDGE, E.G., JAGANNATHAN, R., MAHADEVEN, P.R. & YEAP, S.K. 1988. The identification of novel tyrosinase inhibitors with *in vitro* activity against *Mycobacterium leprae*. *Proceedings of the 4th European Leprosy Symposium on Leprosy Research. Health Cooperation Papers OCSI No. 7*, pp. 259−270.

HUGO, W.B. & LONGWORTH, A.R. 1965. Cytological aspects of the mode of action of chlorhexidine diacetate. *Journal of Pharmacy and Pharmacology* **17**, 28−32.

JENSEN, R. & WOOLFOLK, C.A. 1985. Formation of filaments by *Pseudomonas putida*. *Applied and Environmental Microbiology* **50**, 364−372.

KATCHMAN, B.J., SPOERL, E. & SMITH, H.E. 1955. Effects of cell division inhibition on phosphorus metabolism of *Escherichia coli*. *Science, New York* **121**, 97−98.

LEWIS, P.R. & KNIGHT, D.P. 1977. *Staining Methods for Sectioned Material*, Vol. 5, Part I, *Practical Methods in Electron Microscopy*, ed. Glauert, A.M. Oxford: North Holland Publishing Company.

LICKFELD, K.G. 1976. Transmission electron microscopy. In *Methods in Microbiology*, Vol. 9, ed. Norris, J.R. pp. 127−176. London: Academic Press.

LORIAN, V. & ATKINSON, B. 1976. Effects of subinhibitory concentrations of antibodies on cross walls of cocci. *Antimicrobial Agents and Chemotherapy* **9**, 1043−1053.

MIRELMAN, D., YASHOUV-GAN, Y. & SCHWARZ, U. 1977. Regulation of murein biosynthesis and septum formation in filamentous cells of *Escherichia coli* PAT 84. *Journal of Bacteriology* **129**, 1593−1600.

NEWTON, B.A. 1956. The properties and mode of action of the polymyxins. *Bacteriological Reviews* **20**, 14−27.

NORRIS, J.R. & SWAIN, H. 1971. Staining Bacteria. In *Methods in Microbiology*, Vol. 5A, ed. Norris, J.R. & Ribbons, D.W. pp. 105−134, London: Academic Press.

PATON, A.M. & JONES, S.M. 1971. Techniques involving optical brightening agents. In *Methods in Microbiology*, Vol. 5A, ed. Norris, J.R. & Ribbons, D.W. pp. 135−144. London: Academic Press.

QUESNEL, L.B. 1971. Microscopy and micrometry. In *Methods in Microbiology*, Vol. 5A, ed. Norris, J.R. & Ribbons, D.W. pp. 1−103. London: Academic Press.

REYNOLDS, P.E. 1985. Inhibitors of bacterial wall synthesis. In *The Scientific Basis of Antimicrobial Chemotherapy*, ed. Greenwood D. & O'Grady, F. pp. 13−40. Society for General Microbiology Symposium No. 38. Cambridge: Cambridge University Press.

RICHARDS, R.M.E. & CAVILL, R.H. 1976. Electron microscope study of effect of benzalkonium chloride and edetate sodium on cell envelope of *Pseudomonas aeruginosa*. *Journal of Pharmaceutical Sciences* **65**, 76−80.

SERRY, F.E.M., DENYER, S.P. & HUGO, W.B. 1986. Variations in *Escherichia coli* cell morphology induced by 2-chloroacetamide. *Proceedings, 14th International Congress of Microbiology (Microbe 86)*, Manchester, PG9−65.

SILVA, M.T., SOUSA, J.C.F., MACEDO, M.A.E., POLONIA, J. & PARANTE, A.M. 1976. Effects of phenethyl alcohol on *Bacillus* and *Streptococcus*. *Journal of Bacteriology* **127**, 1359−1369.

SPRAY, G.H. & LODGE, R.M. 1943. The effects of resorcinol and of *m*-cresol on the growth of *Bact. lactis-aerogenes*. *Transactions of the Faraday Society* **39**, 424−31.

TSUCHIDO, T., AHN, Y-N. & TAKANO, M. 1987. Lysis of *Bacillus subtilis* cells by glycerol and sucrose esters of fatty acids. *Applied and Environmental Microbiology* **53**, 505−508.

VAN ITERSON, W. (ed.) 1984a. *Inner Structures of Bacteria. Benchmark Papers in Microbiology Series*, Series ed. Umbreit, W.W. New York: Van Nostrand Reinhold Co.

VAN ITERSON, W. 1984b. *Inner Structures of Bacteria. Benchmark Papers in Microbiology Series*, Series ed. Umbreit, W.W. pp. 213−214. New York: Van Nostrand Reinhold Co.

WALKER, P.D., BATTY, I. & THOMPSON, R.O. 1971. The localisation of bacterial antigens by the use of the fluorescent and ferritin labelled antibody techniques. In *Methods in Microbiology*, Vol. 5A, ed. Norris, J.R. & Ribbons, D.W. pp. 219–254. London: Academic Press.

Interaction of Biocides with Model Membranes and Isolated Membrane Fragments

P. GILBERT[1], JILL BARBER[1] AND J. FORD[2]

Department of Pharmacy, University of Manchester, Oxford Road, Manchester M13 9PL, UK; and Department of Pharmacy, Liverpool Polytechnic, Byrom Street, Liverpool L3 3AF, UK

Many antimicrobial agents, used as preservatives of cosmetic and pharmaceutical products, including the biguanides, phenolic compounds, alcohols, ethers and surfactants, interact with bacteria at the level of the membrane. Such action can lead to alterations in membrane permeability, deficiencies in osmoregulatory function and inhibition of membrane-associated enzymes and transport systems. Confirmation of membrane action *in vivo* has often been gained by measuring the loss of intracellular components to suspension supernatant fractions (Denyer & Hugo, this book), and *in vitro* by the functioning of membrane-associated enzymes (Fuller, this book) and transport and respiratory components (Kroll & Patchett and Phillips-Jones & Rhodes Roberts, this book). Traditional methods of study, however, give little information concerning the molecular basis for such action.

Membrane lipids can be extracted and purified. When they are dispersed in buffer solutions the lipid molecules take up a number of configurations which in many respects resemble the natural membranes themselves. These model systems permit the study of not only the properties of the individual lipids but also of the effects upon them of the environment and antimicrobial agents. Model systems do have severe limitations, however, in that they do not accurately reflect the asymmetries of natural membranes. The models may be composed of pure, single or mixed lipids or of lipids isolated directly from the bacterial cell. They may exist as monolayers on aqueous or organic solvents, as bilayers, or vesicles or as multi-lamellar liposomes. The use of reconstituted membrane vesicles and advanced physico-chemical techniques of analysis offers the possibility of gaining detailed intermolecular and intramolecular information on biocide action.

Since other contributions to this book deal with the use of reconstituted membrane vesicles in the study of membrane function (Chopra and Phillips-Jones & Rhodes-Roberts), this chapter will concentrate upon monolayer and

Mechanisms of Action of
Chemical Biocides

bilayer studies, thermal analysis and nuclear magnetic resonance (NMR) spectroscopy as tools for the study of drug−membrane interactions. The preparation of liposomes for the latter two techniques will also be addressed. Space will not permit discussion of techniques such as electron spin resonance (ESR), or the use of fluorescent probes; for this, readers are directed to texts edited by Andrioli *et al.* (1980) and Conti *et al.* (1985).

Phospholipid Monolayer and Bilayer Studies

Monolayer troughs

Phospholipids will, spontaneously, form monomolecular films at air−water or hydrocarbon−water interfaces with their polar head groups facing the aqueous phase and the hydrocarbon chains extending either into the air or into the hydrocarbon phase such that the hydrocarbon chains lie parallel to each other and perpendicular to the interface. In simple terms such monomolecular layers may be considered as half of a unit biological membrane. It is assumed that the lipid configuration in these is similar to that in natural membranes. There are a number of limitations to the application of monolayer models. First, in natural membranes the hydrocarbon chains are not necessarily ordered and parallel. Secondly, neither integral proteins nor any function which relies upon membrane asymmetry may be modelled by a half-membrane.

Formation of a monomolecular film at an air−water interface is relatively simple. If lipid molecules in solution are injected beneath a water surface or if they are taken up in an organic solvent and added dropwise to the surface then, as these amphipathic molecules reach the surface or as the solvent evaporates, a monolayer will form (Gershfield 1974). Monomolecular layers of mixtures of lipids may be made in a similar fashion by injecting or dissolving more than one lipid at a time. Alternatively, the second or subsequent components may be injected beneath the surface of a preformed monolayer and the interactions allowed to equilibrate. This applies equally well to the addition of antibacterial agents, proteins or additional lipids.

The simplest arrangement for the study of the physical properties of monolayers is the fixed-area trough (Gershfield 1974). This consists of a tank, deep enough to allow for heat control and mixing, without disturbing the monolayer itself, and fitted with a means of monitoring surface pressure in the surface film. The latter is commonly a dipping blade arrangement connected either to a sensitive balance or tension transducer and a recorder. Surface pressure (π) is defined as the change in surface tension (ψ) of the film on addition of the amphipathic species (i.e. $\pi = \psi_0 - \psi_a$; where ψ_0 and ψ_a are the surface tensions in the absence and presence of the amphipath, respectively). Often the trough is fitted with a movable beam which can be adjusted to alter the area of the surface film. The device should be mounted in a vibration-free area and protected from dust and air currents and thoroughly cleansed with organic solvents and 70% nitric acid prior to commencing a set of measurements.

The equipment may be used to monitor either the area occupied by each molecule in the monomolecular layer or the surface pressure within the film. If a known molar concentration of lipid is applied to the surface of the trough and the solvent allowed to evaporate to form a lipid monolayer, then the formation of the layer can be followed by monitoring the surface pressure in the film via the hanging slide arrangement. In infinitely dilute monolayers the individual surface molecules can then be treated as independent particles whose behaviour obeys the ideal gas law, viewed in two dimensions. Thus, as the surface film becomes more concentrated, π increases. If the concentration of lipid is altered or the area of the film changed by means of the movable beam then surface pressure will also alter as the distance between adjacent lipid molecules in the surface film changes. Force−area diagrams may then be constructed (Fig. 1a, b). These indicate the collapse pressure at which the monolayer deforms. Compression of the film beyond the collapse pressure results in multi-layer formation. The area per molecule at the collapse pressure relates to a close pack arrangement and probably most closely models that in natural membranes. It should be borne in mind, however, that a number of other properties will affect π. These include the temperature and ionic strength of the subsolution. With many lipid materials force−area curves reveal multiple changes in the slope of the curve. These probably correspond to alterations in the orientation of the lipids as the film becomes more compressed (Fig. 1c). The behaviour of biocides which interact with membrane layers may be studied by monitoring changes in π following their addition into the subsolution of films held close to their collapse pressures or alternatively from force−area curves constructed for lipid/biocide monolayers (Kaye & Proudfoot 1971; Proudfoot & Davdani 1974, 1975; Denyer et al. 1986). When such measurements are made for a variety of lipids then insight may be gained as to the likely action in vivo.

There have been a number of studies performed where enzymes were incorporated into the monolayers and their activity assessed. This is particularly important for membrane-bound enzymes, as in the glycosyltransferase system where, for incorporation into a hydrophobic environment, it is imperative for the enzymes to assume a functional comformation (Romeo et al. 1970). In such systems, substrates and inhibitor may then be added to the subsolution and activities determined. Alternatively the orientation of such proteins in the membrane and therefore their accessibility to attack can be assessed by proteolytic cleavage within the bilayer. In these instances parts of the protein deep within the monolayer are protected (Bangham & Dawson 1960).

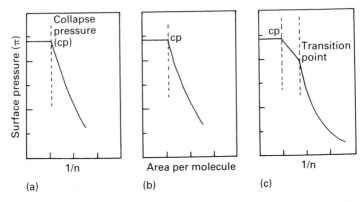

FIG. 1. Force—area curves for compressed lipid monomolecular films. *n*, number of lipid molecules applied to a fixed surface area; π, surface pressure. (a and b) show a collapse point corresponding to the formation of a close packed monolayer whilst (c) shows a complex situation where re-orientation of the molecules in the surface film occurs after collapse.

'Black' lipid bilayers

Some of the limitations of monolayer studies can be overcome by creating lipid bilayers. These allow conductivity measurements to be made across the membranes and the transport and catalytic properties of integral proteins to be assessed. Whilst a brief account of bilayer studies will be given here, for a detailed account readers are directed to the review by Fettiplace *et al.* (1975).

Bilayers are produced by drawing solutions of lipid(s)/protein, in appropriate organic solvents, over a small hole within a Teflon or polytetrafluoroethylene (PTFE) septum. The septum separates two aqueous phases. As the organic solvent diffuses into the aqueous phase and the lipid film drains and thins, then the lipids assume a bilayer arrangement with their polar head groups orientated outwards towards the aqueous compartments and the hydrocarbon chains directed inwards towards each other. As the film thins further, then London van der Waals forces cause the hydrocarbon chains to interchelate to a limited extent. At this point the membrane closely models a natural membrane. Since the thickness of the membrane at this point causes incident light to be totally internally refracted, then the bilayer appears dark when viewed and is thereby termed a 'black' lipid membrane. Indeed its establishment is monitored by an arrangement of illuminating light beams and an inspection microscope. Electrodes placed either side of the membrane permit specific capacitance measurements to be made. Other experimental arrangements permit solute fluxes across the bilayer to be assessed and fluorescence spectroscopy undertaken. Interactive biocides may be incorporated into the aqueous compartments of the apparatus and their effects monitored. Such studies have been particularly informative with respect to the ionophore antibiotics but have seldom been employed for the study of chemical antimicrobial agents.

Thermal Analysis

Thermal analysis has wide application to the study of aqueous dispersions of membranes and lipids and has become a standard technique for studying the thermally induced transitions of biological membranes and bilayers from ordered crystalline states at low temperature, when they are said to be in the gel state, to disordered liquid—crystalline states at higher temperatures. Older thermal analysis equipment for differential thermal analysis (DTA) and differential scanning calorimetry (DSC) suffer from poor sensitivity relating to their small sample sizes ($<100\,\mu l$) and relatively fast scanning rates which cause low-energy transitions to be lost. Modern instruments, however, are capable of greater accuracy and sensitivity (Wendlandt 1986). High-sensitivity calorimeters used with a large cell volume ($>1\,ml$) and lipid concentrations of $0.02-1.0\%$ (w/v) have been recommended for the study of biomembranes (Privalov et al. 1975; Mabrey & Sturtevant 1978; Blume 1988). Each instrument allows heating (or cooling) of the sample in comparison with an inert reference (i.e the aqueous vehicle). Upon heating or cooling through a transition temperature, samples may undergo processes which will either emit or absorb heat, (i.e. latent heats of fusion etc.). High-sensitivity calorimeters (Privalov et al. 1975) detect either excess heat or the corresponding power used to keep the sample and reference at identical temperatures. Two types of commercial DSC instrument exist, heat-flux DSC where the instrument measures the temperature difference between the sample and reference, and converts it to heat flow, and power-compensation DSC where two individual heaters are used to heat the sample and reference and a control system regulates their temperature difference. In both of these instruments the area under the curve of the transition, endotherm or exotherm, relates to the enthalpy of the reaction. In DTA the temperature difference between the sample and reference is measured as each is subjected to a controlled heating or cooling programme. It is more difficult to relate the area of the transition to its enthalpy than is the case with DSC.

A typical endotherm is given in Fig.2. In addition to the area under the curve and hence associated heats of transition, other parameters which may be used to characterize the process are the temperature at the peak (T_m), the onset temperature of the transition (T_o) and even the extrapolated onset temperature (T_e) calculated by the intercept of an extended baseline to the slope of the leading edge of the endotherm. Additionally $\triangle T_{1/2}$ may be determined which is the width of the transition at half peak height. Figure 2 shows no heat capacity change between the pretransition and post-transition baseline. If a heat capacity change occurs great care must be taken in

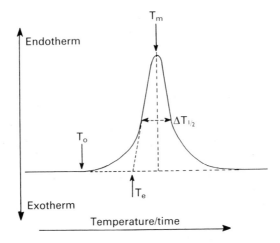

F$_{IG}$. 2. Typical lipid endotherm illustrating measurable parameters. T_m, peak temperature; T_e, extrapolated temperature; T_o, onset temperature; $\triangle T^{1/2}$, half-peak height width, where T = temperature.

determining the true baseline: corrections to be made have been published (Heuvel & Lind 1970).

One advantage of high-sensitivity calorimetry or DSC over DTA is that endotherms may be used to determine cooperativity of a transition. The cooperative unit is defined (Mabrey & Sturtevant 1978) as that quantity of a substance which, if the sample were composed of independent units of that size undergoing a two-state transition, would give the transition curve of the observed shape. The cooperative units are affected by the presence of other chemicals such as proteins or other lipids, ionic strength of solution and the presence of antimicrobial agents. It is these changes that make thermal analysis such a useful tool in determining the sites of action of antimicrobial substances.

Whilst DSC provides a rapid technique which can be used to characterize a system without the modification or attachment of spectroscopic probes and gives quantitative information without disturbing the transitions of interest, it is unable to survey the behaviour of the different parts of the phospholipid molecules, information which is given by ESR and spin labelling.

Pure lipid studies

In general, thermal analysis of phospholipids and membranes will produce an endothermic transition whose T_m varies according to the hydrocarbon chain attached to the phosphate moiety, the head group and the presence of other solutes. Generally an increase in chain length increases the value of T_m whereas an increase in double bonds will decrease the T_m. The gel−liquid crystalline transition that this endotherm represents is a partial melting, representing a trans to gauche rotational isomerization arising from the hydrocarbon chains and involving lateral expansion and a decrease in bilayer thickness with additional changes in van der Waals interaction between the chains and polar interactions at the lipid bilayer−water interface. The pretransition is a change in the polar head groups or lamellar structure and is broader and smaller than the chain melting endotherm. The pretransition is not found for all phospholipids but is present in phosphatidylcholine bilayers.

When phospholipids are dispersed in aqueous solutions and shaken vigorously they arrange themselves in suspension as lipid bilayers or liposomes. Pure lipids when dispersed in water form multi-lamellar liposomes which consist of several concentric circles. On thermal analysis of these phospholipid bilayers, especially phosphatidylcholines, two transitions are apparent (Fig. 3). The first, the pretransition, is due to a rotation of the polar head portion of the lipid molecules and is followed by the major transition which is a gel−liquid crystal transformation (Hinz & Sturtevant 1972). Impurities broaden the transition which in the highest purity lipids is isothermal. The temperature difference between the pretransition and gel−liquid crystalline transition of

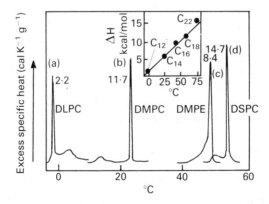

Fig. 3. High-sensitivity DSC traces showing the phase transition of: (a) dilauroylphosphatidylcholine (DLPC); (b) dimyristoylphosphatidylcholine (DMPC); (c) dimyristoylphosphatidylethanolamine (DMPE); and (d) disteroylphosphatidylcholine (DSPC). Note that two transitions are apparent. The transition occurring at the lower temperature is a pretransition and corresponds to rotation of the polar head portion of the molecule prior to the major transition. Inset: enthalpies for the main transitions of phosphatidylcholines with acyl groups containing 12, 14, 16, 18 and 22 carbon atoms plotted against transition temperature. (Reproduced with permission from Mabrey & Sturtevant 1978.)

homologues of the same head group decreases with increasing chain length of the attached fatty acid.

Artificial membranes

Artificial membranes containing more than one component have thermal properties different to the individual ingredients, as may be seen from their phase diagrams. When two phospholipids containing the same head group differ by two carbon atoms in their fatty acids nearly ideal mixing will take place. A difference of four carbon atoms shows deviations from ideality and once the chain length differs by six or more carbons, non-ideality occurs and monotectics may be formed that are indicative of phase separation. It is assumed that phospholipids are fully hydrated and consequently phase diagrams are often regarded as binary systems. Where the ingredients behave ideally the resultant system will be a continuous series of solid solutions. Deviations from ideality produce monotectics, eutectics, and even peritectics and complex formation, all with concomitant broadening of the transition range.

Incorporation of fatty acids (Oritz & Gomez-Fernandez 1987) and/or proteins (Papahadjopoulos *et al.* 1975) into the bilayers modifies the transition and may vastly alter the properties of the proteins. Interactions between proteins and lipid layers commonly result in large depressions in the phase transition temperatures and increases in vesicle permeability, all of which may be detected by DSC (Papahadjopoulos *et al.* 1975)

Drug interaction studies

Physiological adjustment of bilayer fluidity is important, especially when the membrane transition exists at or just below the growth temperature. Bacteria modify their transition temperature by the selective inclusion of different fatty acids. Crystalline arrays in lipids exclude proteins and may lead to permeability disordering and changes in osmotic balance. For *Escherichia coli* the shift in fatty acid spectrum at lower growth temperatures is essential to maintain a functional fluid state (Melchior & Steim 1977). As membranes pass through the transition from high to low temperatures they become more crystalline. This increased order gives rise to aberrant behaviour inducing changes in enzyme kinetics, cell leakage, cessation of cell division and even cell lysis. Many antimicrobial agents will interact with the membrane to bring about such perturbations. Although transitions in whole bacteria are documented, they are too complicated to use in mechanistic studies and consequently artificial membranes containing various phospholipids are used. Since aqueous dispersions of extracted lipids have transitions at the same temperatures as the membranes from which they were extracted (Reinert & Steim 1970; McElhaney

1974), *in vitro* DSC studies utilizing vesicular preparations of isolated lipids or pure lipids yield much information concerning the nature of biocide–membrane interactions. Thus, Polymixin B decreased the endothermic transition of dipalmitoylphosphtidylcholine (DPPC) at 42°C and removed it at 1:1 and 2:1 lipid–drug ratios (Pache *et al.* 1972). ESR, NMR and optical rotary dispersion techniques showed that electrostatic interactions had taken place between the aminogroups of the antibiotic and the phosphate groups of the DPPC, such that the tails of the polymixin penetrated, through electrostatic interactions, into the lipid layer. Although bacterial membranes do not contain DPPC, other negatively charged phospholipids are present and the interactions are probably similar.

The pretransition of DPPC is abolished by gramicidin A even at a 1:200 drug:lipid molar ratio (Chapman *et al.* 1974). At higher concentrations of gramicidin A the peak maximum shifts to lower temperatures and the energy of the transition is lowered. This suggests that packing of the DPPC polar groups is affected. The loss of energy indicates that the gramicidin molecules interdigitate with the lipid fatty acid chains and prevent chain crystallization from occurring. In this instance, whilst the bulk of the lipids below the transition temperature would remain rigid, those immediately adjacent to the gramicidin would remain fluid (Chapman *et al.* 1974).

Ikeda *et al.* (1984) compared the activity of polyhexamethylene biguanide hydrochloride (PHMB) with its monomer diaminohexylbiguanide hydrochloride (DAHB). The possible sites of activity of PHMB are membrane-bound proteins and phospholipids. The neutral lipid phosphatidylethanolamine (PE) constitutes 80% of total lipids in *E. coli* and the acidic phospholipid, diphosphatidyl glycerol (DPG) and its dimer, cardiolipin are present to 10%. PHMB and DAHB were added to liposomes of DPPC, dipalmityldiphosphatidylethanolamine (DPPE), PE or phosphatidylglycerol (PG). The DPPC dispersion gave a sharp endotherm with T_m at 44°C and the presence of 20% PHMB or DAHB did not significantly change T_m or peak shape. DPPE and egg PE dispersions gave endotherms with T_m values at 56° and 16°C, respectively, which were reduced by 1–2°C in the presence of PHMB or DAHB. Egg PG dispersions gave an endotherm at $T_m = -5$°C, with the high PG acyl chain length heterogenicity making it a broad phase transition. Addition of 20% PHMB in this instance depressed T_m to -15°C and caused precipitation whilst addition of DAHB caused depression to -15°C but no precipitation. Mixtures of DPPC and egg PG gave endotherms with an intermediate peak temperature to the pure lipids (e.g. 50:50 DPPC:egg PG gave a peak at $T_m = 27$°C). Addition of PHMB raised this T_m from 27° to 32°C and produced a second endotherm with T_m at -15.5°C (Fig. 4). This corresponded to the PHMB:PG dispersion T_m and suggested, therefore, that PHMB had produced an isothermal phase separation of the mixture into PHMB–PG- and DPPC-

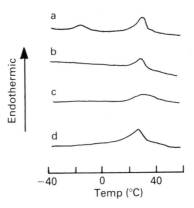

F<small>IG.</small> 4 Effect of various cations on a mixed lipid membrane of dipalmitoylphosphatidylcholine (DPPC) and egg phosphatidylglycerol (PG) (50:50 w/w). (a) 2 mg polyhexamethylenebiguanide; (b) 2 mg diaminohexylbiguanide; (c) 2 mg MgCl$_2$.6H$_2$O; (d) none. 5 mg DPPC and 5 mg egg PG were dispersed in 30 µl of Tris-HCl buffer/ethyleneglycol mixture (1:1w/v) at pH 7.4. (Reproduced with permission from Ikeda *et al.* 1984.)

enriched domains. Addition of DAHB caused only a shift in the T_m to a slightly lower temperature and no new peaks were formed. It would appear therefore that PHMB has a large effect on negatively charged bilayers as compared with neutral lipid bilayers and will interact with negatively charged species in mixed bilayers of neutral and acid phospholipids.

Nuclear Magnetic Resonance Spectroscopy

Nuclear magnetic resonance (NMR) was discovered by physicists in the 1940s and relatively quickly became established as a tool used by chemists in the structural determination of small organic molecules. Although the potential of NMR in biology was realized very quickly, the problems inherent in the technique continue to frustrate and to challenge in equal measure. Nowhere is this more true than in its applications to membrane research.

NMR is one of the few techniques available at present which allow both structural and dynamic information to be obtained, often at atomic resolution. The NMR phenomenon is associated with nuclei which have unpaired protons and/or neutrons and therefore have the property known as nuclear spin. Nuclei with one unpaired proton or neutron have a spin number (I) of ½, those with two unpaired nucleons have $I=1$ and so on. Important nuclei with $I=½$ include ^{1}H, ^{13}C, ^{15}N, ^{17}O, ^{19}F and ^{31}P. Nuclei with $I=1$ include ^{2}H and ^{14}N.

When an external magnetic field (H_0) is applied to a nucleus with spin, the interaction causes the nucleus to precess around the applied magnetic field. If a second, much weaker, magnetic field from a radio frequency source is applied in a plane perpendicular to H_0, the nucleus will attempt to precess about this direction also. Only when the radio frequency is equal to the precessional frequency is energy transferred to the nucleus and resonance occurs. In quantum mechanical terms the radio frequency induces transitions between the allowed energy states of the nucleus. For $I=\frac{1}{2}$, the two spin states $+\frac{1}{2}$ and $-\frac{1}{2}$ are allowed, for $I=1$, the three states -1, 0 and $+1$ are allowed. The spectrometer detects the transition of a nucleus between these states.

An NMR signal is characterized by three parameters, chemical shift, spin−spin coupling and relaxation processes. Chemical shift relates to the precessional frequency of the nucleus which is determined by the identity of the nucleus and by the magnetic field it experiences. This in turn depends upon the applied magnetic field and the local environment of the nucleus. Chemical shift (δ) is generally normalized to the frequency of the spectrometer used and expressed in parts per million, and gives information about the chemical environment of the nucleus. The relaxation parameters of interest are the spin−lattice relaxation time T_1, the time taken for the excited nucleus to lose energy to its surroundings and the spin−spin relaxation time T_2, the time taken for the energy to be redistributed among the excited nuclei. This redistribution limits the lifetime of the excited state and gives rise to line broadening. Short T_2 values, and hence broad lines in the spectrum, constitute the greatest difficulty in using NMR directly upon biological systems. Spin−spin coupling, though of great value to chemists, is therefore not generally of interest in membrane work since its detection requires lines that are narrow. Short T_2 values are a feature of large molecules and of restricted rotation about bonds in these molecules or in small molecules bound to them. A typical spectrum of a membrane is an uninteresting single broad peak. Despite this and despite the inherent insensitivity of the technique, many ingenious methods have been developed for studying membranes by NMR.

Drug interactions

NMR studies on the interactions of antimicrobial agents on membranes have generally been carried out using model membranes of varying complexity. For example, a sonicated aqueous dispersion of phosphatidylinositol 4,5-biphosphate (PIP$_2$) has been employed as a model to study the action of neomycin B. The neomycins are a group of aminoglycoside antibiotics which are believed to interact with membrane-bound PIP$_2$. This interaction has been studied by ^{31}P, ^{1}H and ^{13}C NMR spectroscopy and, because of the relative simplicity of the system, highly resolved spectra were obtained and interpreted in some detail (Hayashi *et al.* 1980; Redi & Gajjar 1987). It is imperative in such studies, in order that T_2 may be extended as much as possible and narrow line spectra obtained, to produce a highly dispersed lipid vesicle system for study. Thus Broxton *et al.* (1984) obtained highly resolved spectra for a number of vesicle preparations of a variety of phospholipids, including acidic phosphatidylglycerol and neutral phosphatidylethanolamine. In the presence of polyhexamethylene biguanides (PHMB), a biocide which interacts specifically with acidic phospholipids to produce domains (Ikeda *et al.* 1984), spectra of the neutral lipids and biocide were unaffected and essentially superimpositions of the individual spectra whilst those for acidic lipid−PHMB combinations showed only the biocide lines (Fig. 5). In conjunction with data from thermal analysis studies this was indicative of PHMB converting the acidic lipid vesicles to the planar lamellar state for which spectral lines would not be apparent.

A relatively simple but very effective technique has been developed for detecting disruption of lipid vesicles (Fernandez *et al.* 1973). When a paramagnetic cation such as praseodymium is added to an aqueous lecithin dispersion, distinct signals due to the $-N^+Me_3$ groups inside and outside the vesicles appear in the ^1H NMR spectrum. When the vesicles are disrupted, for example by ionophores such as alamethacin or by surfactants, the two signals collapse to one as the paramagnetic ion enters the vesicles. This technique has also been used to determine the effect of anaesthetics on ion transport (Viero & Hunt 1985) and has been reviewed recently (Springer *et al.* 1985).

Chemical shift and T_1 information from ^{13}C spectra of antibiotics in artificial membranes has been obtained. Neutral ion carriers were shown to retain a high degree of mobility in the membrane phase (Büchi *et al.* 1976). Changes in the T_1 were also observed in the ^1H NMR spectra of chloroplast thylakoid membranes on treatment with protein synthesis inhibitors (Strzalka *et al.* 1984).

The most widely used NMR technique in the study of membranes and drug−membrane interactions is, however, solid-state ^2H NMR. Deuterium has a spin number of 1 and in ordered systems the transitions $-1 \Leftarrow\Rightarrow 0$ and $0 \Leftarrow\Rightarrow +1$ are observed separately, giving rise to two broad lines, the separation and width of which give information about the order in the system. Natural abundance deuterium is very low and so lipids are specifically labelled with deuterium thus removing problems of assignment. The specific labelling technique allows information from the head groups of phospholipids and each position of the lipid chains to be obtained in separate experiments. The technique has been reviewed extensively (Seelig & Macdonald 1987; Watts 1987; Oldfield 1988). As well as being used to study membrane structure this technique has been used in model membrane systems (bilayers) to study the

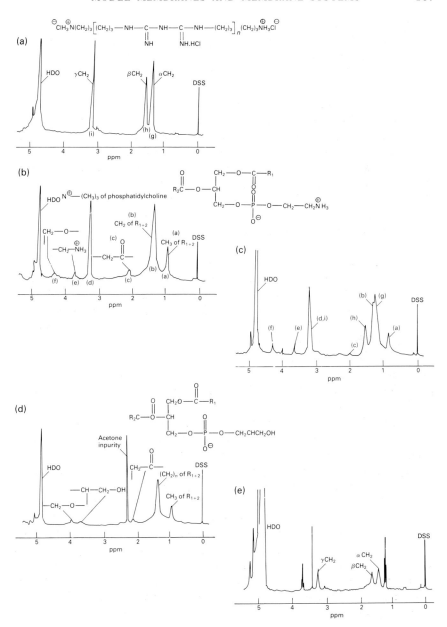

FIG. 5. ^{1}H NMR spectra of (a) polyhexamethylene-biguanide (PHMB); (b) vesicles of phosphatidylethanolamine (PE); (c) mixture of PE and PHMB; (d) vesicles of phosphatidylglycerol (PG); and (e) mixtures of PG and PHMB. (Reproduced with permission from Broxton et al. 1984.)

action of antimicrobial agents. For example polymyxin B has been shown to induce separation of phosphatidylglycerol from phosphatidylcholine lipids (Sixl & Watts 1985). The effect of amphotericin B on cholesterol-containing model membranes has also been studied (Dufourc *et al.* 1984a, b) and T_2 and T_1 measurements suggest that the drug has an overall ordering effect on the membrane.

Many of these studies have been complemented by ^{31}P NMR, but, very unusually in NMR work, the $I=\frac{1}{2}$ nucleus yields less information than the $I=1$ nucleus. An interesting variant on the ^{2}H method is to use ^{14}N NMR, again recording the two signals due to $-1 \Leftarrow\Rightarrow 0$ and $0 \Leftarrow\Rightarrow +1$ transitions (Rothgeb & Oldfield 1981).

Membranes are not easy to study by NMR. None the less, considerable progress has been made, partly in understanding the detailed changes in structure induced by antimicrobial agents, but mainly in understanding gross spectral changes. This is in complete contrast to the more characteristic uses of NMR.

References

ANDRIOLI, T.E., HOFFMAN, J.F. & FANESTIL, D.D. 1980. *Membrane Physiology*. London: Plenum Press.

BANGHAM, A.D. & DAWSON, R. 1960. The physico-chemical requirements for the action of *Penicillium notatum* phospholipase B on unimolecular films of lecithin. *Biochemical Journal* 75, 133−157.

BLUME, A. 1988. Applications of calorimetry to lipid model membranes. In *Physical Properties of Biological Membranes and their Functional Implications*, ed. Hidalgo, C. pp. 71−121. New York: Plenum Press.

BROXTON, P., WOODCOCK, P.M., HEATLEY, F. & GILBERT, P. 1984. Interaction of some polyhexamethylene biguanides and membrane phospholipids in *Escherichia coli*. *Journal of Applied Bacteriology* 57, 115−124.

BUCHI, R., PRETSCH, F. & SIMON, W. 1976. Carbon-13 nuclear magnetic resonance spectroscopic studies on ion-selective liquid membranes. *Helv. Chim. Acta* 59, 2327−2334.

CHAPMAN, D., URBINA, J. & KEOUGH, K.M. 1974. Biomembrane phase transitions: Studies of lipid water systems using differential scanning calorimetry. *Journal of Biological Chemistry* 249, 2512−2521.

CONTI, F., BLUMBERG, W.F., DE GIER, J. & POCCHIARI, F. 1985. *Physical Methods on Biological Membranes and their Model Systems*. NATO ASI Series. London: Plenum Press.

DENYER, S.P., HUGO, W.B. & HARDING, V.D. 1986. The biochemical basis of synergy between the antibacterial agents chlorocresol and 2-phenylethanol. *International Journal of Pharmaceutics* 29, 29−36.

DUFOURC, E.J., SMITH, I.C.P. & JARRELL, H.C. 1984a. Amphotericin and model membranes. The effects of amphotericin B on cholesterol-containing systems as viewed by deuterium NMR. *Biochimica et Biophysica Acta* 776, 317−329.

DUFOURC, E.J., SMITH, I.C.P. & JARRELL, H.C. 1984b. Interaction of amphotericin B with lipids as viewed by deuterium NMR. *Biochimica et Biophysica Acta* 778, 435−452.

FERNANDEZ, M.S., CELIS, H. & MONTAL, M. 1973. Proton magnetic resonance detection of ionophor-mediated transport of praseodymium ions across phospholipid membranes. *Biochimica et Biophysics Acta* **323**, 600−605.

FETTIPLACE, B., GORDON, L.G.M., HLADKY, S.B., REQUENA, J., ZINGSHEIM, H.P. & HAYDON, D.A. 1975. Techniques in the formation and examination of "Black" lipid bilayer membranes. *Methods in Membrane Biology* **4**, 1−75.

GERSHFIELD, N. 1974. Thermodynamics and experimental methods for equilibrium studies with lipid monolayers. *Methods in Membrane Biology* **1**, 69−104.

HAYASHI, F., INOUE, H., AMAKAWA, T. & YOSHIOKA, T. 1980. ^{31}P NMR study of neomycin toxicity. *Proceedings of the Japanese Academy Series B, Physical Biological Sciences* **56**, 597−601.

HEUVEL, H.M. & LIND, K.C.J.B. 1970. Computerized analysis and correction of differential scanning calorimetric data for effects due to thermal lag and heat capacity changes. *Analytical Chemistry* **42**, 1044−1048.

HINTON, J.F., TURNER, G.L. & MILLER, F.S. 1981. A thallium-205 NMR investigation of the thallium (I)-gramicidin complex. *Journal of Magnetic Resonance* **45**, 42−47.

HINTON, J.F., TURNER, G.L., YOUNG, G. & METZ, K.R. 1982. Thallium-205 NMR studies of the thallium (I) ion complexation by gramicidin in non-aqueous and micelle solutions. *Pure and Applied Chemistry* **54**, 2359−2368.

HINZ, H-J. & STURTEVANT, J.M. 1972. Calorimetric study of dilute aqueous suspensions of bilayers formed from synthetic L-α-lecithins. *Journal of Biological Chemistry* **247**, 6071−6075.

IKEDA, T., LEDWITH, A., BAMFORD, C.H. & HANN, R.A. 1984. Interaction of a polymeric biguanide biocide with phospholipid membranes. *Biochimica et Biophysica Acta* **769**, 57−66.

KAYE, R.C. & PROUDFOOT, S.G. 1971. Interactions between phosphatidylethanolamine monolayers and phenols in relation to antibacterial activity. *Journal of Pharmacy and Pharmacology* **23**, 223s.

McELHANEY, R.N. 1974. The effect of alterations in the physical state of the membrane lipids on the ability of *Acholeplasma laidlawii* B to grow at various temperatures. *Journal of Molecular Biology* **84**, 145−157.

MABREY, S. & STURTEVANT, J.M. 1978. High-sensitivity differential scanning calorimetry in the study of biomembranes and related model systems. *Methods in Membrane Biology* **9**, 237−274.

MELCHIOR, D.L. & STEIN, J.M. 1977. Control of fatty acid composition of *Acholeplasma laidlawii* membranes. *Biochimica et Biophysica Acta* **466**, 148−159.

OLDFIELD, E. 1988. Spectroscopic studies of lipids and biological membranes. *Biochemical Society Transactions* **16**, 1−10.

ORITZ, A. & GOMEZ-FERNANDEZ, J.C. 1987. A differential scanning calorimetric study of the interaction of free fatty acids with phospholipid membranes. *Chemistry and Physics of Lipids* **45**, 75−91.

PACHE, W., CHAPMAN, D. & HILLABY, R. 1972. Interaction of antibiotics with membranes; Polymyxin B and Gramicidin S. *Biochimica et Biophysica Acta* **255**, 358−364.

PAPAHADJOPOULOS, D., MOSCARELLO, M., EYLAR, E.H. & ISAC, T. 1975. Effects of proteins on thermotropic phase transitions of phospholipid membranes. *Biochimica et Biophysica Acta* **401**, 317−335.

PRIVALOV, P.I., PLOTNIKOV, V.V. & FILIMONOV, V.V. 1975. Precision scanning microcalorimeter for the study of lipids. *Journal of Chemical Thermodynamics* **7**, 41−47.

PROUDFOOT, S.G. & DAVDANI, B.H. 1974. Interactions of 4-chlorophenol and phenol with phosphatidylethanolamine monolayers in relation to antibacterial action. *Journal of Pharmacy and Pharmacology* **26**, 121P.

PROUDFOOT, S.G. & DAVDANI, B.H. 1975. Interactions of chlorinated phenols with bacterial phosphatidylethanolamine monolayers in relation to antibacterial action. *Journal of Pharmacy and Pharmacology* **27**, 23P.

REDI, D.G. & GAJJAR, K. 1987. A proton and carbon-13 nuclear magnetic resonance study of neomycin B and its interactions with phosphatidylinositol 4,5-biphosphate. *Journal of Biological Chemistry* **262**, 7967–7972.

REINERT, J.C. & STEIM, J.M. 1970. Calorimetric detection of a membrane–lipid phase transition in living cells. *Science, New York* **168**, 1580–1582.

ROMEO, D., GIRARD, A. & ROTHFIELD, L. 1970. Reconstitution of a functional membrane enzyme system in a monomolecular film. *Journal of Molecular Biology* **53**, 475–87.

ROTHGER, T.M. & OLDFIELD, E. 1981. Nitrogen-14 nuclear resonance spectroscopy as a probe of lipid bilayer headgroup structure. *Journal of Biological Chemistry* **256**, 6004–6009.

SEELIG, J. & MACDONALD, P.M. 1987. Phospholipids and proteins in biological membranes. Deuterium NMR as a method to study structure, dynamics and interactions. *Acc. Chem. Res* **20**, 221–228.

SIXL, F. & WATTS, A. 1985. Deuterium and phosphorus nuclear magnetic resonance studies on the binding of polymyxin B to lipid bilayer–water interfaces. *Biochemistry* **24**, 7906–7910.

SPRINGER, C.S., PIKE, M.M., BALSCHJ, J.A., CHU, S.C., FRAZIER, J.C., INGWALL, J.S. & SMITH, T.S. 1985. Use of shift reagents for nuclear magnetic resonance studies of the kinetics of ion transfer in cells and perfused hearts. *Circulation Supplement* **72**, IV89–IV93.

STRZALKA, K., HARANCZYK, H., PAJAK, M. & BLICHARSKI, J.S. 1984. Formation of thylakoid membranes in greening leaves and their modification by protein synthesis inhibitors. 3. Characterisations of the membrane dynamics by proton spin-lattice relaxation studies. *Acta Physica Polonica A* **A66**, 237–244.

VIERO, J.A. & HUNT, G.R.A. 1985. The modulation of ion-channels by the inhalation of general anaesthetics. A proton NMR investigation using unilamellar phospholipid membranes. *Chemical–Biological Interactions* **54**, 337–348.

WATTS, A. 1987. Nuclear magnetic resonance methods to characterise lipid–protein interactions of membrane systems. *Journal of Bioenergetics and Biomembranes* **19**, 625–653.

WENDLANT, W.W. 1986. *Thermal Analysis*. Chemical Analysis Series. Chichester: John Wiley & Sons.

Biocide-Induced Damage to the Bacterial Cytoplasmic Membrane

S.P. DENYER[1] AND W.B. HUGO[2]

[1]Department of Pharmaceutical Sciences, University of Nottingham,
University Park, Nottingham NG7 2RD, UK; and [2]618 Wollaton Road,
Nottingham NG8 2AA, UK

Probably the earliest recognition of the potential sensitivity of bacterial cyto-plasmic membranes to antibacterial agents came from Germany when Kuhn & Bielig (1940) suggested that the quaternary ammonium detergents (QACs) might act on the bacterial membrane in a manner similar to the haemolytic effect of surface active agents on the erythrocyte (Schulman & Rideal 1937). This was to be proved by Hotchkiss (1944) when he was able to detect the leakage of nitrogen- and phosphorus-containing compounds from *Staphylo-coccus aureus* on treatment with a range of agents. Gale & Taylor (1947) confirmed these results when they observed the release of amino acids from *Staph. aureus* and *Streptocococcus faecalis* in the presence of cetytrimethyl-ammonium bromide (CTAB) and phenol. Following this work, Salton carried out an in-depth study of the mode of action of CTAB in work published in the early 1950s. He introduced the technique of growing cells in a medium containing a salt of ^{32}P-labelled phosphate and measured the amount of label released on CTAB treatment (Salton 1950) (later to be extended to the use of ^{14}C and ^{42}K labels by Judis (1962) and Silver & Wendt (1967), respectively). In 1951, Salton (1951) demonstrated the leakage of a wider range of intra-cellular substances following CTAB action. Thus the bacterial membrane became firmly established as a potentially sensitive, and often readily accessible, target for many antibacterial agents and the methods of these earlier workers were to become established as one of the standard probes for investigating biocide mechanism of action.

Recent advances in membrane biochemistry have emphasized the unique osmoregulatory and metabolic significance of this organelle and have under-lined its potential importance as a site for antibacterial action. An interaction at this level may thus lead to specific and non-specific permeability changes, leakage of intracellular material, osmotic lysis and the inhibition of

Mechanisms of Action of
Chemical Biocides

membrane-associated metabolic activity. In this chapter, we will consider the methods by which leakage, permeability changes and lysis may be followed. Other chapters in this book (Kroll & Patchett and Phillips-Jones & Rhodes-Roberts) will deal with membrane-associated metabolic effects.

Routine Preparation of Cells for Experimentation

Most frequently, studies of biocide mechanism of action employ a representative Gram-positive and Gram-negative bacterium, usually *Staph. aureus* and *Escherichia coli*, respectively. These are readily cultured overnight at 35−37°C to high cell numbers on the surface of Nutrient Agar (Oxoid Ltd, Basingstoke, UK) and may then be rinsed off and harvested by centrifugation (5000 *g* for 10 min), washed twice and finally resuspended to an appropriate cell density in the buffer or medium to be employed in the experiment. In general, it is good practice to harvest organisms immediately before experimentation and at the temperature to be employed during the work: in this way excessive loss of intracellular material prior to experimentation may be largely avoided. The experiment is usually initiated in one of two ways, either by the addition of bacterial suspension to the biocide-containing reaction mixture, or by introducing a small volume of concentrated biocide solution to a pre-equilibrated bacterial suspension. In either case, volumes involved must be arranged to ensure that the desired final suspension densities and biocide concentrations are achieved. Adequate mixing following addition is essential.

Alternative micro-organisms and conditions of growth may be employed. It would be usual, however, to retain a washing stage in order to remove possible interference from the carry-over of growth medium.

Experimental Methods

In this summary of methods, we will concentrate on analytical techniques that can be readily performed within the laboratory. To improve the accuracy of such assay methods high numbers of washed bacteria (*c.* 10^9/ml) are generally employed in a suitable buffer system. Controls are an integral part of all experiments. In these studies, suitable controls will include measures of cell behaviour in the absence of biocide, and an assessment of the influence of the biocide, in cell-free systems, on the assay methods employed.

Leakage of intracellular material

The first sign of an increase in membrane permeability is usually provided by the leakage of potassium ions (Lambert & Hammond 1973); other metabolic pool materials that may be released include nucleotides and their component structures (purines, pyrimidines, pentoses and inorganic phosphate) and amino acids. These materials are usually of low molecular weight although the release of proteins, cytochrome C_3 (Postgate 1956) and ribosomes have been reported (Jackson & De Moss 1965).

The rapid leakage of intracellular material has now been observed in the presence of a wide range of antibacterial (biocidal) agents (Table 1), indicating the general utility of the methods outlined below in mode of action studies.

In all circumstances, biocide-induced leakage is assessed by detecting the appearance of intracellular material in the extracellular environment. Frequently, this requires the rapid separation of bacteria from the biocide to ensure suitable conditions for assay and to remove the organism from the leakage-inducing agent. This rapid separation is most satisfactorily achieved by filtration through a 0.2-μm or 0.45-μm pore size membrane filter, although

TABLE 1. *Some examples of biocides causing leakage in bacterial cells*

Substance	Author(s)	Date(s)
Quaternary ammonium compounds (QAC)	Hotchkiss	1944
Phenol, CTAB	Gale & Taylor	1947
CTAB	Salton	1950, 1951
Hexylresorcinol	Beckett et al.	1958, 1959
Sodium dodecyl sulphate	Gilby & Few	1960
Phenols	Judis	1962
Ethanol	Salton	1963
Chlorhexidine	Hugo & Longworth	1964
	Daltrey & Hugo	1974
Tetrachlorosalicylanilide	Woodroffe & Wilkinson	1966
	Hamilton	1968
2-phenylethanol	Silver & Wendt	1967
	Harding et al.	1984
	Denyer et al.	1986
Hexachlorophene	Joswick et al.	1971
Fentichlor	Hugo & Bloomfield	1971b
Dinitrophenol	Allwood & Hugo	1971
A general review	Hamilton	1971
4-hydroxybenzoic acid esters (parabens)	Furr & Russell	1972
4-ethylphenol	Hugo & Bowen	1973
Triclosan	Regos & Hitz	1974
Dodecyldiethanolamine	Lambert & Smith	1976
2-phenoxyethanol	Gilbert et al.	1977b
Polyethoxyalkyl phenols (Tritons)	Lamikanra & Allwood	1977
Phenol	Kroll & Anagnostopoulos	1981a
Polymeric biguanides	Broxton et al.	1983
Chlorocresol	Denyer et al.	1985, 1986
Alexidine	Chawner & Gilbert	1989

procedures involving bench centrifugation (5000 *g* for 10 min) have been employed. The cell-free solution is then subject to analysis. The dynamics of leakage can be followed by the removal of samples for analysis from the biocide/bacterium reaction mixture at timed intervals.

Detection of purines and pyrimidines

These compounds absorb strongly at 260 nm and can be analysed directly by ultraviolet absorbance measurements on the cell-free solution. Occasionally, biocides may also absorb at this wavelength (e.g. phenols) and an appropriate extraction technique must be devised to remove these interfering substances; chloroform extraction often proves useful in this respect (Hugo & Franklin 1968). It is essential to confirm that the extraction procedure does not also remove leaked material.

Detection of pentoses

Pentoses may be determined colorimetrically by the method of Meijbaum (1939).

To 5 ml of the cell-free preparation in a pyrex test tube add 5 ml of orcinol reagent (orcinol (3:5 dihydroxytoluene), 1 g; ferric chloride, 0.1 g; concentrated hydrochloric acid, to 100 ml) and immediately heat in boiling water for 30 min. Cool and read in a spectrophotometer at 660 nm. A calibration curve should be prepared using ribose over the range 0−100µg as standard. High concentrations of phosphate may interfere with this assay.

Detection of inorganic phosphorus (phosphate)

Inorganic phosphorus can be readily determined by the method of Fiske & Subbarow (1925). In this method, the cell-free fluid is reacted with ammonium molybdate in acid solution to give phosphomolybdate. A mixture of sodium bisulphite, sodium sulphite and 1-amino-2-naphthol-4-sulphonic acid is then employed to reduce the phosphomolybdate to form a phosphomolybdenum blue complex. The intensity of the colour at 660 nm is proportional to the inorganic phosphorus concentration and can be compared against an appropriate calibration curve prepared from potassium phosphate solutions over the concentration range equivalent to 0−5 µg/ml inorganic phosphorus. A suitable assay kit is available from the Sigma Chemical Company Ltd, Poole, Dorset.

Detection of amino acids and proteins

Amino acids in the cell-free solution can be determined by the ninhydrin method, using leucine or another appropriate amino acid as standard. Leaked proteins can be determined by the Lowry (Lowry *et al*. 1951) or biuret (Stickland 1951) reactions, with bovine serum albumin as a calibration standard. Reference to these analytical methods is given in most standard texts. Suitable assay kits can be obtained from the Sigma Chemical Company Ltd.

The appearance of intracellular enzymic activity in the suspending medium is a further indication of protein release following membrane damage. Chromogenic reagents can be used such as *o*-nitrophenyl β-D-galactopyranoside for the detection of β-galactosidase enzyme activity. The appearance of such enzymic material usually only occurs after gross membrane damage or lysis.

Detection of released metal ions

Generally potassium is the intracellular ion most frequently studied. Here leakage can be followed within the reaction mixture by the use of an ion-selective electrode. Such a system again requires high numbers of bacterial cells ($c.4 \times 10^9$/ml), this time in a potassium-free buffer system. Care should be taken to ensure that no interfering ions (e.g. sodium) are present if an ion-selective electrode of low specificity is employed. The suspension must be continuously stirred and the control ion flux monitored in the absence of biocide. The electrode can be calibrated by the use of dilutions of potassium chloride from 10^{-1} to 10^{-6} mol/l in the experimental buffer; allowance must be made for the effect of temperature on the electrode response.

Flame photometry can also be employed for following specific ion leakage, but it suffers from the disadvantage of first requiring cell separation. Thus the dynamics of leakage are less readily followed than with ion selective electrode methods.

Cells preloaded with radio-labelled material

Methods have been devised to preload bacteria with radio-labelled material and to follow biocide action and leakage by the subsequent determination of radioactivity appearing in the cell-free solution or by following the amount remaining in treated cells. Radioactive forms of K, Rb^+, phosphate (Silver & Wendt 1967; Harold & Baarda 1968), glucose (Davies *et al*. 1968) and amino acids (Hamilton 1968) have been employed.

Presentation and interpretation of results

In all studies, leakage should be adjusted for control experiments where no biocide is present. Results may be given as absolute values or as a percentage of intracellular pool material. This can be determined by cold (20°C) 5%(w/v) trichloroacetic acid treatment of a bacterial suspension for 2 h to release the soluble pool. Further treatment of the cell pellet with boiling 5% (w/v) trichloroacetic acid for 30 min will release additional intracellular material (Table 2).

The level of leakage observed in the presence of a biocide depends not only on the concentration of agent present but also on the organism used, the conditions under which leakage levels are measured and the leaked species. Loss of metal ions is often rapid and monophasic, while the leakage of higher molecular weight compounds (e.g. purines, pyrimidines, pentoses) is frequently more complex. At physiological temperatures (35−40°C) an initial rapid release of such molecules is often followed by a more gradual secondary leakage (Fig. 1). This secondary release may result from the activation of a latent ribonuclease which causes the breakdown of ribosomal RNA or the operation of other autolytic enzymes. Low temperatures (0−4°C) inhibit this enzyme activity (compare Fig. 2 with Figs 1 and 3). High concentrations of agent which are rapidly bactericidal may progressively inhibit leakage as a result of the inactivation of autolytic enzymes or coagulation of cytoplasmic materials (Figs 1 and 3). Leakage caused by low biocide concentrations may be retarded in the presence of an energy source (Fig. 4) and some recovery of lost pool material may be possible (Fig. 5).

Membrane permeability changes

In addition to following leakage of intracellular contents, biocide action on membrane integrity can also be inferred by the recognition of behaviour indicative of a selective loss of membrane impermeability. Such approaches include the measurement of transmembrane ion flux, sphaeroplast and protoplast lysis in salt solutions, revival and recovery of treated cells on salts media, and dye penetration.

TABLE 2. *Distribution of cytoplasmic material in trichloroacetic acid (TCA) extracts from* Staph. aureus

	Extracted material from 4×10^9 cells/ml	
Extraction method	Inorganic phosphorus (nmol $P_i/4 \times 10^9$ cells)	260 nm absorbing material (OD_{260})
Cold TCA	97.5	0.30
Hot TCA	29.3	2.41
Total TCA extract	126.3	2.71

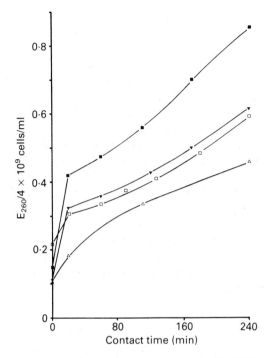

FIG. 1. Time course of tetradecyltrimethylammonium bromide (C_{14}TAB)-induced leakage of 260 nm absorbing material from *Staph. aureus*. C_{14}TAB concentrations: (µg/ml): (△) 10; (▼) 15; (■) 18; (□) 30.

Specific ion fluxes

A delicate balance of ionic gradients exists across the bacterial membrane and any increase in permeability is reflected in a disturbance of these gradients. Kroll & Patchett (this book) highlights methods which may be used to follow changes in cellular energetics associated with transmembrane ion fluxes. These methods may equally well be applied to the detection of permeability changes *per se*. More usually, however, specific changes in ion permeability are followed by the deliberate imposition of ion gradients and subsequent monitoring of their biocide-induced dissipation by ion-selective electrode techniques. These approaches have been applied in particular to the measurement of transmembrane proton and potassium fluxes induced by the addition of protonophoric and ionophoric agents, respectively. The technique can be illustrated by reference to the measurement of proton translocation rates in *E. coli* based on a modification of the method used by Gilbert *et al.* (1977a).

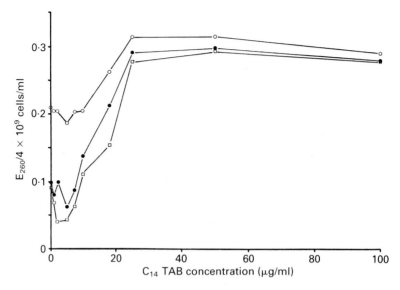

FIG. 2. The effect of C_{14}TAB concentration on the leakage of 260 nm absorbing material from *Staph. aureus* at 4°C after contact times of: (□) 2h; (●) 4h; (○) 24h.

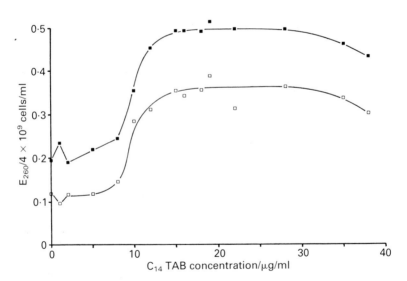

FIG. 3. The effect of C_{14}TAB concentration on the leakage of 260 nm absorbing material from *Staph. aureus* at 37°C after contact times of: (□) 2h; (■) 4h.

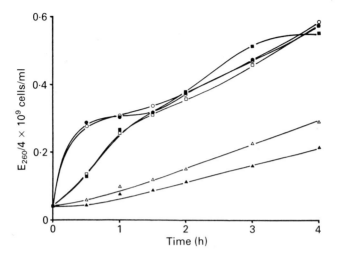

FIG. 4. The effect of 5 mmol/l glucose on the leakage of 260 nm absorbing material from *Staph. aureus* in the presence of the following concentrations of $C_{14}TAB$ (μg/ml): (△) 5; (□) 10; (○) 15. Open symbols, no glucose; closed symbols, glucose present.

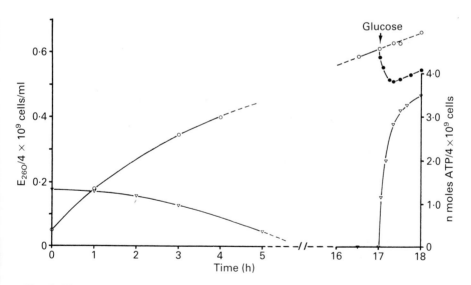

FIG. 5. The recovery of leaked 260 nm absorbing material by cells energized with 5 mmol/l glucose. (○) Leaked material in the absence of glucose; (●) leaked material after addition of glucose. Intracellular ATP content (▽) indicates energy status of cells.

A prewarmed 10-ml suspension of freshly harvested *E. coli* (4×10^9 cells/ml) in 1 mmol/l glycylglycine buffer (pH 6.8) is allowed to equilibrate for 5 min with varying concentrations of biocide. Sufficient 10 mmol/l hydrochloric acid solution (*c.* 450 μl) is then added to lower the cell suspension pH to 4.6–5.0, and the subsequent rate of increase in pH is followed with a glass pH electrode. The suspension should be thoroughly stirred throughout. The translocation rate can be calculated from the rate of change in pH and is expressed as ng ion H^+ per min per 4×10^9 cells, and is adjusted for the translocation rate of untreated control suspensions (Fig. 6). Depending upon the effect of the biocide, translocation is usually followed over a 30-s to 5-min time period. Care must be taken to ensure that the acidification of the suspending medium is not in itself sufficient to cause damage to the membrane. This can be established in preliminary experiments by imposing various pH gradients upon cells in a biocide-free environment.

Sphaeroplast and protoplast swelling and lysis

Sphaeroplasts and protoplasts are osmotically sensitive forms of bacteria partially and completely devoid of cell wall, respectively. When suspended in isotonic solutions of salts or sugars, or in solutions containing high concentrations of solutes which comprise both a permeable and an impermeable

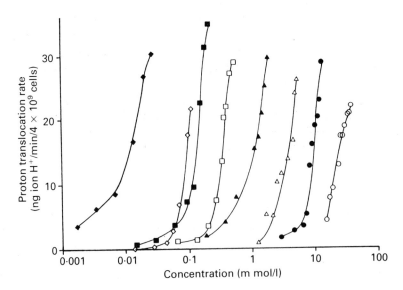

FIG. 6. Proton translocation into *E. coli* following treatment with the following antibacterial agents: (♦) Fentichlor; (◇) 4-*n*-hexylphenol; (■) 4-*n*-pentylphenol; (□) 4-*n*-butylphenol; (▲) 4-*n*-propylphenol; (△) 4-ethylphenol; (●) 4-methylphenol; (○) phenol (from Witham 1983).

ionic species, lysis will not occur. In this latter case, the ready movement of the permeable ion into the cell is retarded as a result of an electrical gradient produced by its corresponding non-permeant ionic partner (Hamilton 1970). If such suspensions are treated in such a way as to cause the breakdown of the specific impermeability to the impermeant ion then both ions can pass into the sphaeroplast. This causes rapid swelling and subsequent lysis due to the concomitant passage of water. Biocide-induced permeability changes to specific ions can thus be investigated using these osmotically sensitive forms. The extent of membrane damage has been related to the size of the newly permeant ionic species (Broxton *et al.* 1983).

The preparations of sphaeroplasts and protoplasts has been described by Williams & Gledhill (this book); the techniques of Hugo & Bloomfield (1971a, b) may also be used. Sphaeroplasts of *E. coli*, prepared by the method of Hugo & Bloomfield (1971a), have been employed below to illustrate the experimental approach and presentation of results.

A concentrated suspension of *E. coli* sphaeroplasts (equivalent to 4.0×10^{10} cells/ml) is prepared in 0.5 mol/l solutions of the chosen salts. A 0.4-ml sample of the suspension is transferred to a 1-cm cuvette containing 3.6 ml of the salt solution pre-incubated at 37°C. The cell is covered and shaken, then placed in a thermostatically controlled (37°C) spectrophotometer for monitoring of the optical density. Using the salt solution as the blank, the absorption is measured at 550 nm over a period of 20 min. The addition of a membrane-damaging biocide will cause swelling and lysis of the sphaeroplasts with a subsequent reduction in the optical density. The effect is illustrated in Fig. 7, following the addition of varying concentrations of 4-*n*-propylphenol to a sphaeroplast suspension in ammonium chloride solution (sphaeroplasts are normally impermeable to Cl^- ions).

An alternative spectroscopic approach, this time following the optical density changes resulting from the deplasmolysis of whole cells, has also been satisfactorily applied to the detection of biocide-induced increases in membrane permeability (Kroll & Anagnostopoulos 1981b).

Salt tolerance

Bacteria subject to sublethal structural damage to their cytoplasmic membrane lose their ability to grow on selective media containing high salt concentrations. This response can be readily employed to follow the onset of biocide-induced membrane damage by viable counting on agar containing high concentrations of salts (Nadir & Gilbert 1982). In this approach, a nutrient-replete agar medium (e.g. tryptone soya agar) is supplemented with increasing concentrations of a salt (e.g. KCl, 0–8% w/v) and the limiting concentration of salt for growth of uninjured cells is determined. Following sublethal biocide

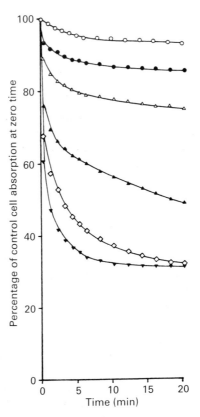

FIG. 7. The permeability of *E. coli* sphaeroplasts to ammonium chloride in the presence of the following concentrations of 4-*n*-propylphenol (µg/ml): (○) 0; (●) 50; (△) 100; (▲) 150; (◇) 200; (▼) 250 (from Witham 1983).

treatment, cells are then plated on to the agar medium with and without this limiting salt concentration and their revival is compared to untreated cells. In this way, loss of salt tolerance can be used to indicate the extent of membrane damage in a population and may also be used to compare the success of biocide-neutralization techniques and to follow bacterial recovery processes.

Dye penetration

Anilino or 2-*p*-toluidinylnaphthylene-6-sulphonate (ANS and TNS; Sigma Chemical Company, Ltd) are dyes which fluoresce strongly when complexed with protein. In the intact cell these dyes are normally efficiently excluded, but following membrane damage they gain access to, and react with, intracellular protein. In general, a washed suspension of bacteria (c. 10^9 cells/ml) will be treated with varying concentrations of the biocide in the presence of the dye $(5-10 \times 10^{-4} \text{mol}/1)$. Measurements can be made directly on the reaction mixture or following separation and resuspension of the cells in fresh buffer (Broxton *et al.* 1983). Fluorescence is determined using a fluorescence spectrophotometer at 440 nm (TNS) or 470 nm (ANS) with excitation wavelengths of 388 or 400 nm, respectively. Suitable blanks can be prepared from dye-free systems, and appropriate controls should be included to account for dye complexation with surface protein. Measurements can be made relative to a standard protein solution (e.g. bovine serum albumin).

Whole-cell lysis

True lysis in bacteria can be seen when the rigid cell wall is wholly or partially dissolved. The cytoplasmic membrane will then rupture in a hypotonic environment due to internal solute pressure and the cell will lyse. Thus, whole-cell lysis is usually indicative of gross cell wall and membrane damage.

The process of lysis can be followed by the rapid appearance of intracellular material (for analytical methods, see earlier) and the reduction in optical density (at c. 500 nm) of the suspension. Lysis can be confirmed by microscopy and the proportion of intact cells remaining can be established from comparison with biocide-free suspensions. Susceptibility to lysis may arise directly through the disruption of cell envelope barriers or, indirectly, by the initiation of autolytic mechanisms or as a result of cell wall changes occurring during growth in the presence of biocide. In growth-dependent lysis, cultures may lyse precipitously following a defined period of incubation in a nutrient medium.

TABLE 3. *Some examples of biocides causing bacterial lysis*

Substance	Author(s)	Date
Formaldehyde	Pulvertaft & Lumb	1948
Phenol		
Mercury (II) chloride		
Sodium hypochlorite		
Merthiolate	Pulvertaft & Lumb	1948
	Delpy & Champsey	1949
	Norris	1957
CTAB	Salton	1957
Sodium dodecyl sulphate	Bolle & Kellenberger	1958
	El-Falaha *et al.*	1989
Mercury compounds	Schaechter & Santomassino	1962
Alcohols	Ingram & Buttke	1984

Examples of biocide-induced whole cell lysis are given in Table 3. It is generally thought that low concentrations of biocides may induce lysis by causing cell wall synthesizing and degrading enzymes to act only in a degradative manner giving rise to weakening and finally dissolution of the cell wall.

Conclusion

The demonstration of leakage will remain an anecdotal event unless it is carefully related to other effects on the cell. In this context, some workers have attempted to correlate leakage with cell death (for example, Gale & Taylor 1947; Salton 1951; Hugo & Longworth 1964; Hugo & Bloomfield 1971b; Gilbert *et al.* 1977b) and potassium leakage has been reported as a lethality index (Kroll & Anagnostopoulos 1981a).

It is important to remember that the effect on viability must occur at the same concentration as an observed biochemical effect and viability studies should be made with extreme precision and with the employment of appropriate neutralizing agents.

Correlations between leakage and death appear to reflect the nature of membrane damage (Broxton *et al.* 1983), but even where there is correlation it is unlikely that leakage *per se* is lethal. However, a concomitant effect on cell metabolism such that the organism can no longer make good its losses may well result in a loss of viability. Lysis is, of course, an assured indicator of cell death.

References

ALLWOOD, M.C. & HUGO, W.B. 1971. The leakage of cations and amino acids from *Staphylococcus aureus* exposed to moist heat, phenol and dinitrophenol. *Journal of Applied Bacteriology* 34, 369−375.

BECKETT, A.H., PATKI, S.J. & ROBINSON, A.E. 1958. Interaction of phenolic compounds with bacteria. *Nature, London* 181, 712.

BECKETT, A.H., PATKI, S.J. & ROBINSON, A.E. 1959. The interaction of phenolic compounds with bacteria. I. Hexylresorcinol and *Escherichia coli*. *Journal of Pharmacy and Pharmacology* 11, 360−366.

BOLLE, A. & KELLENBERGER, E. 1958. The action of sodium lauryl sulphate on *E. coli*. *Schweitzer Zeitung für Pathologie und Bakteriologie* 21, 714−740.

BROXTON, P., WOODCOCK, P.M. & GILBERT, P. 1983. A study of the antibacterial activity of some polyhexamethylene biguanides towards *Escherichia coli* ATCC 8739. *Journal of Applied Bacteriology* 54, 345−353.

CHAWNER, J.A. & GILBERT P. 1989. A comparative study of the bactericidal and growth inhibitory activities of the bisbiguanide alexidine and chlorhexidine. *Journal of Applied Bacteriology* 66, 243−252.

DALTREY, D.C. & HUGO, W.B. 1974. Studies on the mode of action of the antimicrobial agent chlorhexidine on *Clostridium perfringens* II. Effect of chlorhexidine on metabolism and on the cell membrane. *Microbios* 11, 131−146.

DAVIES, A., BENTLEY, M. & FIELD, B.S. 1968. Comparison of the action of Vantocil, cetrimide and chlorhexidine on *Escherichia coli* and its sphaeroplasts and the protoplasts of Gram positive bacteria. *Journal of Applied Bacteriology* **31**, 448–461.

DELPY, P.L. & CHAMPSEY, H.M. 1949. Sur la stabilisation des suspensions sporulées de *B. anthracis* par l'action de certains antiseptiques. *Comptes rendus hebdomadaires des séances de l'Academie des Sciences, Paris* **225**, 1071–1073.

DENYER, S.P., HARDING, V.D. & HUGO, W.B. 1985. The mechanism of bacteriostatic action of chlorocresol (CC) on *Staphylococcus aureus*. *Journal of Pharmacy and Pharmacology* **37**, 93P.

DENYER, S.P., HUGO, W.B. & HARDING, V.D. 1986. The biochemical basis of synergy between the antibacterial agents chlorocresol and 2-phenylethanol. *International Journal of Pharmaceutics* **29**, 29–36.

EL-FALAHA, B.M.A., FURR, J.R. & RUSSELL, A.D. 1989. Effect of anionic detergents on wild-type and envelope mutants of *Escherichia coli* and *Pseudomonas aeruginosa*. *Letters in Applied Microbiology* **8**, 15–19.

FISKE, C.H. & SUBBAROW, Y. 1925. The colorimetric determination of phosphorus. *Journal of Biological Chemistry* **66**, 375–400.

FURR, J.R. & RUSSELL, A.D. 1972. Some factors influencing the activity of esters of *p*-hydroxybenzoic acid against *Serratia marcescens*. *Microbios* **5**, 189–198.

GALE, E.F. & TAYLOR, E.S. 1947. The action of tyrocidin and some detergent substances in releasing amino acids from the internal environment of *Streptococcus faecalis*. *Journal of General Microbiology* **1**, 77–84.

GILBERT, P., BEVERIDGE, E.G. & CRONE, P.B. 1977a. Effect of phenoxyethanol on the permeability of *Escherichia coli* NCTC 5933 to inorganic ions. *Microbios* **19**, 17–26.

GILBERT, P., BEVERIDGE, E.G. & CRONE, P.B. 1977b. The lethal action of 2-phenoxyethanol and its analogues upon *Escherichia coli* NCTC 5933. *Microbios* **19**, 125–141.

GILBY, A.R. & FEW, A.V. 1960. Lysis of protoplasts of *Micrococcus lysodeikticus* by ionic detergents. *Journal of General Microbiology* **23**, 19–26.

HAMILTON, W.A. 1968. The mechanism of the bacteriostatic action of tetrachlorosalicylanilide. *Journal of General Microbiology* **50**, 441–458.

HAMILTON, W.A. 1970. The mode of action of membrane-active antibacterials. *FEBS Symposium* **20**, 71–79.

HAMILTON, W.A. 1971. Membrane-active antimicrobial compounds. In *Inhibition and Destruction of the Microbial Cell*, ed. Hugo, W.B. pp. 77–93. London & New York: Academic Press.

HARDING, V.D., HUGO, W.B. & DENYER, S.P. 1984. An investigation into the mode of action of 2-phenylethanol (PEA) on *Staphylococcus aureus*. *Journal of Pharmacy and Pharmacology* **36**, 58P.

HAROLD, F.M. & BAARDA, J.R. 1968. Inhibition of membrane transport in *Streptococcus faecalis* by uncouplers of oxidative phosphorylation and its relationship to proton conduction. *Journal of Bacteriology* **96**, 2025–2034.

HOTCHKISS, R.D. 1944. Gramicidin, tyrocidin and tyrothricin. *Advances in Enzymology* **4**, 153–199.

HUGO, W.B. & BLOOMFIELD, S.F. 1971a. Studies on the mode of action of the phenolic agent Fentichlor against *Staphylococcus aureus* and *Escherichia coli*. I. The adsorption of Fentichlor by the bacterial cell and its antibacterial activity. *Journal of Applied Bacteriology* **34**, 557–567.

HUGO, W.B. & BLOOMFIELD, S.F. 1971b. Studies on the mode of action of the phenolic agent Fentichlor against *Staphylococcus aureus* and *Escherichia coli* II. The effects of Fentichlor on the bacterial membrane and the cytoplasmic constituents of the cell. *Journal of Applied Bacteriology* **34**, 569–578.

HUGO, W.B. & BOWEN, J.G. 1973. Studies on the mode of action of 4-ethylphenol on *Escherichia coli*. *Microbios* **8**, 189–197.

HUGO, W.B. & FRANKLIN, I. 1968. Cellular lipid and the antistaphylococcal activity of phenols. *Journal of General Microbiology* 52, 365–373.

HUGO, W.B. & LONGWORTH, A.R. 1964. Some aspects of the mode of action of chlorhexidine. *Journal of Pharmacy and Pharmacology* 16, 655–662.

INGRAM, L.O. & BUTTKE, T.M. 1984. Effects of alcohols on micro-organisms. *Advances in Microbial Physiology* 25, 253–300.

JACKSON, R.W. & DE MOSS, J.A. 1965. Effect of toluene on *Escherichia coli*. *Journal of Bacteriology* 90, 1420–1425.

JOSWICK, H.L., CORNER, J.N., SILVERMAN, J.N. & GERHARDT, P. 1971. Antimicrobial actions of hexachlorophene: release of cytoplasmic materials. *Journal of Bacteriology* 108, 492–500.

JUDIS, J. 1962. Studies on the mode of action of phenolic disinfectants. I. Release of radioactivity from carbon-14-labelled *Escherichia coli*. *Journal of Pharmaceutical Sciences* 51, 261–265.

KROLL, R.G. & ANAGNOSTOPOULOS, G.D. 1981a. Potassium leakage as a lethality index of phenol and the effect of solute and water activity. *Journal of Applied Bacteriology* 50, 139–147.

KROLL, R.G. & ANAGNOSTOPOULOS, G.D. 1981b. Potassium fluxes on hyperosmotic shock and the effect of phenol and bronopol (2-bromo-2-nitropropan-1, 3-diol) on deplasmolysis of *Pseudomonas aeruginosa*. *Journal of Applied Bacteriology* 51, 313–323.

KUHN, R. & BIELIG, H.J. 1940. Uber Invertseifen. I. Die Einwirkung von Invertseifen aus Eiweiss-Stoffe. *Berichte der Deutschen Chemischen Gesellschaft* 73, 1080–1091.

LAMBERT, P.A. & HAMMOND, S.M. 1973. Potassium fluxes, first indications of membrane damage in micro-organisms. *Biochemical and Biophysical Research Communications* 54, 796–799.

LAMBERT, P.A. & SMITH, A.R.W. 1976. Antimicrobial action of dodecyldiethanolamine: induced membrane damage in *Escherichia coli*. *Microbios* 15, 191–202.

LAMIKANRA, A. & ALLWOOD, M.C. 1977. Effects of polyethoxyalkyl phenols on the leakage of intracellular material from *Staphylococcus aureus*. *Journal of Applied Bacteriology* 42, 379–385.

LOWRY, O.H., ROSEBROUGH, N.J., FARR, A.L. & RANDALL, R.J. 1951. Protein measurement with the folin phenol reagent. *Journal of Biological Chemistry* 193, 265–275.

MEIJBAUM, M. 1939. Estimation of small amounts of pentose especially in derivatives of adenylic acid. *Hoppe-Seyler's Zeitschrift für Physiologische Chemie* 258, 117–120.

NADIR, M.T. & GILBERT, P. 1982. Injury and recovery of *Bacillus megaterium* from mild chlorhexidine treatment. *Journal of Applied Bacteriology* 52, 111–115.

NORRIS, J.R. 1957. A bacteriolytic principle associated with cultures of *Bacillus subtilis*. *Journal of General Microbiology* 16, 1–8.

POSTGATE, J.R. 1956. Cytochrome C_3 and desulphoviridin; pigments of the anaerobe *Desulphovibrio desulphuricans*. *Journal of General Microbiology* 14, 545–572.

PULVERTAFT, R.J.V. & LUMB, G.D. 1948. Bacterial lysis and antiseptics. *Journal of Hygiene, Cambridge* 46, 62–64.

REGOS, J. & HITZ, H.R. 1974. Investigations on the mode of action of Triclosan, a broad spectrum antimicrobial agent. *Zentralblatt für Bakteriologie und Hygiene, Abt. Orig.* A226, 390–401.

SALTON, M.R.J. 1950. The bactericidal properties of certain cationic detergents. *Australasian Journal of Scientific Research* B3, 45–60.

SALTON, M.R.J. 1951. The adsorption of cetyltrimethylammonium bromide by bacteria, its action in releasing cellular constituents and its bactericidal effect. *Journal of General Microbiology* 5, 391–404.

SALTON, M.R.J. 1957. The action of lytic agents on the surface structures of the bacterial cell. In *Proceedings of the Second International Congress on Surface Activity*, Vol. 11, ed. Schulman, J.H. pp. 245–253. London: Butterworths.

SALTON, M.R.J. 1963. The relationship between the nature of the cell wall and the Gram strain. *Journal of General Microbiology* 30, 233–235.

SCHAECHTER, M. & SANTOMASSINO, K.A. 1962. The lysis of *Escherichia coli* by sulphydryl binding agents. *Journal of Bacteriology* **84**, 318–325.

SCHULMAN, J.H. & RIDEAL, E.K. 1937. Molecular interactions in monolayers. I. Complexes between large molecules. *Proceedings of the Royal Society, London* **B122**, 29–45.

SILVER, S. & WENDT, L. 1967. Mechanism of action of phenylethyl alcohol: breakdown of cellular permeability barriers. *Journal of Bacteriology* **93**, 560–566.

STICKLAND, L.H. 1951. The determination of small quantities of bacteria by means of the biuret reaction. *Journal of General Microbiology* **5**, 698–703.

WITHAM, R.F. 1983. A study of the antimicrobial activity of a homologous series of phenols. *PhD thesis*, University of Nottingham.

WOODROFFE, R.C.S. & WILKINSON, B.E. 1966. The antibacterial activity of tetrachlorosalicylanilide. *Journal of General Microbiology* **44**, 343–352.

Biocide-Induced Perturbations of Aspects of Cell Homeostasis: Intracellular pH, Membrane Potential and Solute Transport

R.G. KROLL AND R.A. PATCHETT

Department of Microbiology, AFRC Institute of Food Research, Reading Laboratory, Shinfield, Reading RG2 9AT, UK

The cytoplasmic membrane of bacteria is the target site of action of several antibiotics and antimicrobial agents. This important cell structure not only delineates the cytoplasm and all the vital processes therein, but is a hydrophobic lipid bilayer through which all the salts and nutrients necessary for growth must be transported. The membrane is also the site of energy transduction and it is now generally accepted that oxidative phosphorylation and the active transport of some solutes is dependent on the formation and maintenance of transmembrane gradients of ions, most notably protons (Mitchell 1973).

There is currently considerable debate about the exact mechanisms and stoichiometries of the processes involved and in particular whether bulk phase or localized proton gradients are energetically important (Ferguson 1985). For present purposes it will be assumed that chemiosmotic mechanisms predominate and thus:

1 the cytoplasmic membrane is poorly permeable to protons, ions and other charged species;

2 oxidation of NADH by the terminal electron acceptor, usually O_2, occurs via the respiratory chain and results in the extrusion of protons from the cell;

3 this forms a transmembrane electrochemical gradient of protons (Δp) composed of an electrical potential ($\Delta \Psi$) and a pH gradient (ΔpH);

4 the energy stored by the Δp can be used by the cell to do useful work. In fermentative organisms the Δp is generated by the hydrolysis of ATP generated by substrate-level phosphorylation via the Mg^{2+}-dependent H^+ translocating ATP-ase, although efflux of fermentation end-products is also thought to contribute (Ten Brinks *et al.* 1985).

In neutrophilic bacteria the cytoplasm is usually negatively charged and alkaline with respect to the environment, the magnitudes of ΔpH and $\Delta \Psi$

Mechanisms of Action of
Chemical Biocides

depending particularly on the external pH (pH_o; Booth 1986). Indeed, it is evident that bacteria go to considerable trouble to control the values of $\Delta\Psi$ and ΔpH, primarily to regulate the intracellular pH (pH_i) and to maintain transmembrane gradients of sugars, amino acids and various ions, notably Na^+ and K^+ (Booth 1988; Higgins & Booth 1988). It is therefore axiomatic that any compounds which can specifically or non-specifically induce the movement of protons or other charged species across the membrane will directly affect the ability of the cell to maintain these gradients and perform other vital functions.

It should be emphasized that this may not necessarily directly lead to measurable effects on the values of $\Delta\Psi$, ΔpH or solute or ion gradients (especially at subinhibitory concentrations of a compound). One feature that characterizes the homeostatic mechanisms for osmotic and pH_i regulation is that initial responses to a stress will bring about changes in the activities of the extant systems (Booth 1988; Higgins & Booth 1988). Only on longer time-scales can changes in gene expression occur to modify the cell's capability to respond. Thus perturbations in ion gradients can be counteracted – up to a certain extent (determined by energy availability, transport capacity etc.).

For instance, at steady-state the rate of H^+ extrusion ($\mathcal{J}_{gen}$) matches that of H^+ in flux ($\mathcal{J}_{dis}$), i.e.

$$\mathcal{J}_{gen} = \mathcal{J}_{dis}.$$

$\mathcal{J}_{gen}$ is composed of $\mathcal{J}_e n$ where $\mathcal{J}_e$ is the rate of electron flow and n the stoichiometry of protons extruded per electron transferred to the terminal oxidant. Furthermore, $\mathcal{J}_{dis}$ is dictated by the magnitude of the Δp generated and the proton conductivity (C) of the membrane (Booth 1988) such that

$$\mathcal{J}_e n = \Delta p C.$$

$\mathcal{J}_e$ appears to be relatively independent of Δp; however, the value of C is dependent on the value of Δp. This non-linear dependence of membrane conductance on the proton motive force is probably a result of a Δp-dependence of the energy transducers in the membrane (Booth 1988). Anti-microbial agents may act to reduce the rate of respiration (decrease $\mathcal{J}_e$) which may lead to a fermentative mode of metabolism in those organisms capable of generating ATP by substrate-level phosphorylation, with generation of Δp by the H^+-translocating ATP-ase. Some compounds may act to increase the permeability of the membrane (increase C) which may lead to the dissipation of Δp. Increasing subinhibitory concentrations of such a compound makes it increasingly difficult for a cell to maintain the various gradients; the expenditure of energy to counteract perturbations in ion and solute gradients is too great, and growth stasis occurs. However, the complete dissipation of Δp may not result in cell death if the extracellular pH, K^+ and amino acid content are favourable. Indeed, with fermentative organisms, complete dissipation of Δp

does not inhibit growth if these conditions are controlled (Harold & Van Brunt 1977). If the environmental conditions are unfavourable, e.g. low pH, low K^+ concentration, then the complete dissipation of Δp can result in cell death, the extent of which will depend on the environmental conditions and the duration of growth stasis. Such considerations will apply only at or below the minimum growth inhibitory concentration (MIC) of a compound. However, with many antimicrobial compounds secondary modes of action of the inhibitor will cause cell death, particularly at concentrations in excess of the MIC.

Methods for the Measurement of Δp

Although originally rather arcane, these methods have been developed to such an extent that they are now routine in many research laboratories. The components of Δp can be measured directly in many eukaryotic cells, without too much damage, with micro-electrodes. Bacteria are too small for impalement (although this has been done with artificially large cells, Felle et al. 1980) and indirect measurements using various probes must be made. Ideally, these would be cheap, non-invasive, allow continuous measurements to be undertaken and give absolute values. None of the present methods fulfil all of these criteria. In general, fairly dense (e.g. > 0.5 mg dry wt/ml) cell suspensions are incubated under physiologically relevant conditions of temperature, ionic strength etc. in the presence of an energy source. When studying the effects of antimicrobial agents it is important that the concentration of the compound should be in the range around the MIC for that organism and that contact times are standardized. When radio-labelled distributions have to be measured the cells are usually separated from their suspending media by either rapid centrifugation or filtration, so that the extracellular and intracellular concentrations of radio-label can be determined. An alternative technique, flow dialysis, has also been successfully applied. Here only the extracellular fluid, which is in equilibrium with another compartment containing the cell suspension, is assayed.

Several reviews have described the current methods available in detail (Kashket 1985; Padan & Schuldiner 1986; Booth 1986; Krulwich & Guffanti 1986) and these will only be summarized here. It cannot be emphasized too much that the proper controls must always be carried out, e.g. compounds which are known to dissipate ΔpH and/or $\Delta \Psi$ should achieve this in the measuring systems under study.

Solute transport

Methods for studying solute and ion transport in bacteria are widely known but the transport of some solutes can be used as an indicator of Δp or Δp components.

Usually a radio-labelled solute is incubated with a cell suspension, the cells are rapidly separated from the suspending medium and the amount of cell-associated and supernatant label is assayed by scintillation counting. It is imperative that the transported solute is not adsorbed by, or incorporated into, the cell material or acted upon by a cell enzyme. This is usually achieved by either using a non-metabolizable analogue of the compound (e.g. α-amino*iso*butyric acid, methylthio-β-D-galactoside) or by the use of a mutant which lacks the enzyme for the substrate and constitutively expresses the transport protein (e.g. lactose and *Escherichia coli* ML308−225; *lac* i$^-$, z$^-$, y$^+$, a$^+$). Therefore the steady-state accumulation levels of compounds that are transported by proton-linked systems can be used to indicate the values of $\Delta\Psi$, ΔpH or Δp depending on the charge on the solute and the H$^+$ stoichiometry (Hamilton 1975). (Similarly, Na$^+$-coupled solutes could be used to indicate Na$^+$ gradients.) It should be emphasized that solute gradients and Δp components may not be in thermodynamic equilibrium (Booth *et al.* 1979) so solute gradients can only be used as indicators of Δp components.

Probes for ΔpH

Measurement of the accumulation of radio-labelled weak acids (pH$_i$ alkaline) or bases (pH$_i$ acidic) is the most commonly used method. In neutrophilic bacteria, intracellular pH (pH$_i$) is usually alkaline with respect to extracellular pH (pH$_o$) and weak acids, usually acetate (4.75), benzoate (4.2), 5,5-dimethyl-2,4,oxazolidinedione (6.3) or salicylic acid (3.0) are used as probes (values in parenthesis are their pK_a values). The method is based on the assumption that the membrane is freely permeable to the uncharged weak acid but is impermeable to the anion.

$$HA \rightleftharpoons H^+ + A^- \qquad \text{in}$$
$$\updownarrow$$
$$HA \rightleftharpoons H^+ \ A^- \qquad \text{out}$$

The accumulation of the weak acid depends on the size of the ΔpH, the pK_a of the weak acid, the pH$_o$ and the amount of acid added, according to the equation

$$\Delta\text{pH} = \log_{10} [(AR) (1 + 10^{pK_a-pH_o}) - 10^{pK_a-pH_o}] \qquad (1)$$

where AR is the accumulation ratio of intracellular to extracellular weak acid. Thus the sensitivity of the method is determined by the value of the pK_a in relation to pH$_o$. For practical considerations the pH$_o$ must always be equal to or higher than the pK_a value. Obviously the accumulation must not be affected by either non-specific binding or active transport of the probe − this does occur with some probe/organism combinations and care is needed. The probe should also not affect cell metabolism at the concentrations used (*cf.* benzoic acid). Weak bases e.g. methylamine or ethylamine (pK_b 10.5−10.7) are used when pH_i is more acidic than pH_o but similar considerations apply (here pK_b should be > pH_o).

Optical probes for pH_i

Several fluorescent probes have been found to be of use with cells having acidic values for pH_i or for everted membrane vesicles prepared from neutralophic bacteria. This is because these probes are weak bases, e.g. 9-aminoacridine, acridine orange, *n*-phenyl-1-naphthylamine. These dyes accumulate in response to the pH gradient resulting in quenching of the fluorescent signal. Generally, these dyes are difficult to calibrate to give quantitative estimates of ΔpH (due to localized phenomena and interaction directly with the membrane) but their major advantage, compared with previously mentioned methods, is that they are extremely useful for following dynamic qualitative changes in ΔpH due to the ability to make continuous measurements. Fluorescein diacetate can be used as a measure of alkaline pH_i but this is dependent on weak acid accumulation and the action of an intracellular enzyme (Slavik 1982).

Use of pH electrodes

In this approach, washed cell suspensions are prepared in a weak buffer solution, rendered anaerobic to inhibit respiration and the pH_o is monitored with an H^+ electrode (Collins & Hamilton 1976; Booth *et al.* 1979). The cells are treated with iodoacetic acid to inhibit substrate-level ATP production from endogenous reserves and carbonic anhydrase is added to rapidly equilibrate CO_2 and bicarbonate. When the pH_o value is steady, respiration is initiated by the addition of O_2. At the end of the burst of respiration and when the pH_o value returns to that before the O_2 addition, the cells are permeabilized with butanol. By measuring the extracellular and intracellular buffering capacity the ΔpH value can be determined from the values of pH_o under energized and de-energized conditions. These experiments are rather tedious to perform but do provide reasonable estimates of ΔpH.

Furthermore, this approach is an excellent method of directly testing whether a particular compound increases the proton permeability of the membrane. For instance, addition of a protonophore speeds up the rate of alkalinization of the pH trace (hence rate of proton entry to the cells) when the O_2 is exhausted or after artificial acidification by the addition of HCl. Obviously for this to be of significance the concentration of the compound must be physiologically relevant.

^{31}P NMR

This method has also been used to measure pH_i directly due to the pH sensitivity of the chemical shifts of intracellular compounds which contain phosphorus — mainly inorganic phosphorus. Unfortunately the pH shift is insensitive at the pH_i values commonly found (because the relevant pK_a for inorganic phosphate is 6.8). However, a synthetic probe, methyl phosphonate (pK_a 7.6) has been shown to give good agreement with other methods for pH_i estimation (i.e. weak acid distribution methods). This method is non-destructive, gives an almost continuous measurement and perhaps is less invasive (despite the need for the artificial probe). The major disadvantages are availability of the equipment, that very dense cell suspensions are needed and aerobiosis can be difficult to ensure.

Measurement of $\Delta\Psi$

The distribution of permeant cations is the most commonly used method for evaluating $\Delta\Psi$. When $\Delta\Psi$ is positive as in everted membrane vesicles or acidophiles, permeant anions are used.

K^+/valinomycin

The bacterial membranes are rendered permeable to K^+ by using the highly specific K^+ ionophore valinomycin. On addition of valinomycin to a bacterial suspension, the K^+ ions should redistribute themselves to an equilibrium determined by the $\Delta\Psi$, which can be calculated directly from the Nernst equation. Intracellular and extracellular K^+ concentrations can be determined by flame photometry or $^{42}K^+$ or $^{86}Rb^+$ isotopes can be used. A disadvantage is that with Gram-negative organisms their outer membrane has to be disrupted with EDTA to allow the valinomycin access to the cytoplasmic membrane, possibly introducing other variables.

Lipophilic cations

The most commonly used probes for $\Delta\Psi$ are lipophilic cations, the accumulation of which can be measured by using radio-labelled compounds or ion-sensitive electrodes. Currently tetraphenylphosphonium ions and tri-phenylmethylphosphonium ions (the former is probably preferable as it seems to diffuse rapidly across membranes, including the outer membrane of Gram-negative organisms) are usually used. However, a considerable problem is that these probes can bind to the cells in the de-energized state and so the difference between energized and de-energized probe accumulation is used to calculate the value of $\Delta\Psi$ from the Nernst equation. This is further complicated however by the possibility of concentration-dependent binding which would render this correction invalid. Thus there are inherent errors in the method and at present it is thought that the values obtained are underestimates (Booth 1988).

Optical probes

Various fluorescent dyes have been found to be quenched when a $\Delta\Psi$ is established across a membrane. Several cyanine dyes, safranine, rhodamine and 1,8-anilino-naphthalenesulphonic acid, have been widely used (Resnick *et al.* 1985) but as with optical ΔpH probes, various artefacts are thought to occur and quantitative values are not reliable: the methods are thus of greatest use for following rapid qualitative changes as continuous measurements can be made.

Carotenoid band shifts

The membranes of photosynthetic bacteria contain carotenoid pigments which shift their light adsorption spectra in response to $\Delta\Psi$. The values obtained are often higher than those obtained by ion distribution methods: the reason for this is not understood.

Reliability of measurements

It is obviously preferable to have independent confirmation of the values of any parameter derived from two different methods. With neutrophiles it is now thought that estimates of pH_i by weak acids are reasonable as ^{31}P NMR data are so similar. It is imperative that with weak acid measurements and with transport experiments, the intracellular volume be estimated under the same experimental conditions as those under which the measurements are made. This is most easily achieved by using radio-labelled non-penetrant markers (Stock *et al.* 1977; Ahmed & Booth 1983). It is currently thought that present methods of estimating $\Delta\Psi$ are unreliable; probably underestimating its true value (Booth 1988).

It should also be mentioned that rather than using whole cells, membrane vesicles or artificial lipid membranes can give valuable information where permeabilities and electrical properties can be determined (Lambert 1978; see also Chopra and Phillips-Jones & Rhodes Roberts (this book) for preparation of vesicles).

Antimicrobial Agents and Δp

Several articles review the effects of antimicrobial agents on membrane functions in more detail than can be given here (Harold 1970; Hamilton 1971; Hugo 1978; Lambert 1978). There are many examples of compounds which will cause gross membrane damage, e.g. chloroform, butanol, toluene, many phenols, hexachlorophane and various detergents such as sodium dodecyl sulphate, deoxycholate, Triton-X100 (see Denyer & Hugo, this book). Such damage will obviously lead to the dissipation of ion gradients and the complete collapse of Δp, and also to the loss of cytoplasmic molecules. This leakage is often seen to be diphasic (e.g. hexachlorophane, Hugo 1978). It can be speculated that the initial leakage is due to the collapse of Δp, either by the inhibition of electron transport (as with hexachlorophane) or by direct dissipation of Δp, and that this then leads to the subsequent leakage of other components (e.g. amino acids, nucleotides) due to the natural turnover of proteins and RNA molecules. However, some membrane-active compounds may increase the membrane permeability to a specific ion or ions leading to specific effects on ΔpH or $\Delta \Psi$, but examples are rather more scarce than those causing general increases in permeability. Obviously the degree and nature of the effects will depend upon the identities of the inhibitor and the target cell, the contact time and the number of molecules per cell (i.e. the relative concentration). For effects on Δp to be considered significant, they must be demonstrable at concentrations of the inhibitor which cause growth inhibition. At higher concentrations, some compounds will affect other targets in the cell. Conversely, other compounds could primarily affect other targets and could cause secondary effects on Δp at higher concentrations. As mentioned, some compounds can interfere specifically with Δp generation (i.e. respiratory inhibitors; Phillips-Jones & Rhodes-Roberts, this book) or Δp dissipation, e.g. N-N'-dicyclohexylcarbodiimide inhibition of the ATP-ase. Similarly, when using solute accumulation as a measure of Δp, some compounds may inhibit the solute carrier protein (e.g. N-ethyl-maleimide and the lactose permease); such effects can easily be misinterpreted as direct effects on Δp and other experimental approaches must be taken to verify the effect on Δp.

Uncouplers

A diverse group of compounds possess the ability to uncouple respiration from oxidative phosphorylation. The classical inhibitors such as 2,4-dinitrophenol (DNP), pentachlorophenol, and carbonylcyanide p-trifluoromethoxyphenylhydrazone (FCCP) are thought to act as mobile carriers of protons across the cytoplasmic membrane and so bring about the dissipation of both ΔpH and $\Delta \Psi$. In order to dissipate Δp by this mechanism uncouplers must be considered as lipophilic weak acids where both HA and A^- are permeable. In practice the initial effect may be to collapse only $\Delta\Psi$, the ΔpH component will dissipate more slowly as large numbers of H^+ need to move to collapse ΔpH.

$$HA \rightleftharpoons H^+ + A^- \quad \text{in}$$
$$\Updownarrow \qquad\qquad \Updownarrow$$
$$HA \rightleftharpoons H^+ + A^- \quad \text{out}$$

In addition, however, many other compounds are able to dissipate Δp and so uncouple respiration from oxidative phosphorylation by more complex mechanisms. This uncoupling activity may occur as a result of non-specific physical damage to the cytoplasmic membrane. Indeed, it is commonly observed that with many antimicrobial compounds, efflux of K^+ is the first indication of membrane damage (Lambert & Hammond 1973). This may be measured by flame photometry or by following ^{42}K efflux, but is most conveniently monitored with a K^+ selective electrode enabling K^+ fluxes to be continuously recorded without the necessity of separating the cells from the suspending medium. It is probable that this movement of K^+ occurs as a result of the inability of the cell to maintain a K^+ gradient in the absence of a Δp, and K^+ efflux occurs in order to maintain electroneutrality in response to the large movement of protons into the cell caused by the collapse of ΔpH.

Weak acids

Several weak acids are widely used as food preservatives (benzoate, propionate, sorbate) and their potency has long been known to increase with decreasing pH. It is now quite clear that their primary effect is to reduce the ΔpH component of Δp. Providing that the dissociated anion remains impermeable weak acids will accumulate in the cytoplasm in accordance with equation (1). The weak acid will dissociate in the cytoplasm to release a proton and will acidify the cytoplasm. The degree of acidification will depend on the cell's capacity to alkalinize the cytoplasm and the external concentration, pH_o, pK_a and the ΔpH such that for a given acid concentration, pH_i will be lowered more at lower values of pH_o. Thus the direct effect is a reduction in pH_i and, in yeasts, growth inhibition has been shown to be due primarily to the inhibition of a specific glycolytic enzyme, phosphofructokinase, as a result of this pH change (Krebs et al. 1983). In bacteria it is not known which enzymes are primarily affected by a lowering of pH_i although there do appear to be secondary effects of weak acids on metabolism, perhaps on energy generation, which contribute to the inhibition. There is, however, a direct relationship between growth rate and pH_i (Salmond et al. 1984). Interestingly, parabens (esters of benzoic acid) do not affect ΔpH at their MIC values (Kroll &

Booth, unpublished results) and the primary mode of action of these compounds is probably inhibition of nucleic acid synthesis (Ness & Eklund 1983).

Ionophores

The ionophores are a group of compounds that are able to promote the specific movement of ions across membranes; for reviews see Harold (1970) and Pressman (1976). Many ionophores are antibiotics, being produced by various fungi or bacteria, although synthetic compounds with similar properties do exist. Most ionophores have found little application as antimicrobial agents due to their poor selective toxicity although monensin, which promotes Na^+/H^+ exchange, is an important coccidiostat. In contrast, however, the ionophores have found widespread application as research tools (Hugo & Denyer 1983). Their effects on Δp depend on the nature of their activity. Valinomycin causes the electrogenic movement of K^+ and as a result causes the collapse of $\Delta\Psi$ whilst increasing ΔpH due to the removal of the potential difference preventing further proton movements. Nigericin, on the other hand, causes the dissipation of ΔpH whilst leaving $\Delta\Psi$ intact by promoting K^+/H^+ exchange. A combination of nigericin and valinomycin in the presence of potassium produces uncoupling activity due to the collapse of both $\Delta\Psi$ and ΔpH as the gradients of both H^+ and K^+ are dissipated. The antimicrobial agent trichlorocarbanilide carries out the exchange of Cl^- and OH^- and may also be used to specifically collapse ΔpH (Ahmed & Booth 1983).

2-phenoxyethanol and phenylethylalcohol

These compounds cause ready efflux of K^+ at concentrations below those having lethal activity in *E. coli* (Silver & Wendt 1967). However, these concentrations also cause disorganization of the outer membrane and gross membrane damage could occur (Gilbert *et al.* 1977; Harding *et al.* 1984). However, the primary effect is thought to be a limited breakdown of the permeability barrier as inhibition has been shown to be reversible.

Lactoperoxidase

Lactoperoxidase catalyses the oxidation of thiocyanate by H_2O_2 to a short-lived intermediate which kills Gram-negative bacteria and causes the rapid leakage of K^+ and amino acids. This unidentified intermediate inhibits Δp generation by D-lactate oxidation but does not appear to increase the proton permeability of the membrane; its action may reflect a direct effect on the lactate dehydrogenase (Law & John 1981).

Other compounds

Fentichlor has been shown to inhibit energy-dependent solute uptake by dissipation of the pH gradient in *E. coli* and *Staph. aureus* (Bloomfield 1974). Similarly, cetyltrimethylammonium bromide has been shown to collapse the ΔpH of *Staph. aureus* at its bacteriostatic concentration but this concentration also caused maximal leakage of 260 nm absorbing material (Denyer & Hugo 1977) thus it is unclear as to what is primarily responsible for growth inhibition. The primary site of action of phenols is the cytoplasmic membrane (Pullman & Reynolds 1965; Hugo & Bowen 1973; Denyer *et al.* 1980) characterized by a rapid and dose-dependent leakage of K^+ (Kroll & Anagnostopoulos 1981). Some anaesthetics reach a similar target site (Silva *et al.* 1979); for instance, amytal inhibits amino acid uptake in *E. coli* but does not inhibit respiration (Boonstra *et al.* 1979). This is due to ΔpH being completely abolished although a slight reduction in $\Delta\Psi$ from 90 to 72 mV was observed.

With the phenols, however, although some uncoupling possibly occurs at low concentrations, more generalized leakage is probably primarily responsible for cell death. Chlorhexidine also induces leakage, but inhibition of the ATP-ase may also occur (Harold 1970).

Some colicins are known to increase membrane permeability by forming voltage-dependent ion channels (Davidson *et al.* 1984). Recently it has been shown that the food-grade antibiotic nisin can also depolarize bacterial membranes in a voltage-dependent fashion (Sahl *et al.* 1987) as can a cationic peptide produced by a staphylococcus (Kordel *et al.* 1988). Whether these effects are the primary mode of action of these substances is not certain and the exact nature of the mechanisms has been questioned (Kell *et al.* 1981).

Effects on solute transport

Obviously dissipation of Δp components affects several vital processes but effects on solute uptake are commonly observed with many compounds. This will often contribute substantially to growth stasis. For example, glutamate uptake in *Staph. aureus* is inhibited by DNP, tetrachlorosalicylanilide and the uptake of several amino acids by Fentichlor (Hugo 1978). DNP will inhibit galactose uptake in *E. coli* and a variety of uncouplers will inhibit the uptake of phosphate, Rb^+, K^+, alanine, glycylglycine and leucine in *Enterococcus* (*Streptococcus*) *faecalis* (Harold 1970). Hexachlorophane or decanoate at their MIC values do not affect rates of electron transport in *Bacillus subtilis* (Levin & Freese 1977) but the transport of amino acids is inhibited because the primary effect of these compounds is to destroy the Δp. The effect of long chain fatty acids has also been studied by Galbraith & Miller (1973).

Just as the transport of different solutes can be used to estimate the values of Δp, $\Delta \Psi$ or ΔpH, the uptake of these solutes will be affected in different ways by different compounds, e.g. lysine uptake will be inhibited by compounds that affect $\Delta \Psi$, while glutamate uptake is related to ΔpH and isoleucine uptake is dependent on Δp and thus will be affected differently (Hamilton 1971, 1975; Hugo 1978). It should be mentioned that some compounds may also inhibit solute uptake without directly affecting Δp. Compounds which can induce chemical changes in enzymes can often directly inhibit membrane carrier proteins (e.g. NEM, bronopol, mercuric salts). The specific inhibition of phosphotransferase systems by vinylglycollic acid and 2-hydroxy-3-butenoic acid is also known (Hugo 1978).

Conclusion

There are only a few well-documented cases where the primary mode of action of chemical antimicrobial agents is on components of the Δp (uncouplers and weak acids). It is quite possible that the primary mode of many other compounds is also on Δp components, causing an effect on Δp-dependent cell functions. These have either not been rigorously investigated yet or, for the few that have, it is difficult to ascribe the effects to primary action on Δp components. Secondary effects, or more usually general permeability increases in the membrane, often appear to be predominant.

References

AHMED, S. & BOOTH, I.R. 1983. The use of valinomycin, nigericin and trichlorocarbanilide in control of the protonmotive force in *Escherichia coli* cells. *Biochemical Journal* 212, 105–112.

BLOOMFIELD, S.F. 1974. The effect of the phenolic antibacterial agent Fentichlor on energy coupling in *Staphylococcus aureus*. *Journal of Applied Bacteriology* 37, 117–131.

BOONSTRA, J., OTTENA, S., SUPS, M.J. & KONNINGS, W. 1979. Uncoupling action of amytal in membrane vesicles from *Escherichia coli*. *European Journal of Biochemistry* 102, 383–388.

BOOTH, I.R. 1986. Regulation of cytoplasmic pH in bacteria. *Microbiological Reviews* 49, 359–378.

BOOTH, I.R. 1988. Control of proton permeability: its implications for energy transduction and pH homeostasis. In *Homeostatic Mechanisms in Micro-organisms*, ed. Whittenbury, R., Gould, G.W., Banks, J.G. & Board, R.G. pp. 1–12. Bath: Bath University Press.

BOOTH, I.R., MITCHELL, W.J. & HAMILTON, W.A. 1979. Quantitative analysis of proton linked transport systems: the lactose permease of *Escherichia coli*. *Biochemical Journal* 182, 687–696.

COLLINS, S.H. & HAMILTON, W.A. 1976. Magnitude of the protonmotive force in respiring *Staphylococcus aureus* and *Escherichia coli*. *Journal of Bacteriology* 126, 1224–1231.

DAVIDSON, V.L., BRUNDEN, K.R., CRAMER, W.A. & COHEN, F.S. 1984. Studies on the mechanism of action of channel-forming colicins using artificial membranes. *Journal of Membrane Biology* 79, 105–118.

DENYER, S.P. & HUGO, W.B. 1977. The mode of action of tetradecyltrimethyl-ammonium bromide in *Staphylococcus aureus*. *Journal of Pharmacy and Pharmacology* 29, 66–70P.

DENYER, S.P., HUGO, W.B. & WHITMAN, R.F. 1980. The antibacterial action of a series of 4-*n*-alkylphenols. *Journal of Pharmacy and Pharmacology* 32, 27P.

FELLE, H., PORTER, J.S., SLAYMAN, C.L. & KABACK, H.R. 1980. Quantitative measurements of membrane potential in *Escherichia coli*. *Biochemistry* 19, 3585–3590.

FERGUSON, S.J. 1985. Fully delocalised chemiosmotic or localised proton flow pathways in energy coupling? A scrutiny of experimental evidence. *Biochimica et Biophysica Acta* 811, 47–95.

GALBRAITH, H. & MILLER, T.B. 1973. Effect of long-chain fatty acids on bacterial respiration and amino acid uptake. *Journal of Applied Bacteriology* 73, 784–789.

GILBERT, P., BEVERIDGE, E.G. & CRONE, P.B. 1977. The lethal action of 2-phenoxyethanol and its analogues upon *Escherichia coli* NCTC 5933. *Microbios* 19, 125–141.

HAMILTON, W.A. 1971. Membrane active antibacterial compounds. In *Inhibition and Destruction of the Microbial Cell*, ed. Hugo, W.B. pp. 77–93. London: Academic Press.

HAMILTON, W.A. 1975. Energy coupling in microbial transport. *Advances in Microbial Physiology* 12, 1–53.

HARDING, Y.D., HUGO, W.B. & DENYER, S.P. 1984. An investigation into the mode of action 2-phenoxyethanol (PEA) on *Staphylococcus aureus*. *Journal of Pharmacy and Pharmacology* 36, 58P.

HAROLD, F.M. 1970. Antimicrobial agents and membrane function. *Advances in Microbial Physiology* 4, 45–104.

HAROLD, F.M. & VAN BRUNT, J. 1977. Circulation of H^+ and K^+ across the plasma membrane is not obligatory for bacterial growth. *Science, New York* 197, 372–373.

HIGGINS, C.F. & BOOTH, I.R. 1988. Molecular mechanisms of osmoregulation: an integrated homeostatic response. In *Homeostatic Mechanisms in Micro-organisms*, ed. Whittenbury, R., Gould, G.W., Banks, J.G. & Board, R.G. pp. 29–40. Bath: Bath University Press.

HUGO, W.B. 1978. Survival of microbes exposed to chemical stress. In *The Survival of Vegetative Microbes*, ed. Gray, T.R.G. & Postgate, J.R. pp. 383–413. SGM Symposium 26. Cambridge University Press.

HUGO, W.B. & BOWEN, J.G. 1973. Studies on the mode of action of 4-ethylphenol on *Escherichia coli*. *Microbios* 8, 189–197.

HUGO, W.B. & DENYER, S.P. 1983. Ionophoretic antibiotics as experimental tools in microbiology. In *Antibiotics: Assessment of Antimicrobial Activity and Resistance*, ed. Russell, A.D. & Quesnel, L.B. pp. 77–91. Society for Applied Bacteriology Technical Series No. 18. London: Academic Press.

KASHKET, E.R. 1985. The proton motive force in bacteria: a crucial assessment of methods. *Annual Review of Microbiology* 39, 219–242.

KELL, D.B., CLARKE, D.J. & MORRIS, J.G. 1981. On proton-coupled information transfer along the surface of biological membranes and the mode of action of certain colicins. *FEMS Microbiology Letters* 11, 1–11.

KORDEL, M., BENZ, R. & SAHL, H.G. 1988. Mode of action of the staphylococcin-like peptide Pep 5: Voltage-dependent depolarisation of bacterial and artificial membranes. *Journal of Bacteriology* 170, 84–88.

KREBS, H.A., WIGGINS, D., STUBBS, M., SOLS, A. & BEDOYA, F. 1983. Studies on the mechanism of the antifungal action of benzoate. *Biochemical Journal* 214, 657–663.

KROLL, R.G. & ANAGNOSTOPOULOS, G.D. 1981. Potassium leakage as a lethality index of phenol and the effect of solute and water activity. *Journal of Applied Bacteriology* 50, 139–147.

KRULWICH, T.A. & GUFFANTI, A.A. 1986. Regulation of internal pH in acidiophilic and alkalophilic bacteria. *Methods in Enzymology* 125, 352–365.

LAMBERT, P.A. 1978. Membrane-active antimicrobial agents. *Progress in Medicinal Chemistry* 15, 88–124.

LAMBERT, P.A. & HAMMOND, S.M. 1973. Potassium fluxes, first indications of membrane damage in microorganisms. *Biochemical and Biophysical Research Communications* **54**, 796−799.

LAW, B.A. & JOHN, P. 1981. Effect of the lactoperoxidase bactericidal system on the formation of the electrochemical proton gradient in *E. coli. FEMS Microbiology Letters* **10**, 67−70.

LEVIN, B. & FREESE, E. 1977. Comparison of the effects of two lipophilic acids, hexachlorophane and decanoate, on *Bacillus subtilis. Antimicrobial Agents and Chemotherapy* **12**, 357−367.

MITCHELL, P. 1973. Performance and conservation of osmotic work by proton-coupled solute porter systems. *Journal of Bioenergetics* **4**, 63−91.

NESS, I.F. & EKLUND, T. 1983. The effect of parabens on DNA, RNA and protein synthesis in *Escherichia coli* and *Bacillus subtilis. Journal of Applied Bacteriology* **54**, 237−242.

PADAN, E. & SHULDINER, S. 1986. Intracellular pH regulation in bacterial cells. *Methods in Enzymology* **125**, 337−352.

PRESSMAN, B.C. 1976. Biological applications of ionophores. *Annual Review of Biochemistry* **45**, 501−530.

PULLMAN, J.E. & REYNOLDS, B.L. 1965. Some observations on the mode of action of phenol on *Escherichia coli. Australian Journal of Pharmacy* **46**, 580−584.

RESNICK, M., SCHULDINER, S. & BERLOVIER, H. 1985. Bacterial membrane potential analyzed by spectrofluorocytometry. *Current Microbiology* **12**, 183−186.

SAHL, H.G., KORDEL, M. & BENZ, R. 1987. Voltage-dependent depolarisation of bacterial membranes and artificial lipid bilayers by the peptide antibiotic nisin. *Archives of Microbiology* **149**, 120−124.

SALMOND, C.V., KROLL, R.G. & BOOTH, I.R. 1984. The effect of food preservatives on pH homeostasis in *Escherichia coli. Journal of General Microbiology* **130**, 2845−2850.

SILVA, M.T., SOUSA, J.C.F., POLONIA, J.J. & MACEDO, P.M. 1979. Effects of local anesthetics on bacterial cells. *Journal of Bacteriology* **137**, 461−468.

SILVER, S. & WENDT, L. 1967. Mechanism of action of phenethyl alcohol: breakdown of the permeability barrier. *Journal of Bacteriology* **93**, 560−566.

SLAVIK, J. 1982. Intracellular pH of yeast cells measured with fluorescent probes. *FEBS Letters* **140**, 22−26.

STOCK, J., RAUCH, B. & ROSEMAN, S. 1977. Periplasmic space in *Salmonella typhimurium* and *Escherichia coli. Journal of Biological Chemistry* **252**, 7850−7862.

TEN BRINKS, B., OTTO, R., HANSEN, U.P. & KONNINGS, W.N. 1985. Energy recycling by lactate efflux in growing and nongrowing cells of *Streptococcus cremoris. Journal of Bacteriology* **162**, 383−390.

Studies of Inhibitors of Respiratory Electron Transport and Oxidative Phosphorylation

MARY K. PHILLIPS-JONES[1]* AND MURIEL
E. RHODES-ROBERTS[2]

[1] Department of Applied Biochemistry and Food Science, School of Agriculture,
University of Nottingham, Sutton Bonington, Loughborough, Leicestershire LE12
5RI, UK; and [2] Department of Biological Sciences, University College of Wales,
Aberystwyth, Dyfed SY23 3DA, UK

Many of the general features of electron transport-dependent ATP synthesis are similar in bacteria, mitochondria and photosynthetic systems (Racker 1970; Haddock & Jones 1977; Stouthamer 1980; Vignais *et al.* 1981). In all cases the components are arranged asymmetrically in a membrane where they catalyse redox reactions which result in a flow of reducing equivalents producing an outward translocation of protons across the membrane (Fig. 1). The precise mechanism of oxidative phosphorylation is still a matter for debate but according to Mitchell's chemiosmotic hypothesis (1966), the protonmotive force generated by proton translocation is great enough to reverse the direction of the proton-translocating ATPase which, in the presence of ADP and inorganic phosphate (P_i), results in a net synthesis of ATP (Fig. 1; Mitchell 1966). Modifications of this mechanism have been proposed including a recent one suggesting that proton translocation is localized, i.e. that the membrane contains an array of small free-energy coupling units made up of carriers and ATPase which operate as local proton microcircuits (Westerhoff *et al.* 1984; Kell 1986, 1988).

Choice of Test Organism

One of the most extensively characterized bacterial species in terms of its electron transport and energy coupling processes is *Paracoccus denitrificans* (formerly *Micrococcus denitrificans*) (John & Whatley 1977; Stouthamer 1980; Vignais *et al.* 1981). Thus it is an ideal test organism to use in studies of

---

* Present address: Department of Molecular Biology and Biotechnology, Biochemistry Section, University of Sheffield, Sheffield S10 2TN, UK.

Mechanisms of Action of
Chemical Biocides

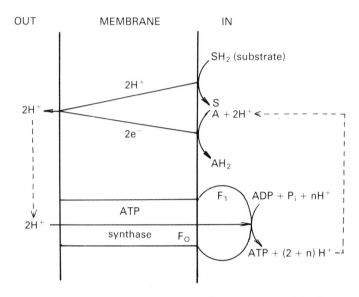

FIG. 1. Diagrammatic representation of a proton-translocating segment of the electron transport chain and ATP synthesis via a reversible ATPase, according to Mitchell (1966). Abbreviations: S, substrate (electron donor); A, electron acceptor.

potential inhibitors of respiration and oxidative phosphorylation. However, it should be borne in mind that the respiratory chain composition of this and other species such as *Escherichia coli* may be diverse, branched and variable depending on the growth conditions (Jones & Redfearn 1967; Haddock & Jones 1977; Vignais *et al.* 1981; Ferguson 1982; Ingledew & Poole 1984); however, enough similarities generally exist between *P. denitrificans* and most other species to enable the extrapolation of many observations to other organisms (Ferguson 1982). Indeed, many of the inhibitors of respiration and oxidative phosphorylation studied in *P. denitrificans* have been shown to inhibit equivalent enzymes in other species. *Paracoccus denitrificans* is an organism which is able to grow heterotrophically on a variety of carbon compounds including methanol, and also autotrophically in the presence of CO_2 and H_2 (Vignais *et al.* 1981). It is non-fermentative but will use nitrate, nitrite and nitrous oxide as terminal electron acceptors. Fig. 2 shows the respiratory chain composition of aerobic-ally grown *P. denitrificans*. It is well known that it has many features in common with its counterpart in mammalian mitochondria, and it is partly for this reason that the organism has been so intensively studied (John & Whatley 1977; Ferguson 1982). This organism is additionally useful for studies of inhibitors because membrane vesicles which exhibit respiratory control can be prepared. This feature has been of great use in determinations of P/O and, to a lesser extent, H^+/O ratios, but it is particularly desirable for the study of inhibitors of ATPase and uncouplers; this is discussed in a later section.

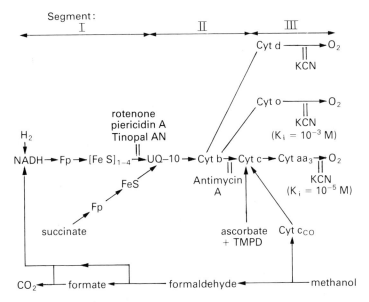

FIG. 2. The aerobic respiratory chain of *P. denitrificans*. Abbreviations: Fp, flavoprotein; FeS, iron−sulphur centre; UQ-10, ubiquinone-10; Cyt, cytochrome; TMPD, N,N,N′,N′-tetramethyl-*p*-phenylene diamine. Taken from van Verseveld (1979) and Vignais *et al.* (1981).

Maintenance of Paracoccus denitrificans

Paracoccus denitrificans NCIB 8944 can be maintained aerobically on a variety of media. We have used succinate−nitrate medium, not only to maintain the organism, but also as a growth medium for respiration experiments which are described in a later section (Burnell *et al.* 1975; Phillips & Kell 1981; Phillips *et al.* 1984). The medium contains (per l): KH_2PO_4, 0.68 g (pH 6.8 with KOH); $(NH_4)_2HPO_4$, 0.60 g (pH 6.8 with HCl); modified Hoagland trace element solution (Collins 1969), 0.1 ml; EDTA (ferric monosodium salt), 12 mg; Na_2SO_4, 54 mg; $CaCl_2.2H_2O$, 25 mg; $MgCl_2.6H_2O$, 25 mg; sodium succinate hexahydrate, 13.5 g; KNO_3, 10.1 g.

For solid medium, 15 g of agar per l is added. Stock solutions of $MgCl_2$ and $CaCl_2$ are autoclaved separately and added when cool.

Inhibitors of Respiration and Oxidative Phosphorylation

Table 1 presents a list of some of the known inhibitors of respiration and oxidative phosphorylation in *P.denitrificans*, other bacteria and mitochondria. Inhibitors of electron transport include those agents which block electron transport at specific points in the chain (Singer 1979). Rotenone and piericidin A

TABLE 1. *Inhibitors of respiration and oxidative phosphorylation in* P. denitrificans, *other bacteria and mitochondria*

Inhibitor	Site of action	Reference
Electron transport inhibitors		
Rotenone	Iron–sulphur centre N-2 of NADH dehydrogenase	Imai *et al.* (1968)
Piericidin A		Scholes & Smith (1968)
		Meijer *et al.* (1978)
		Storey (1981)
		Vignais *et al.* (1981)
Tinopal AN	After cluster N-2 of NADH dehydrogenase	Phillips & Kell (1981, 1982)
		Maguire *et al.* (1983)
Antimycin A	Cytochrome $b-c_1$	Scholes & Smith (1968)
HOQNO (2-*n*-heptyl-4-hydroxyquinoline N-oxide)		Hagihara *et al.* (1975)
		Rieske (1981)
Cyanide	Cytochrome aa_3 and o	van Verseveld & Stouthamer (1978)
		Henry & Vignais (1979)
		Poole (1983)
Uncouplers		
Generally classed as lipophilic, moderately weak acids	Generally act as proton conductors which dissipate the transmembrane protonmotive force	Harold (1970, 1972, 1977)
		Gomez-Pijou & Gomez-Lojero (1977)
		Heytler (1979, 1981)
Halo- and nitrophenols DNP (2,4-dinitrophenol)		Harold (1970, 1972, 1977)

Carbonyl cyanide phenyl hydrazones: FCCP (carbonylcyanide p-trifluoromethoxy-phenylhydrazone)		Phillips & Kell (1981)
CCCP (carbonylcyanide m-chloro-phenylhydrazone)		Heytler (1979)
Dicoumarol (3,3'-methylene bis-4-hydroxycoumarin))		Cunarro & Weiner (1975)
Salicylanilides: TCS (tetrachlorosalicylanilide)		Hamilton (1968)
S13 (2',5-dichloro-3-tert-butyl 4'-nitrosalicylanilide)		Williamson & Metcalf (1967)
Benzimidazoles: TTFB (4,5,6,7-tetrachloro-2'-trifluoromethyl-benzimidazole)		Jones & Watson (1965)
Benzylidenemalononitriles: SF6847 (3,5-di-tert-butyl-4-hydroxybenzylidene-malononitrile)		Heytler (1979)
ATPase inhibitors NBD-Cl (7-chloro-4-nitrobenzo-2-oxa-1,3-diazole)	Modification of phenolic oxygen groups of an essential tyrosine residue in F_1 subunit (mitochondrial studies)	Ferguson et al. (1974)

(continued overleaf)

TABLE 1. *(continued)*

DCCD (N, N¹-dicyclohexylcarbodiimide)	F_0 component in membrane; also F_1 subunit under certain conditions	Harold *et al.* (1969)
Chlorhexidine		Abrams & Smith (1974)
Dio 9		Haddock & Jones (1977)
Azide		Harold (1977)
Aurovertin	ATP synthesis predominantly	Linnett & Beechey (1979)
Citreoviridin		Fillingame (1981)
Oligomycin	Mainly mitochondria only	Azzi *et al.* (1984)
Quercetin		
Venturicidin		

inhibit identical sites in NADH dehydrogenase — more specifically, the iron—sulphur centre cluster N-2 which is bypassed in cells of *P.denitrificans* grown aerobically in the presence of low concentrations of rotenone (Meijer *et al.* 1978). Tinopal AN acts at a similar redox level to rotenone but at a different site, probably after cluster N-2 (Phillips & Kell 1981, 1982; Maguire *et al.* 1983). Antimycin A is a potent inhibitor of electron transport between cytochromes b and c (the concentration required to reduce respiration by 50%, the ID_{50} value, is 0.33 nmol/mg protein in membrane vesicles). 2-*n*-heptyl-4-hydroxyquinoline N-oxide (HOQNO) has a similar mode of action but is approximately 10 times less effective than antimycin A. Aerobically grown cells of *P.denitrificans* are sensitive to cyanide due to the presence of cytochrome aa_3 which acts as the major terminal electron carrier, reacting directly with oxygen to form water. However, van Verseveld & Stouthamer (1978) suggested that cytochrome o, also sensitive to cyanide, is the main terminal oxidase under autotrophic conditions (Fig. 2; for a review, see Vignais *et al.* 1981).

Uncouplers include those agents which dissociate respiration from oxidative phosphorylation by acting as proton conductors which cause proton leakage across, or into, the membrane, hence dissipating any proton gradient and resulting in membrane de-energization (see also Kroll & Patchett, this book). In practical terms, this results in a dramatic reduction in the P/O ratio to zero because there is a decrease in the amount of inorganic phosphate taken up, while respiration, and therefore oxygen consumption, continues in the presence of substrate. Thus, the term 'true uncoupler' has been applied to those agents which bring about such an effect. This distinguishes them from agents such as nigericin and valinomycin, which complex with K^+ and Na^+, and thus allow these ions to equilibrate across the membrane, and also from agents which block phosphorylation directly (ATPase inhibitors). Many true uncouplers are lipid-soluble acids and are very potent, since they are effective at concentrations significantly less than 1 μmol/l (Harold 1972; Heytler 1979; Terada 1981).

All inhibitors of the reversible proton-translocating ATPase may be defined as agents which bind to specific sites in the enzyme which are vital for catalysis (for a review, see Fillingame 1981). Some inhibit both reactions of the enzyme, that is, ATP synthesis and ATP hydrolysis, whilst others, such as aurovertin, appear to affect ATP synthesis more strongly.

Identification of Inhibitors of Respiratory Electron Transport in *P. denitrificans*

The oxygen electrode

Inhibition at any site in the respiratory electron chain will result in a block in respiration. Respiration rates are most conveniently monitored by measurement of oxygen consumption. Traditionally, manometric methods have been used (e.g. the Warburg manometer) (Umbreit *et al.* 1972), but such methods have largely been replaced by the use of the more rapid oxygen electrodes (Beechey & Ribbons 1972). There are many types of electrode available for the measurement of oxygen levels in liquid suspensions ranging from the early open models, designed for immersion in large volumes of liquid, to the coated electrodes which possess a thin layer of protective collodion to maintain rapid response times for use with small volumes of liquid. The ideal electrode for inhibitor studies is the Clark-type membrane-covered electrode (Fig. 3; Beechey & Ribbons 1972; Phillips & Kell 1981). It is convenient to use, robust and commercially available (Rank Bros, Bottisham, Cambridge; Yellow Springs Instrument Co., Ohio). It is ideal for use with small volumes of cell suspensions to which substrates, inhibitors etc. can be added in turn and the response monitored. It consists of a reaction chamber (*c.* 3 ml) with an entry port surrounded by a water jacket which can be used to control temperature. The anode and cathode of the electrode itself are separated from the reaction medium only by a thin semi-permeable membrane, (usually Teflon or poly-ethylene), through which oxygen readily diffuses into the saturated KCl electro-lyte which covers the anode and cathode. Removal of diffusion gradients which will inevitably develop in the chamber is achieved by continuous stirring of the suspension using a small magnetic stirrer and Teflon-coated follower

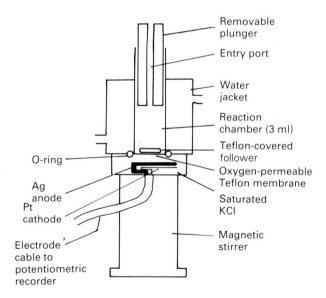

FIG. 3. A Clark-type oxygen electrode and reaction chamber – this design is similar to that of Rank Bros, Bottisham, Cambridge.

(Fig. 3). The oxygen electrode is often associated with an amplification unit and is attached to a suitable potentiometric recorder.

Calibration

Calibration of the oxygen electrode is simple since the relationship between current output and oxygen concentration is linear in most types of electrode. Hence, only two reference concentrations of oxygen are required, the most convenient being that of air-saturated buffer and that of zero oxygen. The former is easily obtained by continuous gentle agitation of the buffer using the magnetic follower which enables a maximum contact with air. Some workers prefer to remove the electrode itself or the entry port (depending on the model) to speed up the process which usually takes a few minutes. The reading on the chart recorder is then adjusted to full-scale deflection (100%), although in practice it is often set at 96% for reasons of accuracy and to check that there is no chart recorder drift. There are a number of methods available to prepare buffer solutions of zero oxygen content (Beechey & Ribbons 1972). The method described by Phillips & Kell (1981) involved the use of sodium dithionite which reacts rapidly with dissolved oxygen resulting in anaerobiosis. Addition of either 0.1 ml of a saturated solution or 1−2 mg of solid sodium dithionite per 3 ml buffer can be followed on the chart recorder which is then usually adjusted to 2% of full-scale deflection, again to be certain that there is no drift.

Determination of respiration rates in whole cells of P. denitrificans

We have used many of the methods outlined below to determine the effect of Tinopal AN on respiratory electron transport (Phillips & Kell 1981, 1982; Phillips *et al.* 1984)

Preparation of whole-cell suspensions

Cells from a mid-exponential culture of *P.denitrificans* grown aerobically at 30°C in succinate−nitrate medium (described above) were harvested at 4°C, washed twice with cold 0.1 mol/l sodium phosphate buffer (pH 7.3) containing 1 mg/ml bovine serum albumin (BSA) and resuspended in the same buffer (lacking BSA) to a final concentration of *c.* 50−100 mg dry wt/ml (McCarthy *et al.* 1981; Phillips & Kell 1981). The stock suspension was kept on ice and samples were removed for respiratory measurements in the oxygen electrode.

Reaction mixes

First, the oxygen electrode is equilibrated at 30°C with 3 ml 0.1 mol/l sodium phosphate buffer (pH 7.3) in the absence (for measurements of endogenous respiration), or the presence of exogenous substrate such as sodium succinate (10 mmol/l). The presence of succinate permits elevated rates of electron transport at the level of NADH, as well as succinate, as a result of the activity of the tricarboxylic acid (TCA) cycle enzymes. With the calibrated potentiometric recorder switched on, cell samples of *c.* 2.5–5 mg dry wt are introduced through the entry port using a microsyringe and oxygen consumption is monitored. A typical trace obtained by Phillips & Kell (1981) is shown in Fig. 4a.

Calculations

A linear trace, indicative of a constant rate of oxygen consumption (and hence respiration), should be obtained. Chart recorder units can be converted to ng atoms or nmol of oxygen, if the oxygen solubility in the buffer used at a specified temperature is known. For instance, in the case described above, the oxygen concentration in 0.1 mol/l sodium phosphate (pH 7.3) at 30°C is 470 ng atom O/ml (= 235 μM). Hence 96 recorder divisions = 470 ng atom O/ml or 1 chart unit = 5 ng atom O/ml.

Respiration rates are often expressed as ng atom O/min/mg dry wt or nmol O_2/min/mg dry wt.

For determining the oxygen content of other air-saturated buffers, measure-

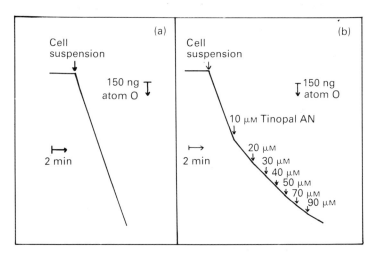

FIG. 4. Respiration of whole cells of *P. denitrificans*. Typical traces were obtained using 2.5 mg cells plus 10 mmol/l disodium succinate; (a) in the absence; and (b) in the presence of successive additions of Tinopal AN.

ment of the decrease in pO_2, caused by the oxidation by membrane vesicles of a known amount of NADH, (whose concentration may be estimated spectrophotometrically), is suitable (Chappell 1964).

Identification of inhibitors of respiratory electron transport

Addition of small amounts $(1-10\,\mu mol/l)$ of a respiratory inhibitor to actively respiring cells of *P. denitrificans* in the oxygen electrode chamber will inhibit electron transport, to a greater or lesser degree, which will result in a decrease in the overall rate of oxygen consumption. Figs 4b and 5 show the effect on respiration of the addition of modest concentrations of Tinopal AN, an inhibitor of NADH dehydrogenase in this organism (Phillips & Kell 1981, 1982).

Locating the site of action in the chain

The effect of a respiratory inhibitor on electron flow through each of the three segments of the electron transport chain (Fig. 2) may be investigated using cytoplasmic membrane vesicle preparations of the organism. Such vesicles lack the cytoplasmic contents of intact cells and no electron transport due to endogenous respiration can therefore occur. Thus, suitable electron donors can be added to vesicle preparations to drive electron transport through selected segments of the chain: e.g. addition of NADH will mediate electron flow through all three segments, while succinate (in the presence of rotenone) allows electron flow only through segments II and III, and artificial electron

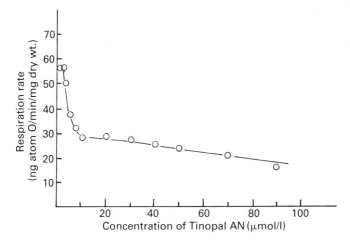

FIG. 5. Inhibition of respiration of intact cells of *P. denitrificans* by Tinopal AN.

donors such as ascorbate in the presence of N,N,N',N'-tetramethyl-*p*-phenylenediamine (TMPD) can be used, in the presence of a segment II inhibitor such as antimycin A, to monitor electron flow through segment III only.

Preparation of cytoplasmic membrane vesicles

Since some of the electron donors used in such studies cannot permeate the cytoplasmic membrane, it is necessary to prepare vesicles which are inside-out relative to the original orientation of the membrane: these are obtained when cells are lysed using lysozyme and exposed to a hypotonic medium. The cytoplasmic membrane bursts and the membrane fragments reform themselves into vesicles of which *c.* 80% are inside-out.

The following method is that of Burnell *et al.* (1975) with modifications by John (1977) and was used by Phillips & Kell (1981) and Phillips (1983) to prepare inside-out vesicles of *P. denitrificans*. Cells from a mid-exponential culture (absorbance at 550 nm of 1.7−1.9) of *P. denitrificans*, grown anaerobically in 2 l of succinate−nitrate medium, are harvested by centrifugation at 5000 *g* for 30 min. Hereafter, all operations, except the lysozyme treatment, must be carried out at 4°C. The cells are washed once in 800 ml 150 mmol/l NaCl containing 10 mmol/l Tris-HCl (pH 7.3) and are resuspended in 400 ml 0.5 mol/l sucrose containing 10 mmol/l Tris-HCl (pH 7.3) so that a 0.1-ml sample of this suspension, when diluted to 2.5 ml with water, has an absorbance at 550 nm of 0.3 (25 mg wet wt cells/ml). Lysozyme is then added at a final concentration of 250 µg/ml, and the suspension is incubated at 30°C for 20−30 min, or until the absorbance of a sample, diluted 1:25 with water, decreases from 0.3 to < 0.05. The protoplasts are then harvested by centrifuging at 40 000 *g* for 10 min and are resuspended in 40 ml of 100 mmol/l Tris-acetate buffer containing 10 mmol/l disodium ATP, with a Potter−Elvehjem homogenizer. Vesicle preparation is now achieved by gently pouring the suspension into 360 ml distilled water to disrupt the protoplasts. After incubation for 20 min, 2 mmol/l magnesium acetate and a trace of deoxyribonuclease are added to digest the released DNA. When the viscosity of the suspension is sufficiently low, the vesicles are harvested by centrifugation at 40 000 *g* for 40 min. The upper (red) layer of the double-layered pellet is kept and resuspended in 400 ml 10 mmol/l Tris-acetate (pH 7.3) containing 1 mmol/l magnesium acetate. The lower (white) layer of poly-β-hydroxybutyrate is discarded. Finally, the vesicle suspension is harvested by centrifugation (40 000 *g* for 40 min) and resuspended in 10 mmol/l Tris-acetate (pH 7.3) containing 1 mmol/l magnesium acetate (vital for membrane stability) to a concentration of *c.* 5−10 mg protein/ml (*c.* 5−10 ml). If stored at 4°C, vesicle preparations will remain stable for up to 3 days after preparation in terms of phosphorylation, but for studies of electron transport, may be used over a much longer period.

Vesicle experiments

To locate the site of inhibition of respiration and to determine whether it is a consequence of a direct block in electron transfer, membrane vesicles of *P. denitrificans* are prepared as above. As described by Phillips & Kell (1981), who investigated the respiratory site of action of Tinopal AN, respiration rates through segment III, through segments II and III or through all three segments of the chain of such vesicles, may be monitored in turn by means of the oxygen electrode. In each of these three cases, the 3-ml reaction mixes contain 0.1 mol/l sodium phosphate buffer (pH 7.3) at 30°C, 5 mmol/l magnesium acetate and 1 mg vesicle protein which is added last. For electron flow through only segment III (comprising cytochrome oxidase), 5 mmol/l sodium D-*iso*ascorbate in the presence of 0.1 mmol/l TMPD hydrochloride is added as an artificial electron donor system, and antimycin A is added to a final concentration of 1 µmol/l to block any residual electron flow due to trace amounts of any other electron donors. When the vesicles have been added and a steady respiration rate has been achieved, the inhibitor under test is added. Only inhibitors of cytochrome c oxidase will cause an immediate inhibition of respiration. Hence, for example, addition of a segment I inhibitor such as Tinopal AN will have no effect (Fig. 6c). Electron flow through segments II and III (from ubiquinone-10) can be investigated with a reaction mixture containing 10 mmol/l disodium succinate as electron donor plus 1 µmol/l rotenone to block any residual electron flow from NADH. The addition of segment II inhibitors such as antimycin A (or a segment III inhibitor) will result in an immediate decrease in the respiration rate whereas the addition of a segment I inhibitor, such as Tinopal AN (Fig. 6b), will again have no effect. Any inhibitor of NADH dehydrogenase (segment I) can now be identified by using a fresh reaction mix, this time containing NADH as substrate. This is achieved by the addition of 1% (v/v) ethanol, 50 µg alcohol dehydrogenase and 0.6 mmol/l NAD$^+$. The NADH-generating mixture is used because NADH, as received, is usually rather impure, and may contain inhibitors of NADH-requiring enzymes. Addition of a segment I inhibitor will cause an immediate inhibition of respiration under these conditions (e.g. Tinopal AN, Fig. 6a; Phillips & Kell 1981).

The vesicle experiments described above will identify inhibitors of NADH dehydrogenase since this is the only enzyme carrier present in segment I. In the other two segments, an inhibited enzyme is more difficult to locate since there are more carriers present (Fig. 2). For example, segment II respiration is inhibited by the succinate dehydrogenase inhibitors thenoyltrifluoroacetone

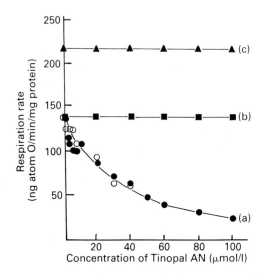

Fig. 6. Effect of Tinopal AN on the respiration rate for three segments of the respiratory chain of cytoplasmic membrane vesicles of *P. denitrificans*. When NADH was the substrate (a) either 0.5 mg (○) or 1 mg (●) membrane vesicle protein was present. Other substrates used were (b) 10 mmol/l disodium succinate in the presence of 1 μmol/l rotenone (■) or (c) 5 mmol/l sodium-D-*iso*ascorbate plus 0.1 mmol/l TMPD hydrochloride in the presence of 1 μmol/l antimycin A (▲) with 1 mg vesicle protein.

and carboxanilide fungicides as well as by antimycin A in such experiments (Ramsay *et al.* 1981). When the *segment* of inhibition has been established, the precise enzyme affected is usually identified by monitoring the effect of the inhibitor on individual enzyme activities. This is conveniently achieved by measuring electron flow at the appropriate redox level in cell extracts using artificial electron donors and acceptors. In the case of succinate dehydrogenase, this can be done using phenazine ethosulphate in the presence of 2,6-dichlorophenolindophenol (Ackrell *et al.* 1980). For an account of appropriate electron donors and acceptors for assays of other oxidoreductase enzymes, see Fleischer & Packer (1978).

Inhibition at the same site as other respiratory inhibitors

Growth studies with segment I inhibitors

The addition of rotenone to log-phase cells of *P. denitrificans*, grown aerobically in succinate-containing media, results in an immediate cessation of growth due to inhibition of electron transport through iron−sulphur centre N-2 of

NADH dehydrogenase (Meijer *et al.* 1978; Phillips & Kell 1982). However, after *c.* 1−2 h, growth is restored to a rate which is *c.* 40% of that before the rotenone addition (Fig. 7). This was shown by electron paramagnetic resonance spectroscopy to be due either to a loss or modification of the rotenone-sensitive centre N-2 which leads to a 'short circuit' of this energy-coupled segment, or to a replacement with a non-phosphorylating, rotenone-insensitive NADH dehydrogenase (Meijer *et al.* 1978). In either case, the result is that electron transport, and hence respiration, recommences albeit with only two sites available for phosphorylation, and that cells are now insensitive to rotenone. Other inhibitors of centre N-2 such as piericidin A will also have no effect upon the respiration of such cells. These observations were used by Phillips & Kell (1982) to show that Tinopal AN, an inhibitor of NADH dehydrogenase, did not act at the same site as rotenone. Cells of *P. denitrificans* were grown aerobically in the succinate−nitrate medium (500 ml) described above at 30°C. When the cells reached early exponential phase, a 100-ml sample was withdrawn (sample 1, Fig. 7), harvested by centrifugation, and washed in preparation for respiration measurements with the oxygen electrode as described previously. When the culture reached early-mid exponential phase, 50 µmol/l rotenone (212 nmol/mg dry wt cells) was added to the remaining 400 ml, causing an immediate cessation of growth (Fig. 7). After 1.75 h, growth resumed

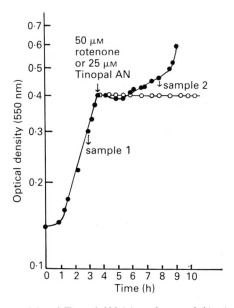

FIG. 7. Effect of rotenone (●) and Tinopal AN (○) on the growth kinetics of *P. denitrificans*.

at *c.* 40% of the rate obtained prior to rotenone addition. A further 100-ml cell sample was taken (sample 2, Fig. 7) and treated as described previously for respiration measurements. The effect of either rotenone or Tinopal AN on the respiration of the two cell samples (one containing rotenone-sensitive cells and the other containing rotenone-insensitive cells) was monitored using the oxygen electrode. As expected, the addition of rotenone to sample 1 (rotenone-sensitive) cells resulted in a marked inhibition in respiration but had no effect on the rotenone-insensitive cells of sample 2 (Fig. 8). Also as expected, the addition of Tinopal AN to the rotenone-sensitive cells caused an inhibition of respiration. However, addition of Tinopal AN to cells unaffected by rotenone, caused a marked inhibition of respiration, showing that Tinopal AN did not share the same binding site in NADH dehydrogenase. In fact, the respiration of rotenone-insensitive cells was even more sensitive to Tinopal AN than that of rotenone-sensitive cells indicating that the removal or modification of the rotenone-sensitive binding site may render the Tinopal AN binding site more accessible to Tinopal AN (Fig. 8; Phillips & Kell 1982).

The use of radio-labelled inhibitors

Competition experiments between the inhibitor under test and a radio-labelled known inhibitor can be carried out to determine whether they share the same

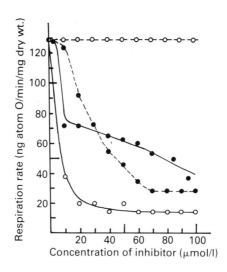

FIG. 8. Effect of Tinopal AN (———) and of rotenone (---) on the respiration of rotenone-sensitive (●) and of rotenone-insensitive (○) cells of *P. denitrificans.*

binding site. Either whole cells or membrane vesicles can be used. However, care must be taken to ensure that any non-specific binding by the labelled inhibitor is reduced: e.g. washing procedures to remove non-specifically bound rotenone are carried out in the presence of 2% (w/v) BSA (Horgan *et al.* 1968). Such experiments have determined whether amytal and piericidin A act at the same site as rotenone in submitochondrial particles (Horgan *et al.* 1968). Aliquots of particles (25 mg) were treated with various amounts of radiolabelled rotenone up to 25 nmol. After extensive washing of each sample with 0.25 mol/l sucrose, 0.025 mol/l sodium phosphate (pH 7.4) containing 2% (w/v) BSA, the amount of bound radiolabel (and hence the amount of bound rotenone) remaining was determined. To investigate the effect of the addition of amytal and piericidin A on the amount of rotenone binding, the experiment was repeated but this time the unlabelled inhibitors were added before the addition of radiolabelled rotenone. A sharp drop in rotenone binding was observed under these conditions, implying that these inhibitors bind to the same site as rotenone (Horgan *et al.* 1968).

Identification of Inhibitors of Oxidative Phosphorylation

Uncouplers

True uncouplers of oxidative phosphorylation uncouple electron transport from ATP synthesis by de-energization of the membrane, dissipating the proton gradient across or in the membrane (John & Whatley 1977; Terada 1981). In whole cells or membrane vesicles of *P. denitrificans*, which exhibit respiratory control, this usually results in a stimulation of the respiration rate as respiratory control is lost. Other effects include the suppression of both ATP synthesis and active transport of ions. The increased respiration rate can be monitored using the oxygen electrode with membrane vesicles of *P. denitrificans* and NADH as substrate as described below and by John & Whatley (1977). They carried out their experiments over a wide range of pH values to show that a true uncoupler induces respiratory stimulation over a wide pH range, hence eliminating the possibility that the transmembrane pH equilibration, which accompanies the action of true uncouplers, is not itself affecting the kinetics of electron transport in some way. For this purpose, they used a 3-ml reaction mix containing 10 mmol/l Tris-phosphate buffer adjusted to various pH values, 5 mmol/l magnesium acetate, 30 μl ethanol, 0.3 mg alcohol dehydrogenase, 0.6 mmol/l NAD^+ and membrane particles (0.08–0.12 mg membrane protein). Respiration rates were monitored at 30°C before the addition of 1–10 μmol/l uncoupler: the results are shown in Fig. 9. The amount of uncoupler added is important, as high levels may inhibit respiration. Thus, respiratory release data can be misleading if the critical range of

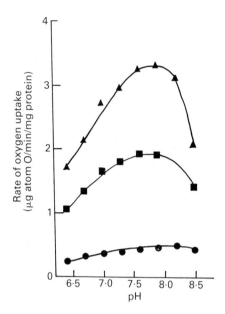

FIG. 9. Effect of pH on respiratory control in *P. denitrificans* vesicles. NADH was used as substrate, in the absence of uncouplers (●), in the presence of 10 μmol/l FCCP (■), and in the presence of 0.3 μg/ml gramicidin D + 15 mmol/l ammonium acetate (▲). (Reproduced from John & Whatley 1977 with permission from Elsevier.)

concentrations is exceeded (Heytler 1979). The importance of concentration has also been recognized for biocide testing and is discussed by Denyer (1989).

Strictly, a true uncoupler is an agent which is able to reduce P/O ratios to zero. Since measurements of P/O ratios are time-consuming, measurements of inhibition of ATP synthesis (by net Pi uptake and ^{32}P-ATP exchange) are often undertaken in addition to the respiratory stimulation experiments described above (Heytler 1979).

Proton-translocating ATPases

Inhibitors of the proton-translocating ATPase can be broadly divided into two main groups – those that interact directly with the ATPase molecules and those that react with other membrane components of the enzyme complex (Linnett & Beechey 1979). In both cases, the effect of such inhibitors is, in general, to inhibit both the synthesis and the hydrolysis of ATP by this reversible enzyme. ATPase inhibitors abolish ADP-stimulated respiration in vesicles of *P. denitrificans*, usually without significantly affecting the respiration rate observed prior to ADP addition. Studies by Ferguson *et al.* (1974) showed the effect of 7-chloro-4-nitrobenzo-2-oxa-1, 3-diazole (NBD-Cl) on the respiration rates in *P. denitrificans*. Vesicles (1.8 mg protein/ml) were pre-incubated in 50 mmol/l Tris-acetate (pH 8.0) for 20 min at 20°C in the presence or absence of 0.2 mmol/l NBD-Cl. Respiration rates were then monitored with the oxygen electrode in a 3-ml reaction mixture of 0.1-ml vesicle sample, 10 mmol/l Tris-phosphate (pH 7.3), 5 mmol/l magnesium acetate, 0.2 mg yeast alcohol dehydrogenase, 30 µl ethanol, and 0.6 mmol/l NAD$^+$, in the presence or absence of 0.2 mmol/l ADP used to stimulate respiration. The NAD$^+$ was added to start the reaction: NBD-Cl, an inhibitor of ATPase, abolished any stimulation of respiration by ADP (Ferguson *et al.* 1974). Confirmation that this agent was indeed an ATPase inhibitor was sought by measuring levels of liberated phosphate produced as a result of ATP hydrolysis. Again the vesicles (1.8 mg protein/ml) were pre-incubated in the presence or absence of inhibitor under the conditions described above. After 20 min at 20°C, ATPase activity was assessed by measuring the amount of phosphate released in an assay medium containing 5 mmol/l ATP, 5 mmol/l magnesium chloride, 20 mmol/l Tris-acetate, and 150 mmol/l sodium bicarbonate (pH 8.0). The presence of sodium bicarbonate has been found to stimulate ATPase activity although the reason for this is not understood. The amount of phosphate liberated was determined by the method of Fiske & Subbarow (1925). By using this approach Ferguson *et al.* (1974) showed that NBD-Cl markedly decreased the amount of P$_i$ liberated due to ATP hydrolysis and therefore concluded that this agent was indeed a true inhibitor of ATPase.

Acknowledgement

We thank Dr D.B. Kell and Professor W.M. Waites for helpful discussions and critical reading of the manuscript.

References

ABRAMS, A. & SMITH, J.B. 1974. Bacterial membrane ATPase. In *The Enzymes*, 3rd edn, Vol. X, ed. Boyer, P.D. pp. 395–429. London: Academic Press.

ACKRELL, B.A.C., BALL, M.B. & KEARNEY, E.B. 1980. Peptides from complex II active in reconstitution of succinate–ubiquinone reductase. *Journal of Biological Chemistry* **255**, 2761–2769.

AZZI, A., CASEY, R.P. & NALECZ, M.J. 1984. The effect of dicyclohexyl-carbodiimide on enzymes of bioenergetic relevance. *Biochimica et Biophysica Acta* **768**, 209–226.

BEECHEY, R.B. & RIBBONS, D.W. 1972. Oxygen electrode measurements. In *Methods in Microbiology*, Vol. 6B, ed. Norris, J.R. & Ribbons, D.W. pp. 25–54. London: Academic Press.

BURNELL, J.N., JOHN, P. & WHATLEY, F.R. 1975. The reversibility of active sulphate transport in membrane vesicles of *Paracoccus denitrificans*. *Biochemical Journal* **150**, 527–536.

CHAPPELL, J.B. 1964. The oxidation of citrate, *iso*citrate and *cis*-aconitate by isolated mitochondria. *Biochemical Journal* **90**, 225–236.

COLLINS, V.G. 1969. Isolation, cultivation and maintenance of autotrophs. In *Methods in Microbiology*, Vol. 3B, ed. Norris, J.R. & Ribbons, D.W. pp. 1–52. London: Academic Press.

CUNNARO, J. & WEINER, W.M. 1975. Mechanism of action of agents which uncoupled oxidative phosphorylation: direct correlation between proton-carrying and respiratory-releasing properties using rat liver mitochondria. *Biochimica et Biophysica Acta* **387**, 234–240.

DENYER, S.P. 1989. ATP bioluminescence and biocide assessment: effect of bacteriostatic levels of biocide. In: *ATP Luminescence: Rapid Methods in Microbiology*, SAB Technical Series 26, eds Stanley, P.E., McCarthy, B.J. & Smither, R. pp. 189–195. Oxford: Blackwell Scientific Publications.

FERGUSON, S.J. 1982. Aspects of the control and organisation of bacterial electron transport. *Biochemical Society Transactions* **10**, 198–200.

FERGUSON, S.J., JOHN, P., LLOYD, W.J., RADDA, G.K. & WHATLEY, F.R. 1974. Selective and reversible inhibition of the ATPase of *Micrococcus denitrificans* by 7-chloro-4-nitrobenzo-2-oxa-1,3-diazole. *Biochimica et Biophysica Acta* **357**, 457–461.

FILLINGAME, R.H. 1981. Biochemistry and genetics of bacterial H^+-translocating ATPases. *Current Topics in Bioenergetics* **11**, 35–106.

FISKE, C.H. & SUBBAROW, Y. 1925. The colorimetric determination of phosphorus. *Journal of Biological Chemistry* **66**, 375–400.

FLEISCHER, F.S. & PACKER, P.L. (eds) 1978. *Methods in Enzymology*, Vol. LIII, *Biomembranes*. Part D, *Biological Oxidations: Mitochondrial and Microbial Systems*. London: Academic Press.

GOMEZ-PIJOU, A. & GOMEZ-LOJERO, C. 1977. The use of ionophores and channel formers in the study of the function of biological membranes. *Current Topics in Bioenergetics* **6**, 222–251.

HADDOCK, B.A. & JONES, C.W. 1977. Bacterial respiration. *Bacteriological Reviews* **41**, 47–99.

HAGIHARA, B., SATO, N. & YAMANAKA, T. 1975. Type b cytochromes. In *The Enzymes*, 3rd edn, Vol. XI, ed. Boyer, P.D. pp. 549–593. London: Academic Press.

HAMILTON, W.A. 1968. The mechanism of the bacteriostatic action of tetrachlorsalicylanilide. *Journal of General Microbiology* **50**, 441–458.

HAROLD, F.M. 1970. Antimicrobial agents and membrane function. *Advances in Microbial Physiology* **4**, 45–104.

HAROLD, F.M. 1972. Conservation and transformation of energy by bacterial membranes. *Bacteriological Reviews* **36**, 172–230.

HAROLD, F.M. 1977. Membranes and energy transduction in bacteria. *Current Topics in Bioenergetics* **6**, 84–139.

HAROLD, F.M., BAARDA, J.R., BARON, J.C. & ABRAMS, A. 1969. Dio 9 and chlorhexidine: inhibitors of membrane bound ATPase and of cation transport in *Streptococcus faecalis*. *Biochimica et Biophysica Acta* **183**, 129–136.

HENRY, M.F. & VIGNAIS, P.M. 1979. Induction by cyanide of cytochrome d in the plasma membrane of *Paracoccus denitrificans*. *FEBS Letters* **100**, 41–46.

HEYTLER, P.G. 1979. Uncouplers of oxidative phosphorylation. In *Methods in Enzymology*, Vol. LV, *Biomembranes*, Part F, *Bioenergetics: Oxidative Phosphorylation*, ed. Fleischer, F.S. & Packer, P.L. pp. 462–472. London: Academic Press.

HEYTLER, P.G. 1981. Uncouplers of oxidative phosphorylation. In *Inhibitors of Mitochondrial Functions, International Encyclopedia of Pharmacology & Therapeutics*, Section 107, ed. Erecinska, M. & Wilson, D.F. pp. 199–210. Oxford: Pergamon Press.

HORGAN, D.J., SINGER, T.P. & CASIDA, J.E. 1968. Studies on the respiratory chain-linked reduced nicotinamide adenine dinucleotide dehydrogenase. *Journal of Biological Chemistry* **243**, 834–843.

IMAI, K., ASANO, A. & SATO, R. 1968. Oxidative phosphorylation in *Micrococcus denitrificans*. *Journal of Biochemistry* **63**, 207–218.

INGLEDEW, W.J. & POOLE, R.K. 1984. The respiratory chains of *Escherichia coli*. *Microbiological Reviews* **48**, 222–271.

JOHN, P. 1977. Aerobic and anaerobic bacterial respiration monitored by electrodes. *Journal of General Microbiology* **98**, 231–238.

JOHN, P. & WHATLEY, F.R. 1977. The bioenergetics of *Paracoccus denitrificans*. *Biochimica et Biophysica Acta* **463**, 129–153.

JONES, C.W. & REDFEARN, E.R. 1967. The cytochrome system of *Azotobacter vinelandii*. *Biochimica et Biophysica Acta* **143**, 340–353.

JONES, O.T.G. & WATSON, W.A. 1965. Activation of 2-trifluoromethyl-benzimidazoles as uncouplers of oxidative phosphorylation. *Nature, London* **208**, 1169–1170.

KELL, D.B. 1986. Localized protonic coupling: overview and critical evaluation of techniques. In *Methods in Enzymology*, Vol. 127, *Biomembranes*, Part 0, *Protons and Water: Structure and Translocation*, ed. Packer, P.L. pp. 538–557. London: Academic Press.

KELL, D.B. 1988. Protonmotive energy-transducing systems: some physical principles and experimental approaches. In *Bacterial Energy Transduction*, ed. Anthony, C.D. pp. 429–490. London: Academic Press.

LINNETT, P.E. & BEECHEY, R.B. 1979. Inhibitors of the ATPase synthetase system. In *Methods in Enzymology*, Vol. LV, *Biomembranes*, Part F, *Bioenergetics: Oxidative Phosphorylation*, ed. Fleischer, F.S. & Packer, P.L. pp. 472–518. London: Academic Press.

McCARTHY, J.E.G., FERGUSON, S.J. & KELL, D.B. 1981. Estimation with an ion-selective electrode of the membrane potential in cells of *Paracoccus denitrificans* from the uptake of the butyltriphenyl phosphonium cation during aerobic and anaerobic respiration. *Biochemical Journal* **196**, 311–321.

MAGUIRE, J.J., HARTZOG, G.A. & PACKER, L. 1983. Action of Tinopal AN, a complex I inhibitor, on submitochondrial particles. *Biophysical Journal* **41**, 325a.

MEIJER, E.M., SCHUITENMAKER, M.G., BOOGERD, F.C., WEVER, R. & STOUTHAMER, A.H. 1978. Effects induced by rotenone during aerobic growth of *Paracoccus denitrificans* in continuous culture. *Archives of Microbiology* **119**, 119–127.

MITCHELL, P. 1966. Chemiosmotic coupling in oxidative and photosynthetic phosphorylation. *Biological Reviews, Cambridge* **41**, 445–502.

PHILLIPS, M.K. 1983. The differentiation of phytopathogenic and saprophytic bacteria especially *Pseudomonas* spp. *PhD thesis*, University College of Wales, Aberystwyth.

PHILLIPS, M.K. & KELL, D.B. 1981. A benzoxazole inhibitor of NADH dehydrogenase in *Paracoccus denitrificans*. *FEMS Microbiology Letters* **11**, 111–113.

PHILLIPS, M.K. & KELL, D.B. 1982. A novel inhibitor of NADH dehydrogenase in *Paracoccus denitrificans*. *FEBS Letters* **140**, 248–250.

PHILLIPS, M.K., KELL, D.B. & RHODES-ROBERTS, M.E. 1984. The antibacterial action of Tinopal AN. *Journal of General Microbiology* **130**, 1999–2005.

POOLE, R.K. 1983. Bacterial cytochrome oxidase. *Biochimica et Biophysica Acta* **726**, 205–243.

RACKER, E. 1970. Function and structure of the inner membrane of mitochondria and chloroplasts. In *Membranes of Mitochondria and Chloroplasts*, ed. Racker, E. pp. 127–171. New York: van Nostrand Reinhold Co.

RAMSAY, A.R., ACKRELL, B.A.C., COLES, C.J., SINGER, T.P., WHITE, G.A. & THORN, G.D. 1981. Reaction site of carboxanilides and of thenoyltrifluoroacetone in complex II. *Proceedings of the National Academy of Sciences, USA* **78**, 825–828.

RIESKE, J.S. 1981. Inhibitors of respiration at energy-coupling site 2 of the respiratory chain. In *Inhibitors of Mitochondrial Functions, International Encyclopedia of Pharmacology & Therapeutics*,

Section 107, ed. Erecinska, M. & Wilson, D.F. pp. 109–144. Oxford: Pergamon Press.

SCHOLES, P.B. & SMITH, L. 1968. Composition and properties of the membrane-bound respiratory chain system of *Micrococcus denitrificans*. *Biochimica et Biophysica Acta* **153**, 363–375.

SINGER, T.P. 1979. Mitochondrial electron-transport inhibitors. In *Methods in Enzymology*, Vol. LV, *Biomembranes*, Part F, *Bioenergetics: Oxidative Phosphorylation*, ed. Fleischer, F.S. & Packer, P.L. pp. 454–462. London: Academic Press.

STOREY, B.T. 1981. Inhibitors of energy-coupling site I of the mitochondrial functions. In *Inhibitors of Mitochondrial Functions, International Encyclopedia of Pharmacology & Therapeutics*, Section 107, ed. Erecinska, M. & Wilson, D.F. pp. 101–108. Oxford: Pergamon Press.

STOUTHAMER, A.H. 1980. Bioenergetic studies on *Paracoccus denitrificans*. *Trends in Biochemical Sciences* **5**, 164–166.

TERADA, H. 1981. The interaction of highly active uncouplers with mitochondria. *Biochimica et Biophysica Acta* **639**, 225–242.

UMBREIT, W.W., BURRIS, R.H. & STAUFFER, J.F. 1972. *Manometric and Biochemical Techniques*, 5th edn. Minneapolis: Burgess Publishing Co.

VAN VERSEVELD, H.W. 1979. Influence of environmental factors on the efficiency of energy conservation in *Paracoccus denitrificans*. *PhD thesis*, University of Amsterdam.

VAN VERSEVELD, H.W. & STOUTHAMER, A.H. 1978. Electron transport chain and coupled oxidative phosphorylation in methanol-grown *Paracoccus denitrificans*. *Archives of Microbiology* **118**, 13–20.

VIGNAIS, P.M., HENRY, M-F., SIM, E. & KELL, D.B. 1981. The electron transport system and hydrogenase of *Paracoccus denitrificans*. *Current Topics in Bioenergetics* **12**, 115–196.

WESTERHOFF, H.V., MELANDRI, A., VENTUROLL, G., AZZONE, G.F. & KELL, D.B. 1984. A minimal hypothesis for membrane-linked free-energy transduction. The role of independent small coupling units. *Biochimica et Biophysica Acta* **768**, 257–292.

WILLIAMSON, R.L. & METCALF, R.L. 1967. Salicylanilides: a new group of active uncouplers of oxidative phosphorylation. *Science, New York* **158**, 1694–1695.

Effect of Biocides on DNA, RNA and Protein Synthesis

T. EKLUND[1] AND I.F. NES[2]

[1] Norwegian Dairies Association, POB 9051 Vaterland, N-0134 Oslo 1, Norway; and [2] Laboratory of Microbial Gene Technology NLVF, POB 51, N-1432, ÅS-NLH, Norway

The desired effect of chemical preservatives is to inhibit the growth of unwanted micro-organisms. Growth inhibition can, in principle, be caused by inactivation of, or interference with, one or more of the following subcellular target groups (Eklund 1989): cell wall; cell membrane; metabolic enzymes; protein synthesis system; genetic material.

This chapter will concentrate on methods to test the effectiveness of biocides acting on protein synthesis and on RNA and DNA synthesis in bacteria, as illustrated here by a study of the paraben preservatives (alkyl esters of p-hydroxybenzoic acid; Nes & Eklund 1983). In addition, the action of the food preservatives benzoic, propionic and sorbic acid have been partly tested on the synthesis systems described, as has the action of the antioxidants butylated hydroxyanisole (BHA) and butylated hydroxytoluene (BHT), both substances having antimicrobial as well as antioxidative properties (Davidson 1983). The effect of organic acids and esters on other subcellular targets has been reviewed elsewhere (Eklund 1989).

While reports on the action of food preservatives on enzyme and membrane processes are abundant, evidence of the direct effect of preservatives on the protein synthesis system is limited to the action of parabens on bacteria (Nes & Eklund 1983). Similarly, only limited knowledge about direct interference with genetic material exists, referring to the action of weak acids on fungi and to the action of parabens on bacteria (Nes & Eklund 1983).

Two tools are described in this paper as methods to determine the preservative inhibition of RNA, DNA and protein synthesis as isolated processes in bacteria. DNA and RNA synthesis has been studied in *Escherichia coli* and *Bacillus subtilis* cells permeabilized by toluene (Matsushita *et al.* 1971; Peterson *et al.* 1971; Moses 1974). This permeabilized system is unsuitable for protein synthesis studies, since toluene destroys the protein synthesizing apparatus. Instead, the well-established cell-free protein synthesis test system (S-30

Mechanisms of Action of
Chemical Biocides

fraction) was used (Nirenberg & Matthaei 1961; Nirenberg 1963; Hirashima *et al.* 1967; Doi 1971).

Experimental Methods

Bacterial strains, growth media and buffers

Bacillus subtilis ATCC 6633 was from the American Type Culture Collection, while *E. coli* ML 308−255 was donated by Dr W. Konings, University of Groningen, The Netherlands. *Escherichia coli* was grown in a medium with the following composition (g/l): KH_2PO_4, 3; K_2HPO_4, 7; sodium citrate. $3H_2O$, 0.5; $MgSO_4.7H_2O$, 0.1; $(NH_4)_2SO_4$, 1; yeast extract, 1; glucose, 5. *Bacillus subtilis* was grown in a medium which contained (g/l): tryptone, 8; NaCl, 5; KCl, 1.9.

The composition of the two buffers employed is as follows: Buffer 1, 50 mmol/l potassium phosphate (pH 7.4); Buffer 2, 20 mmol/l Tris-HCl (pH 7.8); 14 mmol/l $MgCl_2$; 60 mmol/l KCl; 6 mmol/l 2-mercaptoethanol.

DNA and RNA synthesis in toluene-treated cells

Preparation of the cells

The bacteria were grown at 37°C in 100 ml medium in 500-ml Erlenmeyer flasks on a reciprocal shaker. After reaching a concentration of *c.* 5×10^8 cells/ml ($A^{1cm}_{620nm} = 1$, Beckman Model 25 spectrophotometer), the cultures were harvested by centrifugation at 10 000 rev/min in a Sorvall centrifuge (SS-34 rotor) for 10 min at 4°C. The pellet was washed twice with 4 ml of Buffer 1 and resuspended in 7.5 ml of the same buffer. This suspension was transferred to a 100-ml Erlenmeyer flask, 0.075 ml toluene was added, and the flask was gently shaken on a reciprocal shaker for 10 min at 25°C. Thus permeabilized, the toluene-treated cells were rapidly collected by centrifugation (as above, but at 5000 rev/min) and the pellet was thoroughly washed with Buffer 1 to remove traces of toluene. The treated cells were then stored in Buffer 1 at a concentration of $5-10 \times 10^9$ cells/ml in thin-walled plastic vials in liquid nitrogen until required for use.

Assay for DNA synthesis

The assays were performed in 100-μl aliquots in 15-ml glass tubes and gently shaken at 37°C on a reciprocal shaker.

The reaction mixture for DNA synthesis in toluene-treated cells of *E. coli* and *B. subtilis* contained (final concentrations): 67 mmol/l potassium phosphate (pH 7.4); 13.3 mmol/l $MgCl_2$; 10 mmol/l 2-mercaptoethanol; 1.3 mmol/l adenosine 5'-triphosphate (ATP); 33 μmol/l each of 2'-deoxyguanosine 5'-triphosphate (dGTP), 2'-deoxycytidine 5'-triphosphate (dCTP), 2'-deoxyadenosine 5'-triphosphate (dATP) and 2'-deoxythymidine 5'-triphosphate (dTTP), with dTTP as the radioactive substance (^{3}H-methyl-dTTP, specific activity 3.7−18.5 MBq/μmol).

To the reaction mixture were added toluene-treated cells to a final concentration of $1-2 \times 10^8$ cells/ml, and preservatives dissolved either in dimethylsulphoxide (DMSO) (parabens, BHA, BHT) or water (potassium sorbate, sodium propionate, sodium benzoate). Where DMSO was used, the final concentration in the assay mixture was 2.5%, and the same concentration of DMSO was then included in the control. The final volume of the reaction mixture was 250 μl and the mixture was incubated for 30 min at 37°C.

The reaction was stopped by the addition of 5 ml 10% ice-cold trichloroacetic acid (TCA), and the precipitated material thus formed was collected by filtering the mixture through a Whatman GF/C (2.4 cm) glass-fibre filter, subsequently washing three times with 5 ml cold TCA. The filter was dried at 60°C in a vacuum oven, and the radioactivity was determined by scintillation counting, using a standard toluene-based scintillation liquid.

Assay for RNA synthesis

The standard mixture for measuring RNA synthesis in toluene-treated *E. coli* and *B. subtilis* cells contained 67 mmol/l potassium phosphate (pH 7.4); 13.3 mmol/l $MgCl_2$; 10 mmol/l 2-mercaptoethanol; 0.133 mmol/l each of ATP, guanosine 5'-triphosphate (GTP) and cytidine 5'-triphosphate (CTP); 0.067 mmol/l ^{3}H-uridine 5'-triphosphate (^{3}H-UTP); specific activity 3.7−7.4 MBq/μmol). The assay was performed as described above for DNA synthesis, except that the standard reaction time was 15 min.

Cell-free protein synthesis

Preparation of cell-free extracts (S-30)

Cells were grown as described for DNA and RNA synthesis to late exponential phase ($5-10 \times 10^8$ cells/ml), harvested by centrifugation and stored in liquid nitrogen until use. The bacteria (10 g wet wt) were thawed and resuspended in 10-ml Buffer 2. Glass beads (40 g; 0.10−0.11 mm diameter) were added to the cell suspension, and the cells were disrupted in a Braun homogenizer (B. Braun Melsungen AG, Type 853038) for 1 min. The temperature was kept below 5°C by carbon dioxide chilling during the homogenization step. Beads and cell fragments were then removed by centrifugation (15 000 g for 10 min at 4°C), and the pellet was washed twice with 10 ml of Buffer 2. The supernatant fractions from the three centrifugations were combined (total volume

25 ml), supplied with 0.4 ml 140 mmol/l ATP, 0.6 ml 75 mmol/l phosphoenolpyruvate and 0.1 ml phosphoenolpyruvate carboxylase (2.3 mg/ml; Sigma
Chemical Company Ltd, Poole, UK), and incubated for 25 min at 35°C. The
extract was centrifuged (30 000 g for 15 min at 4°C) and dialysed against 2 l of
Buffer 2 (twice for 5 h at 4°C).

The dialysed cell extract (S-30 fraction) was kept in liquid nitrogen until
use for cell-free protein synthesis. The S-30 fractions contained $21-23$ mg
protein/ml as determined by the method of Lowry et al. (1951) using bovine
serum albumin as standard.

Assay for cell-free protein synthesis

The assay employed was in general accordance with the procedures described
by Nirenberg (1963) and Doi (1971). The method determines polyuridylic
acid (poly(U))-dependent protein synthesis.

The assays were performed in 100-µl reaction volumes containing
100 mmol/l Tris-HCl (pH 8.0); 14 mmol/l $MgSO_4$; 50 mmol/l KCl; 2 mmol/l
2-mercaptoethanol; 1 mmol/l ATP; 0.03 mmol/l GTP; 2 µmol/l ^{14}C-phenyl-
alanine (uniformly labelled, specific activity 18.5 MBq/mole); 0.25 mmol/l
each of the other 19 amino acids; 7.5 mmol/l phosphoenolpyruvate; 0.033
mg/ml phosphoenolpyruvate carboxylase; $0.2-0.8$ mg/ml poly(U) (Sigma);
S-30 fraction (final concentration 0.25 mg protein/ml from *E. coli* and 1.3 mg
protein/ml from *B. subtilis*). As for the DNA/RNA synthesis assays, DMSO
was used as solvent for some of the preservatives tested, with a final concentration of 2.5%, which was then also included in the control.

The reaction mixture was incubated with gentle shaking on a reciprocal
shaker at 30°C for 15 min. The reaction was stopped by the addition of 100 µl
0.1 mol/l KOH followed by 3 ml 10% TCA. The precipitate was collected by
filtering the mixture through 2.4-cm nitrocellulose membrane filters (Gelman
Metricel GN-6), washed three times with 10% TCA, dried and counted as
above.

Presentation and Interpretation of Results

Paraben inhibition of DNA and RNA synthesis

The influence of three different parabens at various concentrations on DNA
(Fig. 1) and RNA (Fig. 2) synthesis in toluenized *B. subtilis* and *E. coli* cells is
summarized in Table 1 and compared with paraben concentrations achieving
50% growth inhibition (Eklund 1980). Patterns of macromolecule synthesis
inhibition are broadly similar for both organisms, with 50% inhibition being
achieved at paraben concentrations approximately two- to fourfold that required
to inhibit cell growth to the same extent.

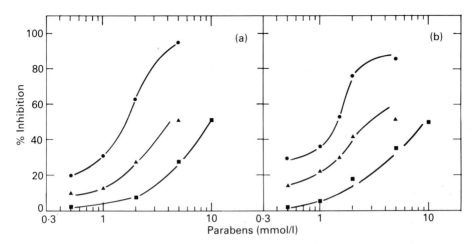

FIG. 1. The effect of parabens on the incorporation of ³H-dTTP into the DNA of toluene-treated cells of; (a) *E. coli*, and (b) *B. subtilis*. In the absence of parabens 25 nmol/l ³H-dTTP and 4 nmol/l ³H-dTTP were incorporated in the DNA of *E. coli* and *B. subtilis*, respectively. The reaction mixture and assay conditions were as described in Experimental Methods. (■) Methyl paraben; (▲) propyl paraben; (●) butyl paraben.

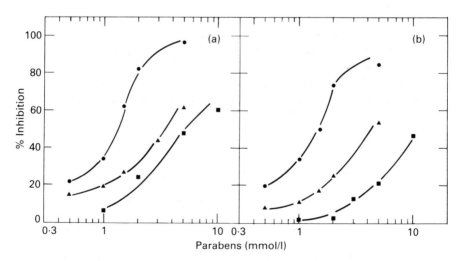

FIG. 2. The effect of parabens on the incorporation of ³H-UTP into the RNA of toluene-treated cells of; (a) *E. coli*, and (b) *B. subtilis*. In the absence of parabens 55 nmol/l ³H-UTP and 80 nmol ³H-UTP were incorporated in the RNA of *E. coli* and *B. subtilis*, respectively. The reaction mixture and assay conditions were as described in Experimental Methods. (■) Methyl paraben; (▲) propyl paraben; (●) butyl paraben.

TABLE 1. *Concentration of various parabens causing 50% inhibition of DNA and RNA synthesis in toluenized cells and 50% growth inhibition in whole cells of* B. subtilis *and* E. coli

Paraben	DNA synthesis	RNA synthesis	Growth (Eklund 1980)
	Concentration (mmol/l) achieving 50% inhibition of:		
Methyl	10	5–10	4.3–5.5
Propyl	5	3–4	0.9–1.1
Butyl	2	1.5	0.4–0.46

Benzoate, propionate and sorbate influence on DNA and RNA synthesis

The effects of sodium benzoate and propionate, and of potassium sorbate were tested individually on RNA and DNA synthesis in toluenized *E. coli* cells.

None of these compounds showed any inhibitory effect on RNA synthesis at concentrations up to 100 mmol/l. Sodium benzoate at concentrations exceeding 25 mmol/l actually stimulated RNA synthesis by 15–20%. When DNA synthesis was measured, benzoate and propionate did not affect nucleotide incorporation at concentrations below 50 mmol/l. At 100 mmol/l, however, both benzoate and propionate caused approximately 40% inhibition of DNA synthesis. In a similar manner to RNA synthesis, sorbate had no inhibitory effect on DNA synthesis.

BHA and BHT inhibition of DNA and RNA synthesis

Figure 3 shows the effects of BHA and BHT on DNA and RNA synthesis in toluenized cells of *B. subtilis*. For BHA, the effects on both DNA and RNA synthesis appear similar to the inhibition caused by butyl paraben. The data for BHT acting on DNA synthesis seem to indicate a low inhibitory activity. However, at concentrations above 0.5 mmol/l BHT began to precipitate in the reaction mixture. For the RNA reaction mixture (data not shown), the same inhibition patterns appeared. Similar results were obtained for DNA and RNA synthesis inhibition in toluenized *E. coli* cells (data not shown).

Inhibition of cell-free protein synthesis by parabens and antioxidants

Previous studies have shown that the cellular uptake of amino acids was prevented by the presence of parabens (Freese *et al.* 1973; Eklund 1980). It was thus not unexpected that the incorporation of radioactive amino acids into proteins in whole cells was efficiently inhibited by parabens (data not shown).

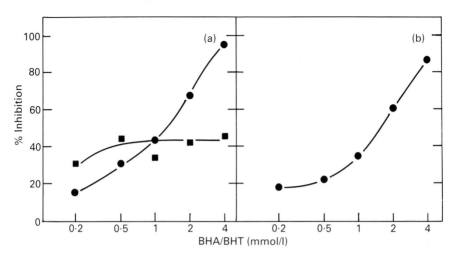

FIG. 3. The effect of antioxidants on the incorporation of ^{3}H-dTTP into the DNA (a), and ^{3}H-UTP into the RNA (b), of toluene-treated cells of *B. subtilis*. The control values for incorporation were as described in the legends of Figs 1 and 2. The reaction mixtures and assay conditions were as described in Experimental Methods. (●) Butylated hydroxyanisole (BHA); (■) butylated hydroxytoluene (BHT).

The activity of poly(U)-directed polyphenylalanine synthesis in cell-free systems was therefore followed at various concentrations of the three parabens. As shown in Fig. 4a, protein synthesis in *B. subtilis* extracts was inhibited by parabens, and 50% inhibition was obtained at concentrations of 4−5 mmol/l, 0.9 mmol/l and 0.6−0.8 mmol/l for the methyl, propyl and butyl esters, respectively.

Thus, in *B. subtilis* protein synthesis was more sensitive to inhibition by parabens than RNA and DNA synthesis. When the same experiments were performed with *E. coli* S-30 extracts, the parabens showed less of an inhibitory effect on protein synthesis (Fig. 4b). These observations suggest that the protein synthesis apparatus of *B. subtilis* contains a more sensitive target for parabens than that present in *E. coli*.

The effects of the antioxidants BHA and BHT were tested with the same cell-free system for possible effects on protein synthesis. It appeared (data not shown) that no inhibitory effect occurred with concentrations below 4 mmol/l. However, a slight inhibition (15−20%) was observed by raising the BHA concentration to 10 mmol/l. As observed with DNA/RNA synthesis experiments, BHT precipitated at relatively low concentrations (*c.* 0.5 mmol/l), but no inhibition by this substance occurred. The observed effects of BHA and BHT were similar for both *E. coli* and *B. subtilis* cell-free protein synthesis systems.

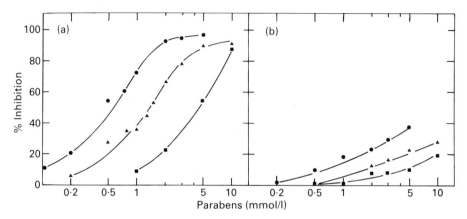

FIG. 4. The effect of parabens on poly(U)-directed polyphenylalanine synthesis in cell-free extracts (S-30) from; (a) *B. subtilis*, and (b) *E. coli*. In the absence of parabens 48 nmol/l poly(U) was formed in the extract from *B. subtilis* and 280 nmol/l poly(U) was formed in the extract from *E. coli* under standard assay and reaction conditions as described in Experimental Methods. (■) Methyl paraben; (▲) propyl paraben; (●) butyl paraben.

Discussion

Earlier investigations on the mode of bacteriostatic action of the preservatives tested have shown the cell membrane to be a prime (although not the sole) target (Davidson 1983; Eklund 1989). The present work, incorporating earlier data (Nes & Eklund 1983), demonstrates that parabens can also inhibit both DNA and RNA synthesis in toluenized *E. coli* and *B. subtilis* cells as well as protein synthesis in cell-free extracts from *B. subtilis* and to a lesser extent, *E. coli*. It seems likely therefore, assuming that the intracellular and extracellular concentrations of inhibitor are the same, that the inhibition of both nucleic acid and protein synthesis can contribute to the observed inhibition of bacterial growth by parabens.

For BHA, nucleic acid synthesis inhibition may be part of the bacteriostatic mechanism of action, but probably not for BHT. Neither of these two anti-oxidants seem to cause any appreciable inhibition of protein synthesis. For the organic acids − benzoic, propionic and sorbic acid − inhibition of nucleic acid synthesis may contribute to the growth inhibitory action for benzoate and propionate, since those substances showed a certain inhibition of DNA (but not RNA) synthesis. For sorbic acid no effects were demonstrated on nucleic acid synthesis, indicating that the bacteriostatic mechanism of action should be sought elsewhere.

Conclusion

The effect of chemical agents on protein synthesis and the replication of genetic material is not easily studied by measuring the incorporation of radioactive precursors into RNA, DNA or protein of living, more-or-less intact cells. This is mainly because such inhibitors may interfere with the transport of precursors across the bacterial membrane, as reviewed by Eklund (1989). For RNA and DNA synthesis, this problem can be circumvented by employing permeabilized cells and for protein synthesis by using a cell-free system.

This study does not discriminate between DNA replication and unscheduled DNA synthesis like DNA repair. The present strains of *E. coli* and *B. subtilis* contain abundant DNA polymerase I, which is the major DNA repair polymerase and has been shown to be responsible for more than 90% of the observed DNA synthesis in a permeabilized system. Thus, the effect of preservatives demonstrated here is at the level of DNA polymerase I. In order to look specifically at DNA replication synthesis, one has to study bacterial strains where DNA polymerase I is absent.

The permeabilized system for studying DNA and RNA synthesis is advantageous in two ways. The toluenized bacteria are fully permeable for molecules which are four to five times larger than parabens or BHA/BHT, and the ultimate substrates for DNA and RNA, i.e. the nucleosidetriphosphates, can be supplied directly; no metabolic activity is needed prior to incorporation in the nucleic acids. These techniques may have a general application, therefore, in the study of macromolecule synthesis in the presence of biocides.

Acknowledgement

This work was done at the Norwegian Food Research Institute (Osloveien 1, N-1430 Ås. Norway), while both authors were employed at the Institute. The authors wish to thank the Institute for providing them with the means to perform this research.

References

DAVIDSON, P.M. 1983. Phenolic Compounds. In *Antimicrobials in Food*, ed. Branen, A.L. & Davidson, P.M. pp. 37–74. New York and Basel: Marcel Dekker, Inc.

DOI, R.H. 1971. *Bacillus subtilis* protein synthesizing system. In *Methods in Molecular Biology*, ed. Last, J.A. & Laskin, A.I. pp. 67–88. New York and Basel: Marcel Dekker, Inc.

EKLUND, T. 1980. Inhibition of growth and uptake processes in bacteria by some chemical food preservatives. *Journal of Applied Bacteriology* **48**, 423–432.

EKLUND, T. 1989. Organic acids and esters. In *Mechanisms of Action of Food Preservation Procedures*, ed. Gould, G. pp. 161–200. London: Elsevier.

234 T. EKLUND AND I.F. NES

FREESE, E., SHEU, C.W & GALLIERS, E. 1973. Function of lipophilic acids as antimicrobial food additives. *Nature, London* **241**, 321–325.

HIRASHIMA, A., ASANO, K. & TSUGITA, A. 1967. A cell-free protein-synthesizing system from *Bacillus subtilis. Biochimica et Biophysica Acta* **134**, 165–173.

LOWRY, O.H., ROSEBROUGH, N.J., FARR, A.L. & RANDALL, R.J. 1951. Protein measurement with the Folin-phenol reagent. *Journal of Biological Chemistry* **193**, 265–275.

MATSUSHITA, T., KALPANA, P.W. & SUEOKA, N. 1971. Chromosome replication in toluenized *Bacillus subtilis* cells. *Nature New Biology* **223**, 111–114.

MOSES, R.E. 1974. DNA synthesis in toluene-treated cells of *Escherichia coli.* In *Methods in Enzymology*, Vol. XXIX, ed. Grossman, L. & Moldave, K. pp. 219–224. New York & London: Academic Press.

NES, I.F. & EKLUND, T. 1983. The effect of parabens on DNA, RNA and protein synthesis in *Escherichia coli* and *Bacillus subtilis. Journal of Applied Bacteriology* **54**, 237–242.

NIRENBERG, M.W. 1963. Cell-free protein synthesis directed by messenger RNA. In *Methods in Enzymology*, Vol. VI, ed. Colowick, S.P. & Kaplan, N.O. pp. 17–23. New York & London: Academic Press.

NIRENBERG, M.W. & MATTHAEI, J.H. 1961. The dependence of cell-free protein sythesis in *E. coli* upon naturally occurring or synthetic polyribonucleotides. *Proceedings of the National Academy of Sciences, USA* **47**, 1588–1601.

PETERSON, R.I., RADCLIFFE, C.W. & PACE, N.R. 1971. Ribonucleic acid synthesis in bacteria treated with toluene. *Journal of Bacteriology* **107**, 585–588.

Biocide-Induced Enzyme Inhibition

S.J. FULLER

Sterling-Winthrop Research Centre, Willowburn Avenue, Alnwick, Northumberland NE66 2JH, UK

Enzymes were considered a target and possibly the key target for antiseptics early in the 1920s. Dehydrogenase enzymes were explored by the recently introduced Thunberg technique which followed enzyme inhibition by the concomitant reduction of methylene blue in an evacuated, or nitrogen-filled, vessel; by the very nature of this technique biocide action was studied under anaerobic conditions. Studies using Warburg and Barcroft respirometry were also undertaken; these involved aerobic environments. No striking differences emerged between the aerobic and anaerobic systems. These early experiments were reviewed by Hugo (1967). It emerged from this work that enzyme inhibition may only be part of the activity of many biocides.

Another approach in this same field was to study the sensitivity of enzymes which contained a thiol group, which was essential for their function (Barron 1951; Hugo 1980). This work suggested that thiol groups were a specific target for some antimicrobial agents, and mercury is classical in this respect (Harold 1970). More recent studies on biocide-inhibited enzyme reactions are found in the work of Stretton & Manson (1973), Gilbert *et al.* (1977), Hammond (1979) and Fuller *et al.* (1985) (see Table 1). These have indicated the potential susceptibility of both cytoplasmic and membrane-bound enzymes.

The specific inhibition of enzyme action by antibacterial agents is rarely a bactericidal event by virtue of the often reversible nature of such inhibitions and the ability of bacteria to adopt alternative metabolic pathways: Furthermore any residual activity which remains in the presence of inhibitor may still allow the metabolic pathway to function at a useful level. Nevertheless, enzyme inhibition can make a significant contribution to the bacteriostatic activity of biocides, thereby strongly influencing bacterial repair and recovery processes.

This account discusses the methods which may be used to investigate enzyme inhibition by biocides and its quantification. Much useful information on enzyme inhibition can be gained if the raw data are subject to the correct mathematical treatment, and detailed reviews on the subject include those by

Mechanisms of Action of
Chemical Biocides

TABLE 1. *Examples of enzyme inhibition by antimicrobial agents*

Enzyme	Inhibitor(s)	Reference
Adenosine triphosphatease (ATP-ase)	Chlorocresol Efrapeptin, quercitin, Dio 9, 4-chloro-7-nitrobenzofuran 1,2-benzisothiazolin-3-one	Denyer *et al.* (1986) Hammond (1979) Fuller *et al.* (1985)
Various thiol-containing enzymes	Ethylene oxide, glutaraldehyde, hypochlorites, iodine, mercurial compounds, β-propriolactone, silver (I) salts, bronopol	Hugo & Russell, (1987)
Glyceraldehyde-3-phosphate dehydrogenase	Bronopol, *para*-chloromercuribenzoate, iodosobenzoate, iodoacetate 1,2-benz*iso*thiazolin-3-one	Stretton & Manson (1973) Fuller *et al.* (1985)
Malate dehydrogenase	Phenoxyethanol	Gilbert *et al.* (1977)
Various dehydrogenases	Toluene, phenol, detergents, 2-phenoxyethanol, propanol, cyclohexanol, benzene, acetone, thymol, formaldehyde, mercury (II) chloride	Hugo (1967)

Michal (1978), Dixon & Webb (1979) and Price & Stevens (1982). For methods dealing with the preparation and determination of specific enzymes the reader is referred to the extensive series of volumes edited by Colowick & Kaplan (1955 onwards). For instruction on the disruption of bacterial cells, and subsequent separation and fractionation of enzymic material therefrom, the reader should consult Williams & Gledhill (this book), and Hugo (1954).

Enzyme Kinetics

Theoretical considerations

Enzymes cause the catalytic acceleration of biochemical reactions. These may involve one, two or more substrates (S) and the mathematics vary accordingly. Single substrate reactions occur via the formation of an enzyme−substrate complex (ES) which then breaks down to product (P) and free enzyme (E):

$$E + S \rightleftharpoons ES \rightarrow P + E. \tag{1}$$

When practical, determinations are performed with enzyme concentrations usually much lower than the concentration of substrate ($[S]$). In addition, the rate of formation of the enzyme−substrate complex is often much greater than the decomposition to enzyme and product. Under these conditions the rate of reaction (V) is described by the Michaelis−Menten equation:

$$V = \frac{V_{max}}{1 + K_m/[S].} \tag{2}$$

K_m is the Michaelis constant and is equal to the substrate concentration at which half the maximum velocity (V_{max}) of the reaction, is achieved.

Using this equation, special states can be described when the substrate is in great excess and $K_m/[S]$ is negligible (i.e. $V = V_{max}$), when the substrate concentration equals K_m (i.e. $V = V_{max}/2$) and when the substrate concentration is much lower than K_m (i.e. $V = (V_{max}/K_m) \times [S]$). In this latter case, the reaction rate is directly proportional to the substrate concentration.

The majority of enzyme-catalysed reactions, however, involve two (or more) substrates. These proceed by one of two general mechanisms. The first involves the formation of a complex between the enzyme and both substrates which may bind in either a random order or, alternatively, binding may always occur in the same ordered sequence. The second general mechanism proceeds via the formation of a complex between the enzyme and one of the substrates. This then degrades to generate a product and an altered form of the enzyme. The second substrate then complexes with the altered enzyme before a further degradation to a second product and the unaltered enzyme. The mathematical equations describing two-substrate reaction are more complex than for single-substrate mechanisms, but the same principles and assumptions apply.

When an enzyme is mixed with its substrate there follows a pre-steady-state period, lasting for only fractions of a second, during which the predominant reaction is the saturation of enzyme with substrate and the formation of the enzyme−substrate complex. Following this is a period of steady-state kinetics where the reaction rate changes relatively slowly. It is during this period when the initial reaction rate (V_i) is determined. As time continues the reaction rate decreases as the levels of substrate are depleted. The progress of a reaction is illustrated by a plot of the amount of substrate transformed with time (Fig. 1). A tangent to the curve drawn through the origin is used to determine the initial reaction rate.

For single-substrate reactions a plot of initial reaction rate against substrate concentration yields the curve shown in Fig. 2. From this plot K_m may be determined by the measurement of the substrate concentration required to achieve half the maximum reaction rate. This may be difficult to obtain accurately from such a plot and an alternative presentation of data is often preferred. The common approaches are the Lineweaver−Burk plot which sets the reciprocals of the initial reaction rate against that of the substrate concentration (Fig. 3a), and the Eadie−Hoftsee approach which plots the initial

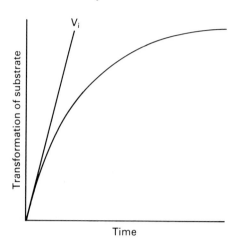

FIG. 1. Progress curve of an enzyme-catalysed reaction.

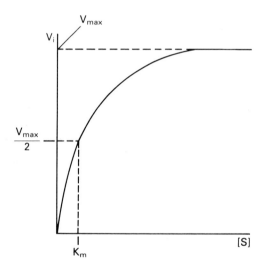

FIG. 2. Plot of initial reaction rate as a function of substrate concentration.

reaction rate as a function of itself divided by the substrate concentration (Fig. 3b). Both produce straight lines from which K_m and V_{max} are readily obtainable.

Two K_m values may be determined for two-substrate reactions, one for each substrate. To obtain K_m for substrate 1, the concentration of substrate 2 is held constant and at a level much higher than its K_m. In a similar way, by holding the concentration of substrate 1 at a level much greater than its K_m,

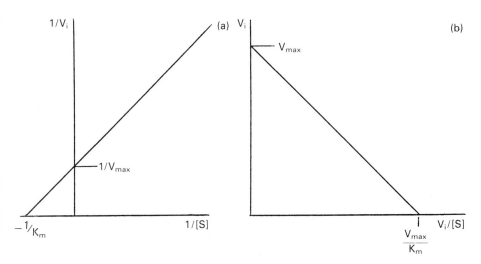

FIG. 3. Lineweaver−Burk (a), and Eadie−Hoftsee (b) plots.

the Michaelis constant for substrate 2 can be determined. Procedures for estimating K_m values when high substrate concentrations are not attainable have been outlined by Michal (1978).

Changes in the environment e.g. fluctuations in pH or temperature, will influence the enzyme activity and consequently the values of K_m and V_{max}. The reaction conditions should, therefore, be held constant during a series of determinations and should be stated when quoting such values. Enzyme activity may also be influenced by chemical inhibitors, and their effect upon the kinetic parameters can provide information on the type of inhibition manifested.

The kinetics of chemical inhibition

Inhibitors, and inhibition, are described as being irreversible or reversible. The former involves the formation of a permanent complex between inhibitor and enzyme which prevents any further enzyme activity. Reversible inhibitors are very generally classed as being competitive, non-competitive or uncompetitive. The kinetics associated with reversible inhibitors are best illustrated using single-substrate reactions.

Competitive inhibition is considered to occur through competition between the substrate and inhibitor for the active site on the enzyme. The affinity of the enzyme for the substrate is thus affected and a change in K_m is observed. The inhibition may be overcome by saturation with substrate hence V_{max} remains the same. Non-competitive inhibition is manifest when the inhibitor combines with the free enzyme or the enzyme−substrate complex at a position other than the active site. This results in a reduction in the rate of formation and decomposition of the enzyme–substrate complex. V_{max} is reduced although K_m remains constant. Uncompetitive inhibition is rare in single-substrate reactions and is thought to occur when the inhibitor reacts with the enzyme–substrate complex to prevent further degradation to products. Both V_{max} and K_m are affected.

Lineweaver–Burk and Eadie–Hoftsee plots may be applied to identify the type of inhibitor and then can be used to arrive at a measure of the inhibitor constant (K_I) (Fig. 4). Dixon (1953) has described the determination of K_I from plots of the reciprocal of the initial reaction rate as a function of inhibitor concentration (Fig. 5). This approach is only valid for competitive and non-competitive inhibition (Dixon & Webb 1979).

The mathematics describing the inhibition of two-substrate reactions is extremely complex because of the different mechanisms and types of inhibition that may occur. The approach of maintaining one substrate in great excess while varying the concentration of the other in order to determine the kinetic parameters, may still be applied, but the inhibitory characteristics observed are likely to be different with respect to each substrate. Cleland (1963a,b,c) has discussed the theory behind these inhibitions and Gilbert et al. (1977) have shown how inhibition may vary depending on which substrate concentration is held constant.

Methods for Studying Enzyme Inhibition

The purpose of this section is not to provide an extensive review of the methodology available for studying enzyme inhibition, but to suggest general approaches.

The activity of an enzyme is estimated by studying the progress of the reaction being catalysed. This is achieved by following the loss of a substrate or the formation of a product, or a change in the redox state of a coenzyme, usually in a quantitative manner, although some qualitative or semi-quantitative approaches are available. Enzyme inhibition is studied by comparing enzyme activity in the presence and absence of inhibitor. It is important to realize that many factors other than the presence of inhibitors may influence the activity of an enzyme. All other variables should therefore be kept constant to allow true comparisons of inhibited and uninhibited reactions.

The methods outlined are illustrative of several applied by the author which have proved to be generally useful in the study of antibacterial action. In many instances, they are modifications of established techniques and may thus need further modification to conform with particular experimental requirements.

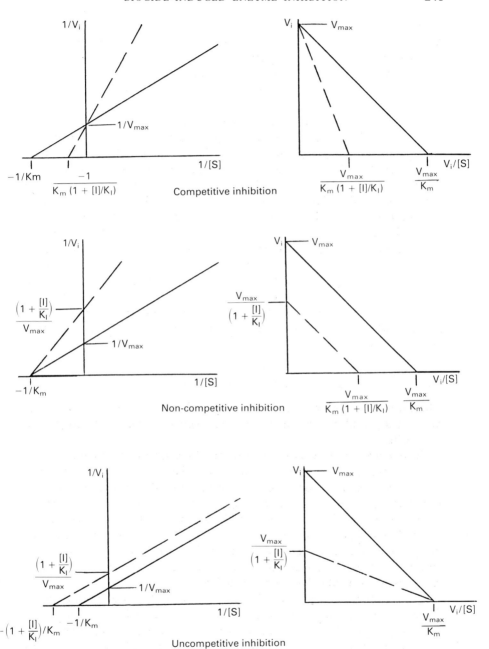

FIG. 4. The effect of different types of reversible inhibition on the Lineweaver–Burke and Eadie–Hoftsee plots. Broken lines indicate inhibited reactions.

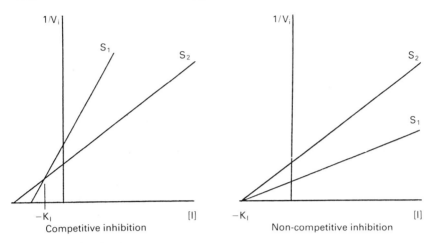

FIG. 5. Dixon plots for the determination of K_I. S_1 and S_2 are different substrate concentrations.

Qualitative and semi-quantitative techniques

The methods described involve the visual detection of a coloured product and can be employed as preliminary screening techniques. They are modifications of methods originally designed to determine the presence of a given enzyme. If these methods are to be used to study the inhibition of enzyme action then it is important to remember that reversible inhibition will not prevent the completion of the reaction, only the rate at which it is achieved. Thus product formation must be followed as a function of time and a comparison between inhibited and uninhibited reactions made after a specified time interval; if both reactions are allowed to go to completion the two systems will be indistinguishable. In addition, while the amount of substrate present must be sufficient to allow the generation of enough product for the detection of enzyme activity in the untreated sample, the amount of inhibitor present should also be sufficient to overcome any nullification of competitive inhibition by the presence of excessive quantities of substrate.

The API–ZYM kit

The API–ZYM kit has been described by Humble *et al.* (1977). It provides a rapid method for the detection of enzymes in whole cells or in disrupted cell preparations. The kits are available from API, Basingstoke, UK.

The system consists of a series of depressions called cupules moulded in a plastic strip. These contain a dehydrated buffer and an appropriate substrate for a specific enzyme. Each cupule is heavily inoculated with 0.04 ml of a washed suspension of untreated organisms (2×10^9 cells/ml), or organisms treated with inhibitor, in a weakly buffered aqueous medium. The strip is placed in a humidifying tray and incubated for 4 h at 37°C. One drop of ZYM A (trihydroxymethylaminomethane 25.0% (w/v); HCl 10 M, 11% (v/v); sodium lauryl sulphate 10% (w/v) in distilled water) and ZYM B (0.35% Fast Blue in 2-methoxyethanol) reagents (provided with the kit) are then added to each cupule and the strip is left for 5 min in bright light for the colour to develop. The colour intensity in each cupule is compared with the reference colour chart and estimated on a scale of 0−5. The level of activity of each enzyme in the presence and absence of inhibitor is thus determined and comparisons drawn.

At present the kit allows the detection of alkaline and acid phosphatases, butyrate esterase; caprylate esterase; myristate lipase; leucine, valine and cystine aminopeptidases; trypsin; chymotrypsin; phosphoamidase; α- and β-galactosidase; β-glucuronidase; α-glucosidase; β-glucosaminidase; α-mannosidase and α-fucosidase. The inhibition pattern amongst the enzymes may highlight a common target e.g. thiol-containing enzymes, which could suggest a mode of action worthy of further investigation.

Bacterial dehydrogenase activity

This method is a modification of that described by Kersters (1967).

The organisms (4×10^{11} cells/ml) are disrupted by sonication in 0.01 mol/l phosphate buffer (pH 7.4) or by another appropriate method (see Chapter 5 and Hugo 1954). Intact cells and unwanted cell debris are removed by centrifugation for 15 min at 1400 g. The supernatant fluid is then centrifuged for 2 h at 25 000 g. Both processes are performed at 4°C. The soluble fraction and the particulate (pellet) fraction are then separated and enzyme activity explored by the following methods.

Soluble fraction. The soluble fraction is assayed by exposure to substrate and cofactor NAD or NADP. Dehydrogenase activity is detected by following the enzyme-catalysed transfer of reducing equivalents from substrate to cofactor. Reduced cofactor is distinguished from the oxidized species by its fluorescence under ultraviolet light.

A filter paper is soaked in 0.01 mol/l phosphate buffer (pH 8.0) containing 10^{-3} mol/l magnesium chloride and dried in air. A pencilled grid pattern is ruled on to the paper and at the intersects 0.01 ml of 0.4 mol/l substrate solutions are applied. Suggested substrates include lactate, succinate, malate, *iso*citrate, glyceraldehyde-3-phosphate and glucose-6-phosphate. Reaction mixtures are then prepared containing soluble fraction, 0.3 ml, NAD or NADP solution (0.05 mol/l), 0.1 ml, and inhibitor and/or buffer to a total volume of 0.8 ml. These may be pre-incubated if required to allow reaction between enzyme and inhibitor. The reaction mixtures (0.1 ml) are then added to each substrate spot and the filter paper clamped between two glass plates, to prevent evaporation, and the whole incubated at room temperature for a suitable time period (*c.* 15 min). The filter papers are then removed and allowed to dry before viewing under ultraviolet light (360 nm). Enzyme activity is indicated by the fluorescence of reduced cofactor NADH or NADPH. The intensity of fluorescence may be allocated a numerical value which will relate to the level of enzyme activity thereby allowing the effect of inhibitor to be estimated.

Pellet fraction. Dehydrogenase activity in the particulate fraction is estimated by mixing the fraction with substrate and an artificial acceptor of reducing equivalents, 2′6-dichlorophenol indophenol (2′6-D). The activity of the substrate dehydrogenase causes the transfer of reducing equivalents to the 2′6-D which is observed visually by a loss in colour from the dye.

The pellet is resuspended in 4.5 ml of 0.01 mol/l phosphate buffer (pH 7.4). Equivalent volumes of either buffer or inhibitor solution are then added to aliquots of the suspension. 2′6-D, 0.15 ml, and substrate solutions (0.5 mol/l), 0.05 ml, are mixed in a series of small test tubes (Durham tubes). The same substrates used in the soluble fraction assays may be employed with the exception of glyceraldehyde-3-phosphate which turns the solutions pink. Particulate (pellet) fraction, 0.05 ml, is then added to the Durham tubes which are briefly shaken to ensure adequate mixing. The degree of bleaching of 2′6-D in each tube is compared at suitable time intervals with a blank tube (no substrate). The rate and extent of bleaching indicates the level of dehydrogenase activity and comparisons can be made between inhibited and uninhibited samples.

Quantitative techniques

These techniques involve the quantitative determination of the amount of either substrate or cofactor transformed or product generated, at a series of time intervals throughout the course of a reaction. This allows the construction of a curve, as shown in Fig. 1, from which the initial velocity may be taken. Repeating this at various substrate concentrations and in the presence and absence of inhibitor allows the application of enzyme kinetics as outlined earlier (see also Dixon & Webb 1979 and Price & Stevens 1982). Alternatively a simpler presentation of data may be adequate, in which the extent of the reaction at a single time interval for a single substrate concentration in the presence of a range of inhibitor concentrations is determined. This will allow the calculation of a percentage inhibition under the conditions so defined, a method used by earlier workers (reviewed by Hugo 1967).

Two approaches may be used for quantitatively studying enzyme activity and its inhibition; these are sampling and continuous methods.

Sampling method

Sampling techniques involve the removal of sample from the reaction mixture at intervals during the reaction. Enzyme activity in the samples is then rapidly quenched, usually by the addition of an agent which is rapidly toxic to the enzyme (e.g. 5% trichloroacetic acid). The samples are then assayed for the chosen product or substrate.

Adenosine triphosphatase (ATP-ase) activity is often studied by such a sampling technique (Denyer *et al.* 1986). The principle of the method is to detect inorganic phosphate produced through the catalytic hydrolysis of ATP. Reaction mixtures are prepared containing the following final concentrations of ingredients: ATP-ase 0.1 u/ml; KCl, 0.1 mol/l; $MgCl_2$, 5 mmol/l, and graded concentrations of inhibitor in a suitable buffer (not phosphate) at pH 7.4. The reactions are initiated by the addition of ATP to 5 mmol/l. Samples are removed at suitable time intervals and the reactions quenched by the addition of 1 ml acid molybdate solution (ammonium molybdate 1.25% (w/v) in 1.25mol/l sulphuric acid) to 2 ml of sample. Inorganic phosphate may be determined by the method of Fiske & Subbarow (1925) and used as an estimate of ATP-ase activity. A kit containing materials for this method of phosphate determination is available from the Sigma Chemical Company Ltd, Poole, UK.

It should be noted that inhibition studies undertaken on the isolated, soluble form of the ATP-ase enzyme may not mirror the effect on the membrane-bound enzyme (Harold *et al.* 1969; Hammond 1979). This is a general principle and should be borne in mind in any study of inhibitor action on cell-free enzyme preparations.

Continuous methods

Continuous methods involve the quantitative estimation of substrate lost or product formed whilst the reaction is proceeding. This is usually performed spectrophotometrically with a requirement that the species determined can be accurately estimated without interference.

Dehydrogenases are often studied by a continuous method because their activity frequently involves the oxidation/reduction of NAD or NADP. These cofactors absorb strongly at 340 nm and fluoresce in their reduced, but not in their oxidized, form which enables detection by ultraviolet spectrophotometry or fluorimetry. Reaction mixtures containing cofactor, enzyme and inhibitor are prepared in the photometer cell. The reaction is initiated by the addition of substrate and the change in absorbance at 340 nm monitored. This can be illustrated by reference to the reaction catalysed by lactate dehydrogenase (LDH):

$$\text{Lactose} + \text{NAD}^+ \underset{\text{}}{\overset{\text{LDH}}{\rightleftharpoons}} \text{Pyruvate} + \text{NADH} + \text{H}^+.$$

The enzyme activity is studied by preparing reaction mixtures of lactate dehydrogenase (500 u/ml), NAD^+ (3 mg/ml), and graded concentrations of inhibitor. A suitable buffer system would be that of glycylglycine (pH 7.4) (0.01 mol/l) though any common biological buffer of similar pH may be employed provided that there is no interaction with the inhibitor. The reaction is initiated by the addition of lactate 10 μg/ml and the consequential increase in absorbance at 340 nm followed. The enzyme also catalyses the reverse reaction hence the activity may be determined by preparing reaction mixtures containing enzyme, NADH and inhibitor. The addition of pyruvate (10 μg/ml) then initiates the reaction which is followed by a decrease in absorbance at 340 nm. The latter approach is often preferred as the reaction equilibrium lies to the left.

Coupled reactions

Continuous methods are usually preferred over sampling methods in quantitative enzyme assay because they avoid sampling error and result in economies in time, effort and materials. When the reaction does not involve a species which allows continuous estimation, however, sampling can be avoided by coupling the catalysed reaction to a second 'indicator' reaction which involves a suitable product or substrate. This approach is employed to study hexokinase (HK) which catalyses the phosphorylation of glucose and is typical of a coupled reaction system:

$$\text{Glucose} + \text{ATP} \underset{\text{}}{\overset{\text{HK}}{\rightleftharpoons}} \text{glucose-6-phosphate} + \text{ADP}.$$

The species present do not enable direct continuous estimation. Glucose-6-phosphate dehydrogenase (G6PDH) and NADP are thus included in the reaction mixture. As glucose-6-phosphate is produced, through the activity of hexokinase, a second reaction proceeds, catalysed by G6PDH, with the production of NADPH; this is then estimated continuously at 340 nm:

$$\text{Glucose-6-phosphate} + \text{NADP}^+ \underset{\text{}}{\overset{\text{G6PDH}}{\rightleftharpoons}} \text{gluconate-6-phosphate} + \text{NADPH} + \text{H}^+.$$

Inhibition of hexokinase activity may thus be studied by preparing reaction mixtures containing, typically hexokinase 2 u/ml; ATP 2 mg/ml; NADP^+ 0.8 mg/ml; G6PDH 1 u/ml; and graded concentrations of inhibitor. The reaction is initiated by the addition of glucose in the range 1.3−16 μg/ml and the increase in absorbance followed at 340 nm.

When using these methods the 'indicator' reaction should proceed much more rapidly than the reaction under study; this allows a true indication of the rate of the primary reaction. This may be encouraged by increasing the amount of 'indicator' enzyme and by including an unlimited supply of additional substrates ($NADP^+$ in the example above). It must also be confirmed that the 'indicator' reaction is not influenced by the inhibitor under study and that both enzymes are specific for their respective reactions.

Coupled reactions are also employed where a substrate is unavailable or too unstable to be of practical use. When this is the case the substrate may be generated through a preceding reaction which is coupled to the reaction of interest. This preceding reaction should not be rate-limiting and this is ensured by the use of high enzyme and unlimited substrate concentrations. It is again axiomatic that the enzyme catalysing the preceding reaction must not be sensitive to the inhibitor under investigation. Such an approach is necessary in the study of inhibitor effects of glyceraldehyde-3-phosphate dehydrogenase (G3PDH) which catalyses the reduction of diphosphoglycerate (DPG) :

$$H^+ + NADH + DPG \xrightleftharpoons{G3PDH} NAD^+ + \text{glyceraldehyde-3-phosphate.}$$

DPG is highly labile and is therefore produced *in situ* by coupling the above reaction to a preceding reaction involving the phosphorylation of glycerate-3-phosphate catalysed by phosphoglycerate kinase (PGK):

$$ATP + \text{glycerate-3-phosphate} \xrightleftharpoons{PGK} ADP + DPG.$$

To study the inhibition of G3PDH reaction mixtures are prepared containing: glycerate-3-phosphate (50 mg/ml), 0.2 ml; ATP sodium salt (20 mg/ml), 0.1 ml; EDTA (10 mg/ml), 0.1 ml; $MgSO_4.7H_2O$ (0.1 mol/l), 0.06 ml; NADH sodium salt (10 mg/ml), 0.05 ml; phosphoglycerate kinase (10 mg/ml), 0.01 ml; G3PDH (10 mg/ml), 0.01 ml; and graded concentrations of inhibitor to a total volume of 3.13 ml in 0.01 mol/l phosphate buffer (pH 7.4). The reaction is initiated by the addition of the glycerate-3-phosphate and is followed by a decrease in absorbance at 340 nm. The above is a modification of the method employed by Stretton & Manson (1973) and has been found, in the author's experience, to work well.

If the calculation of kinetic parameters requires the amount of substrate to be controlled accurately, its production should be complete before the initiation of the reaction under study. In the above example all the DPG should be produced before the initiation of its reduction. The amount of glycerate-3-phosphate added should be sufficient to generate the required amount of DPG. G3PDH is thus not included initially in the reaction mixture but is added following the completion of the first DPG-generating reaction. Because

DPG is unstable, the addition of G3PDH should be made as soon as possible after completion of the first reaction. By this sequential addition it is possible to add the potential inhibitor at a stage which will not influence the generation of the labile substrate.

It is possible to combine both coupling techniques, as in the study of 6-phosphogluconolactonase (PGL-ase) activity. PGL-ase catalyses the conversion of 6-phosphoglucono-δ-lactone (PGL) to 6-phosphogluconate (PG; gluconate-6-phosphate), a reaction which constitutes part of the pentose phosphate pathway. The reaction sequence is described below:

$$\text{Glucose-6-phosphate} + \text{NADP}^+ \xrightleftharpoons{\text{G6PDH}} \text{PGL} + \text{NADPH} + \text{H}^+$$

$$\text{PGL} \xrightleftharpoons{\text{PGL-ase}} \text{PG}$$

$$\text{PG} + \text{NADP}^+ \xrightleftharpoons{\text{PGDH}} \text{ribulose-5-phosphate} + \text{NADPH} + \text{H}^+.$$

PGL is extremely unstable and is therefore required to be produced *in situ* by the action of G6PDH on glucose-6-phosphate. In addition the product of PGL-ase activity, PG, cannot be continually estimated and the reaction is therefore coupled to a further process catalysed by 6-phosphogluconate dehydrogenase (PGDH), which results in the reduction of NADP$^+$ to NADPH. The reaction is therefore followed by spectrophotometry at 340 nm.

Both the reactions result in the formation of NADPH and therefore the two cannot proceed simultaneously. The preceding reaction is allowed to reach equilibrium, indicated by a stable absorbance at 340 nm, before the initiation of PGL-ase activity by enzyme addition. This absorbance level is then used as the baseline from which to follow the indictor reaction. In practice, gradual spontaneous hydrolysis of PGL leads to a slow increase in this baseline absorbance value and a correction factor is applied to the estimation of PGL-ase activity.

References

BARRON, E.S. 1951. Thiol groups of biological importance. *Advances in Enzymology* 11, 201–226.

CLELAND, W.W. 1963a. The kinetics of enzyme catalysed reactions with two or more substrates or products. I Nomenclature and rate equations. *Biochemica et Biophysica Acta* 67, 104–137.

CLELAND, W.W. 1963b. The kinetics of enzyme catalysed reactions with two or more substrates or products. II Inhibition: Nomenclature and theory. *Biochimica et Biophysica Acta* 67, 173–187.

CLELAND, W.W. 1963c. The kinetics of enzyme catalysed reactions with two or more substrates. III Prediction of initial velocity and inhibition patterns by inspection. *Biochimica et Biophysica Acta* 67, 188–196.

COLOWICK, S.P. & KAPLAN, N.O. (eds) 1955. *Methods in Enzymology*, Vol. 1 onwards. New York: Academic Press.

DENYER, S.P., HUGO, W.B. & HARDING V.D. 1986. The biochemical basis of synergy between the antibacterial agents, chlorocresol and 2-phenylethanol. *International Journal of Pharmaceutics* **29**, 29–36.

DIXON, M. 1953. The determination of enzyme inhibitor constants. *Biochemical Journal* **55**, 170–171.

DIXON, M. & WEBB, E.C. 1979. *Enzymes*, 3rd edn. London: Longman.

FISKE, C.J. & SUBBAROW, Y. 1925. The colorimetric determination of phosphorus. *Journal of Biological Chemistry* **66**, 375–400.

FULLER, S.J., DENYER, S.P., HUGO, W.B., PEMBERTON, D., WOODCOCK, P.M. & BUCKLEY, A.J. 1985. The mode of action of 1,2-benzisothiazolin-3-one on *Staphylococcus aureus*. *Letters in Applied Microbiology* **1**, 13–15.

GILBERT, P., BEVERIDGE, E.G. & CRONE, P.B. 1977. Inhibition of some respiration and dehydrogenase enzyme systems in *Escherichia coli* NCTC 5933 by phenoxyethanol. *Microbios* **20**, 29–37.

HAMMOND, S.M. 1979. Inhibitors of enzymes of microbial membranes; agents affecting Mg^{2+}-activated adenosine triphosphatase. *Progress in Medicinal Chemistry* **16**, 223–256.

HAROLD, F.M. 1970. Antimicrobial agents and membrane function. *Advances in Microbial Physiology* **4**, 45–104.

HAROLD, F.M., BAARDA, J.R., BARON, C. & ABRAMS, A. 1969. DIO-9 and chlorhexidine: inhibitors of membrane-bound ATPase and of cation transport in *Streptococcus faecalis*. *Biochimica et Biophysica Acta* **183**, 129–136.

HUGO, W.B. 1954. The preparation of cell-free enzymes from microorganisms. *Bacteriological Reviews* **18**, 87–105.

HUGO, W.B. 1967. The mode of action of antibacterial agents. *Journal of Applied Bacteriology* **30**, 17–50.

HUGO, W.B. 1980. The mode of action of antiseptics. In *Wirkungmechanisma von Antiseptika*, ed. Wigert, H. & Weufen, W. pp. 39–77. Berlin: VEB Verlag.

HUGO, W.B. & RUSSELL, A.D. (eds) 1987. *Pharmaceutical Microbiology*, 4th edn. Oxford: Blackwell Scientific Publications.

HUMBLE, M.W., KING, A. & PHILLIPS, I. 1977. API–ZYM, a simple rapid system for the detection of bacterial enzymes. *Journal of Clinical Pathology*, **30**, 275–277.

KERSTERS, K. 1967. Rapid screening assays for soluble and particulate bacterial dehydrogenases. *Antonie van Leeuwenhoek* **33**, 63–72.

MICHAL, G. 1978. Determination of Michaelis constants and inhibitor constants. In *Principles of Enzymatic Analysis*, ed. Bergmeyer, H.U. pp. 33–35. Weinheim: Verlag Chemie.

PRICE, N.C. & STEVENS, L. 1982. *Fundamentals of Enzymology*. Oxford: Oxford University Press.

STRETTON, R.J. & MANSON, T.W. 1973. Some aspects of the mode of action of the antibacterial compound Bronopol (2-bromo-2-nitropropan-1,3-diol). *Journal of Applied Bacteriology* **36**, 61–76.

Mechanisms of Chemical Reactions with Biomolecules

R.D. WAIGH AND P. GILBERT

Department of Pharmacy, University of Manchester, Oxford Road, Manchester M13 9PL, UK

Chemical antimicrobial agents exert their effect upon bacterial cells either through irreversible covalent associations with biomolecular targets resulting in adjunct formation or through reversible interactions of a physico-chemical nature which alter the physical chemistry of the target molecule. In the former instance, an understanding of the mechanisms and range of chemical interactions between biocide and potential targets is crucial to the elucidation of the mechanism of action in the intact cell (Gilbert 1985). Traditional methods for the evaluation of the chemical mechanism of action of reactive antimicrobial compounds have tended to involve two separate stages following exposure of cells to the agent. The first stage is one of separation and purification of the reaction products, often involving chromatography, and the second is the application of spectroscopy of various kinds to determine the molecular structure of the adjuncts. While these methods are still useful, it is becoming possible to carry out direct spectroscopic studies on systems *in vivo* and *in vitro* which are quicker, easier and more elegant and informative. The principal technique for such studies is nuclear magnetic resonance (NMR) spectroscopy, which in recent years has made substantial advances in sensitivity, with accompanying detailed improvements in experimental technique to enhance the information content of the spectra. Potential users of the technique, who have a basic grounding in NMR spectroscopy, will find the recent books by Sanders & Hunter (1987) and Derome (1987) particularly informative with respect to the latest developments. We propose to illustrate the usefulness of NMR spectroscopy as a tool for understanding the mode of action of biocides by reference to *in vitro* studies backed up by more traditional approaches (in the case of bronopol and *iso*thiazolones) and also by reference to direct *in vivo* methodologies (for noxythiolin and taurolin).

Bronopol (2-bromo-2-nitro-propan-1,3-diol)

Bronopol has a broad spectrum of antibacterial activity (Saito & Onoda 1974) and is widely used, at concentrations up to 0.1%, as a preservative of pharmaceutical and cosmetic products (Croshaw *et al* 1964; Storrs & Bell 1983). There have been a number of studies of the mechanism of action of bronopol, all of which conclude that activity relates to interaction with essential thiols within the cell (Stretton & Manson 1973; Bryce *et al*. 1978; Wong & Preece 1985). Such interaction is thought to lead to oxidation of thiols through a radical anion intermediate (Russell & Danen 1967). Unlike other thiol-interactive antimicrobial agents (e.g. thiomersal), bronopol possesses significant bactericidal activity which cannot be explained solely in terms of thiol oxidation.

Earlier studies on the mode of action have shown that in aqueous solution cysteine is rapidly oxidized to cysteine in the presence of bronopol (Stretton & Manson 1973). This experiment is easy to repeat, by using thin-layer chromatography as the analytical method. In such systems, however, bronopol is not easy to detect and is even harder to quantify by this means. When the bronopol–cysteine reaction is carried out inside the spectrometer (Fig. 1) it is possible, not only to follow the disappearance of the cysteine and the formation of cystine but also to observe the bronopol quantitatively (Shepherd *et al*. 1988). The spectra in Fig. 1 show very clearly that the bronopol is scarcely consumed in this reaction, while the cysteine is rapidly oxidized. When the reactions were monitored by oxygen electrode it was apparent that the reaction mixture, and indeed bacterial suspensions, were rapidly depleted of oxygen upon bronopol addition, irrespective of the bronopol: thiol ratio. The bronopol is therefore acting as an oxidative catalyst in the presence of oxygen.

In the absence of air (Fig. 2) the reaction is much slower and the bronopol disappears at a comparable rate to the cysteine (Shepherd *et al*. 1988). While the reaction is far too complex to allow the direct determination of the structures of the reaction products, the experiment does indicate that different modes of action must apply under oxic and anoxic conditions. Subsequent work with cysteine methyl ester, involving solvent extraction and chromatographic separation of the reaction products, showed that the thiol had been extensively degraded, under anaerobic conditions, by an oxidative mechanism to elemental sulphur. In this case the bronopol itself must be chemically reduced since there is no oxygen available.

Such chemical information is compatible with the observed biological effects of bronopol. Following the addition of bronopol to actively growing cultures of bacteria, growth ceases immediately for a period dependent upon the concentration applied. After this induced bacteriostasis, growth proceeds at an inhibited rate. Bactericidal concentrations (100–500 μg/ml) are considerably in excess of the minimum growth inhibitory concentration (MIC; 10–15 μg/ml). Bactericidal activity, but not growth inhibitory actions, may be

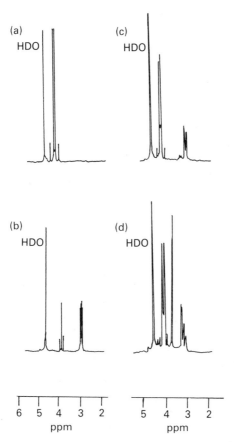

FIG. 1. 80-MHz ^{1}H NMR spectra in deuterium oxide of; (a) bronopol, (b) cysteine, (c) equimolar mixtures of bronopol (20 mg) and cysteine (17 mg) reacted, in air at room temperature, within the NMR tube, and (d) cystine. Note that (c) shows the continued presence of the bronopol doublet whilst cystine is a major product. (For a detailed assignment of the peaks readers are directed to Shepherd *et al.* 1988.)

significantly reduced by the exclusion of air or inclusion of the enzymes catalase or superoxide dismutase in cell suspensions. It is apparent that bronopol undergoes two distinct types of reaction with accessible thiols within cells. Under aerobic conditions, bronopol catalyses the oxidation of thiols such as glutathione and cysteine to their disulphides, utilizing atmospheric oxygen as the oxidant and generating an anoxic state. Further oxygen diffusing into the system will be used catalytically in this manner so long as bronopol remains. Such reactions will bring about the immediate cessation of bacterial growth. By-products or intermediates in this aerobic reaction are active oxygen species such as superoxide and peroxide. These are directly responsible for

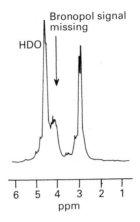

FIG. 2. 80-MHz ^{1}H NMR spectrum of equimolar mixtures of bronopol (20 mg) and cysteine (17 mg) in deuterium oxide reacted in the absence of air at room temperature in the NMR tube. Note the loss of the bronopol doublet and the formation of a new product which does not resemble cysteine or cystine (see Fig. 1).

the bactericidal activity of the compound and for the reduced rate of growth following the bacteriostatic period. Once an anoxic state has been created in the reaction mixture it will be maintained by the presence of unreacted bronopol and reduced thiols but it will allow the slower, consumptive reactions of bronopol to predominate until all the bronopol is consumed. Only then may enzymes such as glutathione reductase restore the redox state of the cell and allow growth to resume. Whether this occurs depends upon the extent of free radical damage incurred during the interim period.

Isothiazolone Biocides

Isothiazolone biocides such as bensisothiazolone (BIT), N-methyl isothiazolone (MIT) and 5-chloro-N-methylisothiazolone (Cl–MIT) are widely used as environmental biocides. BIT has been shown to interact oxidatively with accessible thiols and specifically to inhibit glucose transport in vivo (Fuller et al. 1985). Addition of thioglycollate, mercaptoethanol, glutathione or cysteine at equimolar concentrations to all three biocides totally neutralizes their inhibitory effects. For Cl–MIT activity is also reversed in vivo by the addition of valine or histidine.

Conventional spectral and analytical studies have suggested that the reactions of BIT with thiols are as outlined below. Initial reaction leads to the formation of a disulphide conjugate. Reaction of the conjugate with further thiols leads to the formation of a thiol dimer and a ring-opened form of the biocide which itself could serve as a further source of interactive thiol to give a dimerized biocide as an additional product (Fuller *et al.* 1985). Cl−MIT and MIT are thought to act similarly to BIT but whilst BIT is a hypersensitizing agent, Cl−MIT is both a primary skin irritant (>25 μg/ml; Weaver *et al.* 1985) and Ames positive (Monte *et al.* 1983). Cl−MIT has reported bactericidal activity, unlike BIT which is primarily bacteriostatic in action. Cl−MIT is antibacterial at considerably lower concentrations than BIT. The reasons behind these fundamental differences in activity were unclear until NMR spectroscopy studies were undertaken.

Reactions of BIT with cysteine were examined by ^{1}H NMR spectroscopy with a Bruker WP80 spectrometer and the reaction pathway suggested by Fuller *et al.* (1985) confirmed. When similar studies were undertaken with Cl−MIT, however, (Fig. 3) loss of the downfield proton peak indicated exchange with D_2O and suggested that the ring-opened form of the biocide could tautomerize, to give a highly reactive thio-acid chloride.

Formation of the thio-acid chloride *in vivo* would explain the apparently anomalous toxicological and antimicrobial activity of the chlorinated *iso*thiazolone in that it would possess a far higher reactivity than the parent molecule.

Noxythiolin and Taurolin

Investigations into these and other 'masked formaldehyde' antibacterial agents can be conceptually separated into those studies which deal with the nature of the active antibacterial form and those dealing with the detoxification processes possessed by the organism. In both cases the critical experiments have been conducted using NMR spectroscopy, either for direct observation of chemical equilibria, for which it was superior to alternative methods, or for *in vivo* observation of metabolites, a task for which NMR is uniquely suited.

The toxic intermediates

On a simplistic basis both noxythiolin and taurolin can be considered as

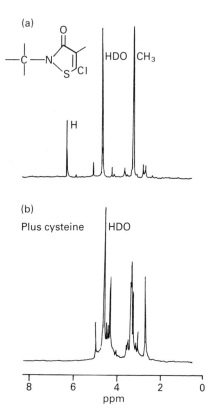

FIG. 3. 80-MHz ^{1}H NMR spectra of; (a) 5-chloro-N-methyl *iso*thiazolone, and (b) equimolar mixtures of 5-choloro-N-methyl *iso*thiazolone (5 mg) and cysteine (10 mg) in deuterium oxide reacted at room temperature in the NMR tube. Note the loss of the downfield proton of 5-chloro-N-methyl *iso*thiazolone indicating exchange with the D$_2$O solvent and therefore isomerization.

formaldehyde-producing antibacterial agents, the overall simplified equations for their aqueous decomposition being as described in the following schemes.

$$HN \diagdown N-CH_2-N \diagup NH \quad +3H_2O$$
$$O_2S \diagdown \diagup N-CH_2-N \diagdown SO_2 \xrightleftharpoons[-3H_2O]{} 2\ H_2NCH_2CH_2SO_2NH_2 + 3\ HCHO$$

Taurolin

A simple chemical experiment (Gidley *et al.* 1981; Gidley & Sanders 1983) demonstrates an important difference in the chemical behaviour of the two compounds. Sodium cyanoborohydride is a reducing agent which is reasonably stable in aqueous solution, and which reacts slowly with formaldehyde to give methanol. (It should be noted that formaldehyde exists largely as the hydrated form in aqueous solution.)

$$HO \diagdown CH_2 \diagup \xrightleftharpoons[+H_2O]{-H_2O} \overset{H}{\underset{H}{\diagdown}} C=O \xrightarrow{NaBH_3CN} CH_3OH$$

When a solution of noxythiolin is treated with reducing agent the only reaction is the slow reduction of formaldehyde to methanol. The reaction tends to show that noxythiolin is truly a source of formaldehyde as the toxic species and it is no surprise that *Escherichia coli* survival curves, after exposure to noxythiolin solutions, are very close to those obtained with formaldehyde itself (Gidley & Sanders 1983). In contrast, treatment of taurolin solutions with the reducing agent gives almost quantitative conversion to an N-methyl intermediate.

$$O_2S \diagup^{HN} N-CH_2-N \diagdown^{NH} SO_2 \rightleftharpoons O_2S \diagup^{HN} N^+ = CH_2 + HN \diagup^{NH} SO_2$$

$$\downarrow NaBH_3CN$$

$$O_2S \diagup^{HN} N-CH_3$$

The methylene iminium ion $R_2N^+=CH_2$ is a more reactive species than formaldehyde towards hydride ions provided by the reducing agent, so that the reaction is chemically quite orthodox, proving the presence of the iminium ion. NMR spectroscopy provides a convenient means of following the reaction as it proceeds without the necessity for repetitious chemical analyses (Gidley *et al.* 1981).

We now have an explanation for the enhanced antibacterial activity of taurolin and for the increased antibacterial activity of formaldehyde in the presence of certain amines. The iminium ion is likely to be more readily attacked than formaldehyde by the biological nucleophile, in an analogous manner to the attack by hydride ions, resulting in more rapid inactivation of the susceptible bacterial system. For systems in which the amine is added separately, the distinction can be made between weak and strong bases, in an exactly comparable way.

$$R_2NH + HCHO \rightleftharpoons R_2NCH_2OH$$
Weak base

$$R_2NH + HCHO \rightleftharpoons R_2NCH_2OH \rightleftharpoons R_2\overset{+}{N}{=}CH_2 + H_2O$$
Strong base   More toxic

In these studies the major role of NMR spectroscopy is as an elegant, non-disruptive, simultaneous assay for formaldehyde and other reaction products or intermediates. An illustration of the extraordinary power of the method, however, is provided in the case of imidazole–formaldehyde mixtures (Gidley & Sanders 1983).

This system does not produce iminium ions in great quantity but was none the less more effective than formaldehyde alone. Another NMR spectroscopy experiment showed that the above equilibrium was capable of producing naked (non-hydrated) formaldehyde about 40 times more frequently than a simple aqueous solution of formaldehyde alone, thus providing a feasible explanation for the enhanced antibacterial activity.

Metabolic studies

In order to study metabolic reactions involving potentially toxic species it is necessary to use concentrations below those which kill the cell. The pathways which are revealed are thus essentially detoxification processes and probably compete with those through which the antibacterial agent exerts its desired effects. Whether comparable studies of the toxic reactions will ever be feasible remains to be seen.

In vivo ^{13}C NMR spectroscopy

While there is no room here for a general discourse on NMR spectroscopy, some explanation of the special attributes of ^{13}C NMR spectroscopy will help to explain how the experiments with formaldehyde were conceived.

One of the most significant features of ^{13}C NMR spectroscopy, compared to ^1H NMR as used in the work described previously, is that ^{13}C is a minor isotope, constituting only 1.1% of natural carbon. If the material whose metabolism is to be studied is labelled with a high concentration of ^{13}C, the peaks for the added material are of greater intensity and can be studied with minimal interference from background natural abundance carbon. In addition, the range of resonance frequencies for ^{13}C is very wide, so that interference between peaks is less likely, even for chemically similar molecules, and the exact resonance frequency (chemical shift) is highly characteristic for any given position in a molecule, provided that pH is held constant. Given that carbon–carbon coupling is not a problem (owing to the low natural abundance), that each carbon resonance can be reduced to a single line, and that efficient techniques are available for the determination of the number of protons attached to the labelled carbon, it can thus be seen that ^{13}C NMR spectroscopy is tailor-made for the problem in hand.

Formaldehyde metabolism by Escherichia coli

The work described by Sanders and co-workers (Hunter et al. 1984, 1985; Mason et al. 1986) examines this subject in great depth, and includes a consideration of deuterium incorporation which can also be measured and provides further insight. The major findings, however, can be simply stated as follows.

A ^{13}C spectrum of an E. coli suspension, treated with ^{13}C-labelled formaldehyde at a sublethal concentration, initially shows only one major peak, corresponding to $^{13}CH_2(OH)_2$, the hydrated form of formaldehyde, at $\delta 83.2$ (Fig. 4a). Three hours later there are five other peaks corresponding to methanol, formate and three rather similar products, namely propane-1,2 diol, propane-1,3-diol and glycerol (Fig. 4b), the latter identified with the aid of bacteria grown on ^{13}C-labelled glucose. Subsequent experiments showed that the first-formed adduct is 5-(hydroxymethyl)-glutathione, formed non-enzymically within a very short time after formaldehyde addition.

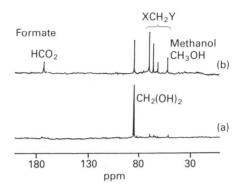

FIG. 4. 100.6-MHz ^{13}C NMR spectrum in deuterium oxide of a non-aerated *E. coli* suspension (10^{12} cells/ml) initially containing 10 mmol/l ^{13}C-labelled formaldehyde. (a) Spectrum obtained during the first 20 min after formaldehyde addition, and (b) 3 h later. A total of 500 transients was collected, with a 2-s relaxation delay and 45° pulse width. (Reproduced with permission from Hunter *et al.* 1984.)

This glutathione adduct, with a labelled ^{13}C resonance at δ66.6, remains until the one-carbon residue is disposed of by metabolism. There is no evidence for incorporation of the label into serine, methionine or other methyl groups, which effectively rules out the incorporation of this exogenous formaldehyde into the tetrahydrofolate pool. Deoxygenation virtually abolishes metabolism, while aeration results in loss of label, presumably through oxidation to bicarbonate and loss of carbon dioxide.

While the identification of metabolites such as methanol and formate follows very simply from measurement of the chemical shift and determination of the number of protons attached to the labelled carbon, the identity of the similar three-carbon products is less easy to establish. The chemical shifts of the labelled carbons are similar at δ68.0, 63.9 and 59.8; all three of these have two attached protons with CH-coupling constants of about 140 Hz. All three are therefore consistent with the unit $R^{13}CH_2OH$. This problem was solved quite elegantly by feeding the bacteria with glucose, uniformly labelled with ^{13}C at a level of 14.3%, compared to the 90% labelling of the formaldehyde. In the spectra obtained it is therefore possible to distinguish carbons arising from glucose (14.3% label) from those arising from formaldehyde (90% label), and to infer the diverse origins of carbons with intermediate levels of labelling. The more immediate intention, however, was to allow the unidentified carbons, labelled from ^{13}C formaldehyde, to interact with their neighbours, which will now be seen in the spectrum. This reveals their chemical shift and gives a clue as to their chemical environment. This concept may be expressed as follows for propane-1,2-diol, one of the previously identified metabolites

(*C=90% label, •C=14% label). Using ^{12}C glucose the ^{13}C NMR spectrum shows

$$HO^*CH_2 - CHOH - CH_3.$$

(CHOH-CH$_3$ is of low relative intensity)

Using partially ^{13}C glucose shows

$$HO^*CH_2 - {}^{\bullet}CHOH - {}^{\bullet}CH_3.$$

*C and •C are coupled, i.e. they each cause splitting of the others' signal. We therefore know the chemical shift of the carbon adjacent to *C and the number of protons attached to it; a great aid to identification. Similar arguments apply to glycerol and propane-1,3 diol, with some subtleties which cannot be expounded here.

While ^{13}C NMR is almost ideal for studies of formaldehyde metabolism, there are limitations to the technique imposed mainly by the inherent lack of sensitivity associated with this nucleus. Even at the relatively high field strength used by Sanders and co-workers, spectrum accumulation normally took 20 min to give acceptable signal-to-noise. In a rapidly changing system this would be too slow. Nevertheless, it is likely that the use of NMR spectroscopy to investigate the mode of action of antibacterial agents will become more common and even more effective.

References

BRYCE, D.M., CROSHAW, B., HALL, J.E., HOLLAND, V.R. & LESSEL, B. 1978. The activity and safety of the antimicrobial agent bronopol (2-bromo-2-nitropropan-1,3-diol). *Journal of Cosmetic Chemistry* **29**, 3–24.

CROSHAW, B., GROVES, M.J. & LESSEL, B. 1964. Some properties of bronopol, a new antimicrobial agent against *Pseudomonas aeruginosa. Journal of Pharmacy and Pharmacology* **16**, 127T.

DEROME, A.E. 1987. *Modern NMR Techniques for Chemistry Research.* Oxford: Pergamon Press.

FULLER, S.J., DENYER, S.P., HUGO, W.B., PEMBERTON, D., WOODCOCK, P.M. & BUCKLEY, A.J. 1985. The mode of action of 1,2-benzisothiazolin-3-one on *Staphyloccocus aureus. Letters in Applied Microbiology* **1**, 13–15.

GIDLEY, M.J. & SANDERS, J.K.M. 1983. Mechanisms of antibacterial formaldehyde delivery from noxythiolin and other 'masked-formaldehyde' compounds. *Journal of Pharmacy and Pharmacology* **35**, 712–717.

GIDLEY, M.J., SANDERS, J.K.M., MYERS, E.R. & ALLWOOD, M.C. 1981. The mode of antibacterial action of some 'masked' formaldehyde compounds. *FEBS Letters* **127**, 225–227.

GILBERT, P. 1985. The revival of microorganisms sub-lethally injured by chemical inhibitors. In *The Revival of Injured Microbes,* pp. 175–197, eds Andrew, M.H.E. & Russell, A.D., London: Academic Press.

HUNTER, B.K., NICHOLLS, K.M. & SANDERS, J.K.M. 1984. Formaldehyde metabolism by *Escherichia coli. In vivo* carbon, deuterium and two dimensional NMR observations of multiple detoxifying reactions. *Biochemistry* **23**, 508–514.

HUNTER, B.K., NICHOLLS, K.M. & SANDERS, J.K.M. 1985. Formaldehyde metabolism by

Escherichia coli. Carbon and solvent deuterium incorporation into glycerol, 1,2-propanediol and 1,3-propanediol. *Biochemistry* **24**, 4148–4155.

MASON, P.R., SANDERS, J.K.M., CRAWFORD, A. & HUNTER, B.K. 1986. Formaldehyde metabolism by *Escherichia coli*. Detection by *in vivo* ^{13}C NMR spectroscopy of *s*-(hydroxymethyl)-glutathione as a transient cellular intermediate. *Biochemistry* **25**, 4504–4507.

MONTE, W.C., ASHOOR, S.H. & LEWIS, B.J. 1983. Mutagenicity of two non-formaldehyde-forming antimicrobial agents. *Food Chemistry and Toxicology*, **21** 695–697.

RUSSELL, G.A. & DANEN, W.C. 1967. Electron transfer processes VIII. Coupling of radicals with carbanions. *Journal of the American Chemical Society* **90**, 347–353.

SAITO, H. & ONODA, T. 1974. Antibacterial action of bronopol on various bacteria, especially on *Pseudomonas aeruginosa*. *Chemotheraphy, Tokyo* **22**, 1466–1473.

SANDERS, J.K.H. & HUNTER, B.K. 1987. *Modern NMR Spectroscopy*. Oxford: Oxford University Press.

SHEPHERD, J.A., WAIGH, R.D. & GILBERT, P. 1988. Antibacterial action of 2-bromo-2-nitro-propan-1,3-diol (bronopol). *Journal of Bacteriology* **32**, 1693–1698.

STORRS, F.J. & BELL, D.E. 1983. Allergic contact dermatitis to 2-bromo-2-nitropropan-1,3-diol. *Journal of the American Academy of Dermatologists* **8**, 157–170.

STRETTON, R.J. & MANSON, T.W. 1983. Some aspects of the mode of action of the anti-bacterial compound bronopol (2-bromo-2-nitro propan-1,3-diol). *Journal of Applied Bacteriology* **36**, 61–76.

WEAVER, J.E., CARDIN, C.W. & MAIBACH, H.I. 1985. Dose-response assessments of kathon biocide (1) Diagnostic use and diagnostic threshold patch testing with sensitised humans. *Contact Dermatitis* **12**, 141–145.

WONG, W.C. & PREECE, T.F. 1985. *Pseudomonas tolasii* in mushroom (*Agaricus bisporus*) crops: Activity of formulations of 2-bromo-2-nitropropane-1,3-diol (bronopol) against the bacterium and the use of this compound to control blotch disease. *Journal of Applied Bacteriology* **58**, 275–281.

Intracellular Delivery of Biocides

S.P. DENYER, D.E. JACKSON AND M. AL-SAGHER

Department of Pharmaceutical Sciences, University of Nottingham, University Park, Nottingham NG7 2RD, UK

Although some lipophilic antibacterial agents with an intracellular target can successfully reach their site of action by passive diffusion, many others of a more hydrophilic nature are excluded by the efficient barrier function of the bacterial cytoplasmic membrane. This may not necessarily mean that no antibacterial activity will result from their presence, but it will necessitate the use of higher applied concentrations to ensure sufficient intracellular levels. Clearly, one approach to overcoming this penetration problem would be to encourage the uptake of antibacterial compounds *via* existing bacterial transport systems. This mechanism of uptake is recognized to occur naturally in the action of certain antibiotics (Chopra & Ball 1982) and has been exploited in the design of synthetic antibacterial peptide analogues (Ringrose 1980).

A natural extension to this approach is to link an antibacterial compound covalently to a molecule that is actively transported by a pre-existing carrier system. This would provide both a transmembrane route of access and a mechanism by which a biocidal agent could be concentrated intracellularly. By necessity, the permeant molecule developed would need to exploit a relatively non-specific transport system and would need to be susceptible to intracellular cleavage to release its antibacterial component. Limited studies have been undertaken with non-antibiotic agents (Table 1) demonstrating the potential applicability of this approach to biocides.

In an attempt to exploit the β-galactoside permease system, we have examined the antibacterial potential and intracellular hydrolysis of 2-nitrophenyl β-D-galactopyranoside (ONPG) and methyl 4-hydroxybenzoate β-D-galactopyranoside (MPHBG; Fig. 1). This study can be used to illustrate some of the chemical and biochemical approaches appropriate to the investigation of these phenomena. An extension of the synthetic programme has resulted in the preparation of a further series of substituted phenyl-β-D-galactopyranosides (Table 2) and their activity against β-galactosidase-positive bioluminescent *Escherichia coli* has been determined.

Mechanisms of Action of
Chemical Biocides

TABLE 1. *Portage transport of antibacterial agents*

Antibacterial agent	Porter compound	Transport system/organism	Reference
Phenylethanol	Galactose	β-galactoside/*E. coli*	Whitehouse & Loyalka (1967) Johnston & Pivnick (1970)
Phenol	Galactose	β-galactoside/*E. coli*	Johnston & Pivnick (1970)
4-chloro-2-cyclopentyl phenol (Dowicide 9)	Galactose	β-galactoside/*E. coli*	Johnston & Pivnick (1970)
4-[N-(2-mercaptoethyl)] aminopyridine-2, 6-dicarboxylic acid	Cysteine-containing mixed di- or tri-peptide	Di- or oligopeptide/*E. coli*	Boehm *et al.* (1983)
Thiophenol	Glycine-containing di-peptide	Di- or oligopeptide/*E. coli*	Kingsbury *et al.* (1984)
Aniline	Glycine-containing di-peptide	Di- or oligopeptide/*E. coli*	Kingsbury *et al.* (1984)
Phenol	Glycine-containing di-peptide	Di- or oligopeptide/*E. coli*	Kingsbury *et al.* (1984)
5-fluorouracil	Glycine-containing di- or tri-peptide	Di- or oligopeptide/*E. coli*	Kingsbury *et al.* (1984)

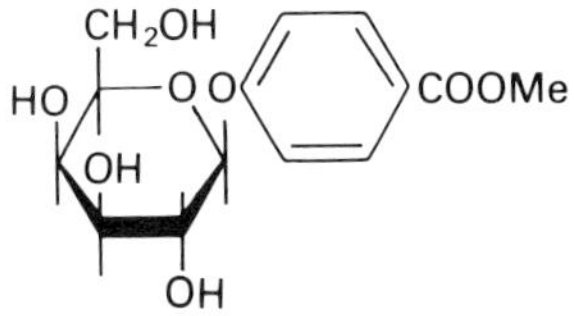

FIG. 1. The structure of methyl 4-hydroxybenzoate β-D-galactopyranoside.

TABLE 2. *Series of phenyl-β-D-galactopyranosides*

Biocide	β-D-galacto-pyranoside (G) derivative	Abbreviation
Phenol	Phenyl-G	PG
4-methylphenol	4-methylphenyl-G	PMPG
4-bromophenol	4-bromophenyl-G	PBPG
3, 4, 5-tribromophenol	3, 4, 5-tribromophenyl-G	TBPG
2, 4-dichlorophenol	2, 4-dichlorophenyl-G	DCPG
4-chloro-2-nitrophenol	4-chloro-2-nitrophenyl-G	PCONPG
Ethyl 4-hydroxy-benzoate	Ethyl 4-hydroxy-benzoate-G	EPHBG

Methods

Organisms

Escherichia coli NCTC 86 was grown in Nutrient Broth (Oxoid, Basingstoke, UK) supplemented with 3.5 mmol/1 *iso*propylthiogalactoside (IPTG) as β-galactosidase inducer. When required as a washed suspension, cells were grown on the above medium supplemented with 1.5% Agar No. 1 (Oxoid) and harvested by centrifugation at 37°C. After twice washing in 0.1 mol/1 phosphate buffer, pH 7.4, (37°C) cells were suspended for use in this buffer at 37°C. Careful temperature control was essential during the preparation of washed suspensions in order to avoid thermal shock and the consequent release of intracellular enzyme.

Bioluminescent *E. coli* pSB100 (harbouring the *lux* plasmid pBTK5; Stewart *et al.*, this book) were grown overnight (18 h) at 30°C in L-broth (yeast extract, 0.5%; tryptone, 1%; sodium chloride, 0.5%, pH 7.0) containing 30 µg/ml ampicillin. The strain was confirmed β-galactosidase-positive by its biochemical profile on API20E.

Chemicals

ONPG was obtained from Sigma Chemical Company Ltd, Poole, UK. MPHBG was synthesized from methyl 4-hydroxybenzoate and tetraacetyl β-D-galactopyranosylbromide (Aldrich, Dorset, UK) according to the procedures of Seidman & Link (1950) and Csuros *et al.* (1964) and finally obtained as pure white crystals (melting point 185−186°C) by catalytic deacetylation (Leaback 1960). Chemical identity and purity were established by spectroscopic methods (^{13}C NMR, ^{1}H NMR and FAB−MS). The substituted phenyl-β-D-galactopyranosides in Table 2 were prepared by the method of Kleine *et al.* (1985) using the appropriate phenol. The purity of the acetylated derivatives was confirmed by ^{1}H NMR spectroscopy and thin-layer chromatography (De Bruyne & Wouters-Leysen 1971) and the galactosides were obtained by deacetylation (Leaback 1960). Chemical identity and purity were established by spectroscopic methods as before.

Antibacterial action

Minimum growth inhibitory concentration

Minimum growth inhibitory concentrations (MICs) for ONPG and MPHBG were obtained by inoculation (with 5×10^{7} cells of *E. coli* NCTC 86) of 2 ml nutrient broth containing varying concentrations of compound under investigation. Growth was assessed visually after 24 h incubation at 37°C. MPHBG was added in dimethylsulphoxide (final concentration not exceeding 5%); control experiments demonstrated that this level of solvent used had no effect on cell growth.

Bioluminescent studies

A 0.1-ml volume of an 18-h culture of *E. coli* pSB100 was used to inoculate 10 ml of fresh L-broth containing varying concentrations of the phenyl-β-D-galactopyranosides dissolved in dimethylsulphoxide (to a final concentration of 2%). The suspensions were incubated statically at 30°C and 25 µl samples were removed at the required times and placed in triplicate in microtitre plate wells. 225-µl quantities of aldehyde−glucose solution (2% sodium azide, 40 µg/ml polymyxin B sulphate, 1% Triton X100, 0.5% dodecanal, 0.2% glucose) were added to each well, mixed, and the bioluminescence measured immediately in an Amerlite luminometer (Amersham International plc, Amersham, UK). The bioluminescent yield remained constant over 5 min and results were recorded as the light output 3 min after addition of the aldehyde−glucose solution.

Bacterial metabolism of galactopyranoside

Hydrolysis of ONPG and MPHBG was examined at 37°C in the presence of both whole-cell washed suspensions of *E. coli* (4×10^9 cells/ml) and cell lysate obtained by sonication. Samples were removed from reaction mixtures at various intervals, filtered through a 0.45-μm pore-size membrane filter, and the presence of free 2-nitrophenol and methyl 4-hydroxybenzoate determined by spectrophotometry and thin-layer chromatography, respectively.

Results and Discussion

Native biocide was released in the presence of both whole cells and cell-free extracts (for example, see Fig. 2), but the antimicrobial activity of the β-D-galactopyranoside was significantly less than the free biocide (Table 3). This was attributed to the time-dependent hydrolysis of the galactopyranosides and to the freely permeable nature of 2-nitrophenol and methyl 4-hydroxybenzoate which may be released readily from the intracellular compartment. For the latter compound, this lends support to the theory that methyl 4-hydroxy-benzoate is sufficiently lipophilic to influence transmembrane proton gradients (Eklund 1980). An extension of these studies to include the effects of other phenyl-β-D-galactopyranosides on *E. coli* growth (as indicated by biolumine-scence; Stewart *et al.*, this book) showed activity to reside also in the 2,4-dichloro-, 4-bromo-, and 3,4,5-tribromophenyl derivatives (Table 4). An observed initial delay (6−18 h) in the onset of action is presumably a consequence of time-dependent hydrolysis.

In principle, portage transport can be considered for a wide range of non-antibiotic agents. It may offer potential in the design of selectively active antibacterial compounds with lower intrinsic mammalian toxicity, and may also find application in the development of selective microbiological culture media. Successful exploitation of biocide portage, however, will require evidence of the intracellular location of the antibacterial event. In our studies, we have

TABLE 3. *Antibacterial activity of 2-nitrophenol and methyl 4-hydroxybenzoate and their respective β-D-galactopyranoside derivatives, ONPG and MPHBG*

Compound	MIC (mmol/l)
2-nitrophenol	3
ONPG	20
Methyl 4-hydroxybenzoate	4.5
MPHBG	100

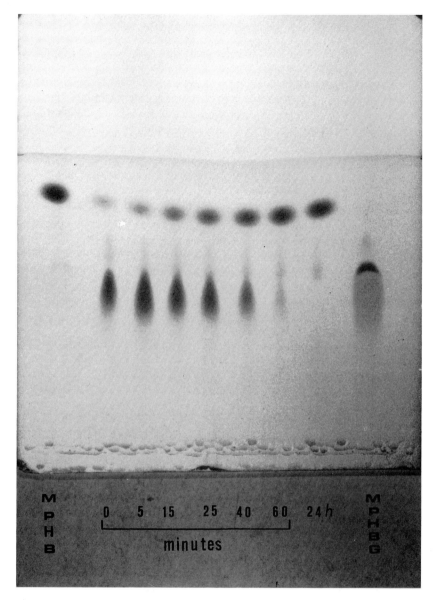

FIG. 2. Hydrolysis of MPHBG by *E. coli* NCTC 86 whole cells. Samples were removed at various time intervals and hydrolysis assessed by thin-layer chromatography (TLC). Standard compounds are represented at the extremes of the TLC. MPHB, methyl 4-hydroxybenzoate; MPHBG, methyl 4-hydroxybenzoate β-D-galactopyranoside.

TABLE 4. *Bioluminescence from* E. coli, *pSB100 growing in the presence of selected phenyl-β-D-galactopyranosides*

Galactopyranoside*	Concentration (mmol/l)	Bioluminescence as % of control at:		
		6 h	18 h	24 h
PG	1.2	136	99	118
PMPG	1.1	132	112	126
PBPG	0.89	173	85	62
TBPG	0.61	156	14	6
DCPG	0.92	169	1	1
PCONPG	0.45	99	106	123
EPHBG	0.91	110	109	112

* For abbreviations see Table 2.
Control cells were grown in the presence of 2% dimethylsulphoxide.

clearly demonstrated that the action of methyl 4-hydroxybenzoate is not enhanced by the active transport of the agent into the cell, lending credence to a possible cytoplasmic membrane target in *E. coli*. Portage transport studies may thus contribute to our further understanding of mechanisms of antibacterial action.

References

BOEHM, J.C., KINGSBURY, W.D., PERRY, D. & GILVARG, C. 1983. The use of cysteinyl peptides to effect portage transport of sulfhydryl-containing compounds in *E. coli*. *Journal of Biological Chemistry* 258, 14850–14855.

CHOPRA, I. & BALL, P. 1982. Transport of antibiotics into bacteria. *Advances in Microbial Physiology* 23, 183–240.

CSUROS, Z., DEAK, G. & HARASZTHY-PAPP, M. 1964. Correlation of the optical rotation of aromatic galactosides with the dissociation constants of the corresponding phenols. *Acta Chimica Academiae Scientiarum Hungaricae* 42, 263–267.

DE BRUYNE, C.K. & WOUTERS-LEYSEN, J. 1971. Synthesis of substituted phenyl β-D-galacto-pyranosides. *Carbohydrate Research* 18, 124–126.

EKLUND, T. 1980. Inhibition of growth and uptake processes in bacteria by some chemical food preservatives. *Journal of Applied Bacteriology* 48, 423–432.

JOHNSTON, M.A. & PIVNICK, H. 1970. Use of autocytotoxic β-D-galactosides for selective growth of *S. typhimurium* in the presence of coliforms. *Canadian Journal of Microbiology* 16, 83–89.

KINGSBURY, W.D., BOEHM, J.C., PERRY, D. & GILVARG, C. 1984. Portage of various compounds into bacteria by attachment to glycine residues in peptides. *Proceedings of the National Academy of Sciences, USA* 81, 4573–4576.

KLEINE, H.P., WEINBERG, V.D., KAUMAN, R.J. & SIDHU, R.S. 1985. Phase-transfer-catalyzed synthesis of 2, 3, 4, 6-tetra-O-acetyl-β-D-galactopyranosides. *Carbohydrate Research* 142, 333–337.

LEABACK, D.H. 1960. Deacetylation of glycoside polyacetates. *Journal of the Chemical Society*, 3166.

RINGROSE, P.S. 1980. Peptides as antimicrobial agents. In *Microorganisms and Nitrogen Sources*, ed. Payne, J.W. pp. 641–692. London: John Wiley & Sons.

SEIDMAN, M. & LINK, K.P. 1950. *o*-Nitrophenyl-β-D-galactopyranoside and its tetracetate. *Journal of the American Chemical Society* 72, 4324.

WHITEHOUSE, F. & LOYALKA, S. 1967. Antimicrobial properties of phenethyl alcohol and phenethyl-β-D-galactopyranoside. *Antimicrobial Agents and Chemotherapy* **1966**, 555–562.

Microbial Adherence and Biofilm Production

S.P. GORMAN

School of Pharmacy, Medical Biology Centre, The Queen's University of Belfast, Belfast BT9 7BL, UK

Micro-organisms may adhere to a vast array of surfaces and may proceed, under suitable conditions, to form a biofilm. Adherence and biofilm formation on materials of industrial significance, and biocide effects thereon, are well-known phenomena and have recently been extensively reviewed (Gilbert & Herbert 1987; Sharma *et al.* 1987). Examination of bacterial adherence and the investigation of effects of agents on adherence leads to an understanding and control of the adhesion process. The effects of macromolecules (Olsson *et al.* 1980), polypeptides (Lamberts *et al.* 1985), proteins (Fletcher 1976), enzymes (Ridgway *et al.* 1984), glycoconjugates (Ludwicka *et al.* 1985), surfactants (Paul & Jeffrey 1985; Humphries *et al.* 1987), non-antibiotic agents (Gorman *et al.* 1987a) and antibiotics (Shibl 1985) on the adhesion process and/or biofilm formation have all been described.

Antimicrobial agents are generally to be defined as those entities which adversely affect the viability (microbiocidal) or growth (microbiostatic) of a micro-organism. Increasingly, however, the recognition that other adverse effects may be exerted on micro-organisms at concentrations below the minimum growth inhibitory concentration (subMIC) of some agents implies that the label 'antimicrobial' requires broader definition. This is clearly demonstrated, for example, by the ability of numerous antimicrobial agents to alter the adherence of microbes to surfaces. Furthermore, an ever growing group of substances which do not possess intrinsic microbiocidal or microbiostatic activity is being shown to exert an 'antimicrobial' effect through the interference with the microbial adhesion process. The influence of antimicrobial agents on microbial adherence merits close examination and quantification as an alternative possibility for prophylactic or therapeutic interference with the infectious process and in the industrial control of microbial biofilms. This chapter provides a description of methods which may be used to determine the effects of biocides on the adherence process. It will concentrate on

Mechanisms of Action of
Chemical Biocides

microbial adherence within environments of a clinical nature but many of the methods are also applicable to non-clinical studies.

Methods for Determining Bacterial Adherence to Epithelial Cells

Exfoliated epithelial cells

Bacterial adherence to epithelial cells may be influenced by several experimental factors in the methodology which in turn may dictate the extent of antiadherence activity demonstrated by an antimicrobial agent. Assay conditions which may influence the level of adherence and which should be considered in the light of previous experience (Kimura & Pearsall 1980; Funfstuck *et al.* 1987) include:

1   Bacteria used and culture conditions – choice of clinical isolate or laboratory strain, single or multiple challenge, growth medium, medium pH and osmolality, incubation temperature, microbial growth phase.

2   Epithelial cells – cell viability should be ascertained. Source-related factors known, or suspected, to alter adherence include smoking, chronic obstructive pulmonary disease, diabetes mellitis, immobility and incontinence. Drugs known to, or suspected to, alter adherence include diuretics, steroids, antiasthmathics, anticholinergics and antibiotics. Cells should not be obtained from patients in any of the above categories.

3   Adherence assay – specific ion concentrations, salivary proteins, incubation time and temperature, concentration ratios of epithelial cells and bacteria.

The adherence assay involves consideration of three main stages:

1   Isolation/identification of bacteria and culture conditions. Single strains of clinical isolates are grown in a selected medium to the desired growth phase. Bacterial cell concentrations are determined by optical density measurements and are confirmed by viable counts.

2   The attachment of bacteria to epithelial cells has often been studied by incubating washed bacterial suspensions with buccal, pharyngeal or vaginal epithelial cells obtained by scraping the appropriate tissue surface. Uroepithelial cells, also frequently used, are obtained by centrifugation of mid-stream urine samples. Epithelial cells may be obtained from an individual or collected from a number of volunteers and pooled. Following at least two washes by centrifugation (150 rev/min, 10 min, 20°C) in 0.01 mol/l phosphate buffered saline (PBS) (pH 7.3) the cells are suspended in PBS at a given concentration, though generally at a level of 10^5 cells/ml. The cell concentration is adjusted after counting by light microscopy in a haemocytometer. Cell viability (i.e. percentage of live cells) may be estimated by application of trypan blue dye. Equal volumes of trypan blue dye (0.01%) and cell suspension are mixed and incubated at 24°C for 10 min, placed on slides and examined microscopically. Exclusion of the dye by the cell indicates viability.

Valentin-Weigand *et al.* (1987) have further refined this preparative method by layering the collected epithelial cells on top of a Percoll gradient contained in polypropylene tubes of 14 ml capacity. The gradient consists of 3 ml 30% Percoll (Pharmacia, Freiburg, FRG) in PBS (density, 1.035 g/ml) at the bottom and of 3 ml 15% Percoll in PBS (density, 1.020 g/ml) at the top. After centrifugation (30 s at 9000 g), the epithelial cells are removed from the interface between 15 and 30% Percoll. The cells are then washed twice in PBS for 30 min at 1800 g and are adjusted to the required cell concentration in a haemocytometer.

3   Adherence assays are essentially as described by Svanborg-Eden (1978). 1-ml volumes each of bacterial suspension (*c.* 10^8 bacteria/ml) and epithelial cells (10^5 cells/ml) are mixed and incubated with shaking at 37°C for a period of time (e.g. 1 h). Epithelial cells are recovered by centrifugation and unattached bacteria are washed free with two cycles of centrifugation (150 rev/min, 10 min) and washing in 3 ml PBS. The epithelial cell/bacterial preparation is then fixed by air-drying to a glass slide and is stained. The numbers of bacteria adhering to each of 50 (minimum) epithelial cells are counted by light microscopy at a magnification of ×1000. Electron microscopy may also be used to view microbial adherence. Figure 1 shows attachment of *Candida ablicans* blastospores to human buccal epithelial cells.

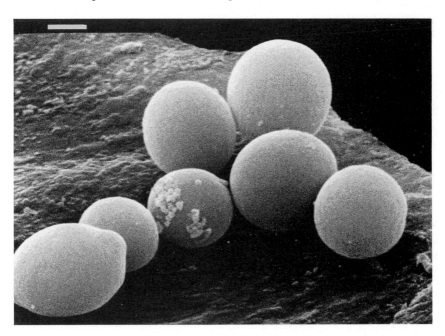

FIG. 1. Scanning electron micrograph of *Candida albicans* blastospores adhering to a buccal epithelial cell. (Bar marker=1.0 μm.)

A widely used variation of this adherence assay is to include a filtration step following (or replacing) the centrifugation/washing cycles to remove unattached bacteria. If filtration is to follow centrifugation, the non-adherent bacteria in the supernatant liquid are discarded. The pellets are then re-suspended in, and washed with, 50 ml PBS over polycarbonate filters having a pore diameter in the order of 12 μm. Capillary pore filters are superior to matrix pore filters as the former promote laminar flow through the filters with fewer non-adherent bacteria being trapped. Filters with epithelial cells and adherent bacteria are stained (normally with methylene blue or crystal violet) and are viewed microscopically. Table 1 describes typical data obtained from such adherence assays. Blastospores of *C. albicans* grown to either exponential or stationary phase and having no treatment (i.e. water as control) are observed to adhere in significantly higher numbers to buccal epithelial cells than do blastospores treated with various antimicrobial agents.

TABLE 1. *The effect of treatment of* C. albicans* blastospores with taurolidine, chlorhexidine and povidone-iodine on adherence to human buccal epithelial cells*

Treatment (30 min, 37°C)	No.[†] of *C. albicans* adhering/epithelial cell		Decrease in adherence compared to control[†]	
	Stationary	Exponential	Stationary	Exponential
Water	3.57±0.39	3.47±0.31		
Taurolidine (2%)	1.59±0.16	2.07±0.18	$P < 0.001$	$P < 0.001$
Water	3.57±0.39	3.47±0.31		
Chlorhexidine (0.05%)	1.70±0.21	1.97±0.24	$P < 0.001$	$P < 0.001$
Water	3.57±0.39	3.47±0.31		
Chlorhexidine (0.02%)	1.82±0.16	2.14±0.23	$P < 0.001$	$P < 0.001$
Water	3.57±0.39	3.47±0.31		
Povidone-iodine (0.075%)	1.79±0.16	2.04±0.18	$P < 0.001$	$P < 0.001$

* Oral isolate grown at 37°C.
[†] Mean ± s.e. of blastospores adhering.
[‡] Determined using a two-tailed unpaired *t*-test.

Counting methods

The majority of adherence studies have employed a direct light microscopic method utilizing simple staining techniques to obtain the number of adherent bacteria. Bacteria that touch the border or rest within the boundary of the epithelial cell are counted as adherent. An epithelial cell is normally considered for counting if it:

1 excludes viability stain;
2 presents no folding on itself;
3 is a complete entity with no fragmentation;
4 does not overlap other cells;
5 is in a field free of background bacteria.

In many studies, direct observation offers distinct advantages over other methods in the type of information gathered. For example, the number of bacteria on each epithelial cell, giving the distribution, can be quantified. Viable epithelial cells only may be counted and background bacteria can be accurately assessed. A double staining technique such as that described by Reid & Brooks (1982) advances this method to some degree. The general method is, however, tedious and time-consuming. The subjectivity of the visual counting assay prompted Kozody et al. (1985) to develop a radioactive assay involving direct ^{125}I-labelling of the bacterial external surface. This is a further refinement of the radioactive adherence assays using ^{14}C-labelled and [^{3}H] uridine-labelled micro-organisms developed by Parsons et al. (1979) and Schaeffer et al. (1981), respectively.

Although assays using radio-labelling have been developed for certain enteric bacteria it has not been possible to apply them to streptococci. These organisms tend to clump and form chains making it difficult to separate unattached bacteria quantitatively from epithelial cells by either differential centrifugation or filtration. Centrifugation of mixtures of [^{3}H] thymidine-labelled streptococci and epithelial cells in 50% Percoll to form a density gradient has recently been shown to readily separate epithelial cells having adhered bacteria (near the top) from unattached bacteria (near the bottom). The epithelial cells are collected on membrane filters and the number of adherent bacteria is then determined by scintillation counting (Tylewska & Gibbons 1987). The development in our laboratory of an adherence assay method using an electronic particle counter (Coulter Electronics Ltd, Luton, UK) allows rapid counting, in the order of seconds, providing ease of repetition and statistical confidence in the high counts obtained (Gorman et al. 1986). Typical data obtained for adherence of *Escherichia coli* to buccal and uroepithelial cells are presented in Table 2. Instrument settings are selected to count microorganisms at the minimum value above the electronic noise level. As two quite different cell sizes (micro-organism and epithelial) are involved,

TABLE 2. *Adherence of* E. coli *determined by electronic counting*

	Adherence components (controls)			Adherence mixture		Adherence	
	A	B	C	D	D–C	A–(D–C)	A–(D–C)/B
	*Organism count after 2h incubation †11/16 A1/2	Epithelial count after 2h incubation using haemocytometer	Epithelial count after 2h incubation †11/16 A1/2	Organism count after 2h adherence †11/16 A1/2	True organism count	Total organism epithelial adherence	Adherence epithelial cell
Escherichia coli and buccal epithelial cells	52 025 ±533	65 ±19	18 991 ±734	69 371 ±624	50 380	1645	25.5 ±3.5
Escherichia coli and uroepithelial cells	52 025 ±533	183 ±20	25 281 ±856	72 365 ±901	47 084	4941	27 ±0.3

* ± s.e. of mean of at least six counts. A coincidence factor of 2.5 used for correction of all Coulter counts. Microscopic assay adherence per buccal epithelial cell: 21.5±2.4 at 2h (i.e. 26.5–5 commensal background count). Microscopic assay adherence per uroepithelial cell: 23±1.2 at 2h.

† Background count (0.9% w/v sodium chloride) of 4376±868 taken from all readings at these settings. A, Amplification; I, aperture current. Viable count, 1.15 × 10^8 ml.

Buccal and uroepithelial haemocytometer count 1.3 × 10^5/ml and 3.66 × 10^5/ml, respectively.

Epithelial count in adherence mixture equivalent to epithelial count in control B.

contributions from either at particular settings should preferably be negligible. The Coulter Counter detects particles by the volume of electrolyte displaced by the particle and expresses this in terms of the equivalent spherical diameter. The morphology of the cell types is therefore important. Epithelial cells present difficulties in sizing due to their flexibility and changing morphology thus direct counting of these in a haemocytometer is required.

Fluorescent antibody staining techniques (Reid & Brooks 1985; Sveum *et al.* 1986) or a fluorescent dye such as fluorescein *iso*thiocyanate (Valentin-Weigand 1987) may also be applied to the bacterial cells in the adherence assay. In the latter, the stained bacteria are washed four times (until the supernatant becomes colourless) in PBS (0.15 mol/l, pH 7.4) prior to inclusion in the adherence assay. Epithelial cells with adherent fluorescent bacteria are washed twice, sedimented by centrifugation and resuspended in 1 ml PBS. Subsequently, 2.5 ml of 0.5 mol/l NaOH is added for extraction of fluorescein. The extract is then centrifuged (3 min, 5000 *g*) and the fluorescein contained in the supernatant liquid measured in a spectrofluorimeter. The measurements are expressed as a percentage of the total emission obtained from all bacteria used in the assay thus indicating the degree of adherence. Direct counting of adherent bacteria in a fluorescence microscope may also be undertaken. The use of the fluorochrome, acridine orange, in our laboratory has proved to be similarly useful. Further benefit from acridine orange use derives from its ability to distinguish between viable and non-viable adherent bacterial cells as in the direct epifluorescence filter technique (DEFT). In studies involving antimicrobial agents it is particularly useful to know not only the mean number of adherent micro-organisms but also the relative proportions of viable and non-viable adherent microbes. The frequency distribution plot in Fig. 2a describes the adherence to human mucosal epithelial cells of viable and non-viable blastospores within a late exponential phase population of an oral isolate of *C. albicans*. Treatment of this population with an antimicrobial agent possessing anti-adherence activity (e.g. chlorhexidine at sublethal concentration) radically affects the distribution of adherent viable and non-viable blastospores (Fig. 2b).

Statistical evaluation of data

The importance of correct statistical methodology in evaluating data from adherence assays has been emphasized by Rosenstein *et al.* (1985). This is particularly the case where a decrease in adherence is observed following treatment of microbial or epithelial cells with a chemical agent. A study by Woolfson *et al.* (1987), in our laboratories, demonstrated that application of parametric (unpaired *t*-test) or non-parametric (Mann-Whitney *U*-test) methods to such data gave similar results, although there were some minor

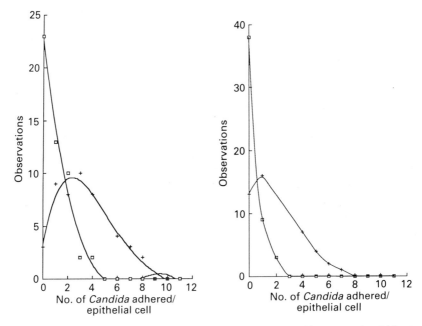

Fig. 2. Frequency distribution plot showing adherence of *C. albicans* blastospores (□, viable, +, non-viable) to human buccal epithelial cells as determined by acridine orange staining. (a) No treatment. (b) Treatment with subMIC chlorhexidine.

differences in the levels of significance achieved. The effect of the agent on the deviation of adherence data from normality may also be quantified from calculation of the skewness coefficient. A significant anti-adherence effect appears to result in a decrease in the skewness of the adherence assay data. This provides further information on the nature of the anti-adherence activity of the agent as a larger number of epithelial cells will have no microbial cells adhering following treatment.

Monolayer assay

A drawback to the use of exfoliated epithelial cell preparations in adherence studies is the presence of non-viable cells in the mixture. Thus, variation in the number of adherent micro-organisms is always observed. The epithelial cell preparations may also vary according to the donor, the time of sampling, the extent of colonization by the normal flora and the degree of exposure to various secretions (Douglas 1987). To overcome these difficulties, methods for measuring microbial adherence to more uniform populations such as cell monolayers have been developed. Provided that the kinetics of the monolayer assay show good linearity with respect to incubation time and to the number of added bacteria the results can be normalized to a common bacterial density and the adherence of different bacterial species to a common type of monolayer can be compared.

A tissue culture cell line such as the Intestine 407 line (ATLC CCL6, Flow LABS, Irvine, UK) used by Vosbeck *et al.* (1979) is maintained in Minimal Essential Medium containing 10% calf serum and monolayers are prepared in multiwell dishes with 3×10^5 cells used as the inoculum for each monolayer. Monolayers are confluent after 20 h of growth and are washed twice with Hepes−Hank solution (Hank's balanced salt solution buffered with Hepes) immediately before use. To each well 0.5 ml of Hepes−Hank solution is also added. The bacterial suspension is grown in broth containing a radioactive label such as [^{14}C] acetate 0.37 MBq/ml) and standardized to contain the desired number of bacteria/ml. For adherence tests with bacteria grown in the presence of a subMIC of a given antimicrobial agent, the latter is added to the growth medium to give the appropriate concentration at the beginning of the incubation period. Several washes with Hepes−Hank solution remove antibiotic from the final bacterial growth prior to standardization.

In the adherence assay, 0.5 ml of bacterial suspension are added to each monolayer to give a total volume of 1.0 ml. The monolayer plates are then shaken at 120 rev/min on a reciprocating shaker at 37°C. After incubation for a predetermined time (e.g. 30 min) unbound bacteria are removed by washing of the monolayer with 1.2 ml Hepes−Hank solution dispensed from an automatic syringe. Sodium dodecyl sulphate (1.5 ml of a 0.5% w/v solution) is then added with further incubation on the shaker at 37°C for at least 3 h. Aliquots (0.75 ml) of the solubilized mixture are then assessed for radioactivity in a scintillation counter. Results are calculated as the percentage of radioactivity bound to the monolayer and normalized to an original bacterial concentration of 10^8 ml.

Experimental tissue

Jacques *et al.* (1985) describe a method whereby rabbit mesentery samples are fixed on glass slides. These are then immersed vertically in the bacterial suspension which is gently agitated (100 rev/min) for 1 h at 37°C. The slides are then removed, washed with distilled water and stained for microscopic examination.

In an alternative method, the tissue is mounted in a perfusion chamber and infected with the bacteria for a specific time prior to washing, homogenization and examination by scanning electron microscopy (Marcus & Baker 1985).

Methods for Determining Bacterial Adherence to Solid Surfaces

Biofilm formation and slime production

Bacterial populations may form a biofilm by adhering to surfaces using fimbriae and exopolysaccharides. The cells become enveloped in a matrix of hydrated exopolysaccharides termed a glycocalyx (Costerton *et al.* 1981; Fig. 3). The glycocalyx matrix, often appearing as a slime, alters the environment of the adherent bacteria by concentrating nutrients and protecting the micro-organisms from adverse conditions including attack by antimicrobial agents.

Several studies have shown that micro-organisms may, under suitable conditions, grow in clumps in liquid medium or produce 'sticky colonies' on solid growth medium. These microbial strains often produce mucoid growth in the form of extracellular slime which, in combination with the clumping characteristic, confers resistance to many antiseptics and disinfectants (Kolawole 1984; Bolton *et al.* 1988). Slime-producing ability within a micro-organism is readily tested by visual assessment of adherence to the

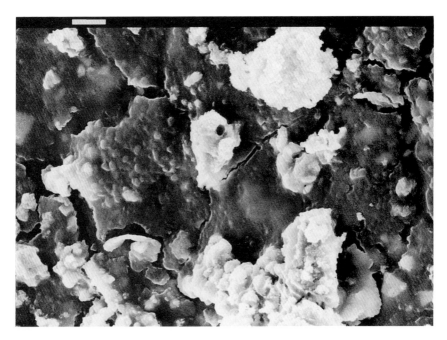

FIG. 3. Scanning electron micrograph of a urinary catheter surface showing the development of a thick bacterial biofilm. (Bar marker=1.0 μm.)

walls of a glass test tube following (for *Staphylococcus epidermidis* an 18-h incubation period would be appropriate, for example) static incubation in 10 ml Tryptone Soya Broth (Difco Laboratories Surrey, UK) at 37°C. The culture tubes are emptied of their contents and stained with trypan blue or safranin (0.1% w/v). Slime production is judged to have occurred if a visible film lines the walls of the tube. Ring formation at the liquid—air interface is judged not to be indicative of slime formation (Christensen *et al.* 1982).

Adherence of bacterial cells to synthetic polymer surfaces, especially to biomedical materials, is of considerable clinical importance. The formation of a biofilm is a two-stage process requiring:

1 effective adherence of the bacterium to the substrate;
2 suitable environmental conditions enabling multiplication of the micro-organism to proceed to biofilm formation.

Inhibition of biofilm formation may thus be possible with suitable agents through an effect at either of these stages. In addition, antimicrobial agents should be examined for activity against micro-organisms embedded in biofilms (sessile) in comparison with free-floating organisms (planktonic). The methods of study appropriate to these stages are considered below.

Adherence of bacteria to substrate

The majority of methods for estimating the number of bacterial cells adhered to a solid surface have been based on microscopic examination.

Light microscopy

Static system. The examination by McCourtie *et al.* (1986) of the effects of chlorhexidine, amphotericin B and nystatin on adherence of *Candida* spp. to denture acrylic illustrates the application of light microscopy to this area. Acrylic strips (5 mm², 0.5 mm thick) are incubated in a solution of the anti-microbial agent at the appropriate temperature and time before performing the adherence assay. Control strips are similarly treated with distilled water. The strips are placed vertically in the wells of a serology plate to which is added standardized micro-organism suspension in PBS (0.4 ml) and the plate is then shaken gently on an orbital shaker for a predetermined time. The strips are removed and washed five times with PBS. Attached micro-organisms are fixed in methanol, stained with Gram crystal violet and examined under a microscope. Thirty fields are counted on each acrylic strip and a minimum of 12 strips used in each assay.

Continuous flow system. A quantitative study of adhesion requires consideration of parameters such as the poorly controlled hydrodynamics and irreproducible rinsing conditions which may occur under static conditions of assay (Pratt-Terpstra *et al.* 1987); these are more easily accounted for in a continuous flow approach. Furthermore, an advantage of this system is the ability to coat the substratum surface with various substances, e.g. protein, prior to the adherence assay in order to mimic a particular *in vivo* situation. The substrata are then exposed to a flowing bacterial suspension containing 10^9 cells/ml for various time intervals up to 75 min. Substrata are then rinsed for 1 min with buffer, fixed for 2 min with 2% (v/v) glutaraldehyde and rinsed with buffer for a further 1 min. Subsequently the substrata are removed from the flow cell, air-dried and stained with crystal violet before examination in the microscope for adherent bacteria.

Other microscopic methods employed to measure adherence of bacteria to solid surfaces include those of Marshall *et al.* (1971) using phase-contrast microscopy for cell counts in wet preparations, and the use of image analysis by Verran *et al.* (1980) based on a method for measurement of absorbance due to stained cells *in situ* on glass (Rutter & Abbott 1978). The last method measures percentage coverage of surface by cells and also mean clump size of cells.

Electron microscopy

The scanning electron microscope (SEM) offers a direct and visually effective means of investigating bacteria adhering to surfaces. Edwards & Jeffryes (1987) described a method using the SEM to examine streptococci adhering to pellicle-coated dental enamel. In this study the GTGO−AD procedure of Gamliel *et al.* (1983) was used. This has the advantage that critical point drying or freeze-drying need not be employed and thus both the spatial and structural integrity of the adherent streptococci and the pellicle are maintained. Bacterial adherence is achieved by immersing 5-mm^2 sections of solid material in washed suspensions of micro-organism for 2 h followed by three rinses in sterile de-ionized water to remove loosely or non-adherent cells. The material sections are fixed overnight in 2% glutaraldehyde and are rinsed in PBS before mordanting in a mixture of 2% tannic acid and 2% guanidine hydro-chloride (Sigma Chemical Company Ltd, Poole, UK) in PBS for 1 h. After another 1-min rinse in PBS, the sections are immersed in 2% osmium tetroxide in PBS for 1 h. The sections are washed in de-ionized water and then passaged through a series of increasing concentrations of absolute ethanol in distilled water; a 10-min contact period is allowed in each solution. The fixed, dehydrated specimens are stored in 100% Freon 113 prior to gold coating and microscopic examination.

Fluorescence microscopy

Acridine orange, a fluorochrome dye buffered at low pH, has been used to detect bacteria adherent to intravascular catheters (Zufferey *et al.* 1988) and for determining adherence of bacteria to polymers (Verrier *et al.* 1987). The method is simple and rapid requiring a brief (2−5 min) staining of bacteria adhered to the material with 0.01% acridine orange followed by rinsing and examination with an epifluorescence microscope. Attachment of an image analyser to the microscope further enhances the usefulness of this method (Khan *et al.* 1988).

Spectrophotometry

A rapid screening method developed by Cowan & Fletcher (1987) to screen bacterial mutants for altered adherence ability may also be applied for the determination of antimicrobial effects on adherence. The wells in 96-well polystyrene microtitre plates are used as the attachment surface. Numbers of adhered bacteria are measured by staining them with congo red, eluting the stain with ethanol and measuring the absorbance (490 nm) of the eluted stain in the wells with a microtitre plate reader.

Bioluminescence

The above methods may be time consuming and subject to analytical limitations. Furthermore, they may not be applicable to material such as catheter tubing having irregular or rounded surfaces. A rapid bioluminescent assay performed in a single cuvette and specifically designed by Ludwicka *et al.* (1985) for the measurement of bacterial adherence to polyethylene overcomes these shortfalls. Polyethylene is cut into segments of surface area $0.1 \, cm^2$, five of which are incubated with $250 \, \mu l$ of bacterial suspension (10^8 cfu/ml). The segments are then washed with 10 ml of PBS to remove loosely or non-adhered bacterial cells, shaken to remove excess PBS and transferred to cuvettes, each containing $50 \, \mu l$ of 2.5% trichloroacetic acid (TCA), to extract bacterial ATP. Rapid shaking of the cuvette ensures complete mixing and the TCA also inactivates ATP-degrading enzymes so allowing extracts to be kept at room temperature for several hours. ATP is assayed after addition of 1 ml of reconstituted (in Tris-EDTA buffer) ATP Monitoring Reagent (LKB-Wallac, Finland) by measuring light emission in the cuvette. The number of attached cells per cm^2 is calculated from standard curves prepared with known amounts of bacterial cells in suspension.

Agar overlay method

A relatively simple method for the assessment of staphylococcal adherence to plastic surfaces is described by MacKenzie & Rivera-Calderon (1985). Bacterial suspensions (10 ml) are placed in Petri dishes and left for 5 h at ambient temperature. The inoculum is then removed by suction and the dish washed three times with PBS (pH 7.2). After the final wash, 10 ml of agar at 45°C is poured over the plate and allowed to set. The agar contains Tryptone Soya Agar (Difco Laboratories), 1% glucose and 0.015% neutral red. The overlaid plates are incubated at 37°C for 48 h by which time colonies have developed from the adherent bacteria. These colonies take up the neutral red and may be readily counted. Other materials may be fixed to the bottom of the Petri dish prior to addition of the bacterial suspension. The method has the advantage of measuring the viability of the adherent bacteria, allowing evaluation of biocidal activity.

Biofilm formation

A strain of *Serratia marcescens* whose planktonic cells were sensitive to 0.1% chlorhexidine was resistant to 2.0% of the antiseptic when its cells grew in a thick biofilm on the surface of a plastic storage vessel (Marrie & Costerton 1981). A similar effect was noted with *Pseudomonas cepacia* (Hugo *et al.* 1988). This illustrates the importance of testing antimicrobial agents on both planktonic and sessile bacterial populations. Several methods are currently employed for biofilm formation with the intention of stimulating the *in vivo* situation. One popular method uses the Robbins device to sample sessile biofilm populations of bacteria. This has been used with success, particularly in industrial settings, to examine the activity of biocides in penetrating and killing biofilms (Costerton & Lashen 1984). The device has also been applied in clinical settings where in place of the removable metal studs applicable to industrial situations, there may be inserted discs of catheter material on which the biofilm forms. Nickel *et al.* (1985) examined the activity of the antibiotic tobramycin against a biofilm formed by a uropathogenic strain of *Ps. aeruginosa* on this biomaterial. Twelve hours contact with 1000 µg/ml tobramycin did not kill the biofilm cells whereas 50 µg/ml for 8 h was sufficient to allow a complete kill of the planktonic bacteria.

Criticism of the Robbins device has come recently in a report by La Tourette Prosser *et al.* (1987). These authors argue that when determining the efficacy of antibiotics in penetrating and killing bacteria in a biofilm, the Robbins method is cumbersome and is unable to control the large numbers of planktonic bacteria which can inactivate the agent. As an alternative they describe a simple method for studying the effect of antimicrobial agents on established thick biofilms. In this, *E. coli* cells grown overnight on Mueller−Hinton agar at 37°C are scraped from the agar surface and suspended in Hepes−Hank buffer (pH 7.4) to an OD_{540} of 8.0. The cell suspension is dispensed in 80-μl amounts on to ethylene oxide sterilized 0.5-cm^2 discs of silicone latex catheter material. The discs are incubated for 1 h at 37°C, washed once with buffer and transferred to Petri dishes containing broth for continued incubation at 37°C for 20−22 h. The discs are then washed in buffer, placed in broth alone or in broth containing antimicrobial agent, incubated at 37°C for 6 h, washed in buffer and placed in fresh broth or broth containing antimicrobial agent. This procedure is repeated after 24 h. At each time interval, some discs are removed and the surface film scraped with a sterile scalpel into 5 ml of PBS. Each disc plus scrapings are placed in a vial, vortexed for 1 min, and gently sonicated in a sonic cleaner before determining the viable count. Discs are also removed for examination by light microscopy, after staining with 0.4% methylene blue, and for scanning electron microscopy.

Christensen *et al.* (1985) described a quantitative model for adherence based on the differing optical densities of adherent biofilms produced under different conditions or resulting from various treatments. The wells of flat-bottom tissue culture plates are inoculated with 0.2 ml of a 1:100 diluted stationary phase bacterial culture and incubated for 18 h at 37°C. The contents of each well are then gently aspirated with a Pasteur pipette and the wells washed four times with 0.2 ml PBS. Adherent organisms are fixed in place with Bouin fixative (71% v/v saturated aqueous picric acid, 24% v/v formalin and 5% v/v acetic acid) and stained with crystal violet. Excess stain is washed off under running water and, after drying, the ODs of the stained adherent biofilms are read with a MicroELISA Reader (570 nm). In addition, Christensen *et al.* (1985) extended their work on slime production described above (Christensen *et al.* 1982) by microscopic examination of the production of slime by adherent biofilms. Biofilms on glass slides are prepared by incubating sterile glass slides in TSB inoculated with the bacterium. The slides are rinsed four times, fixed with Bouin fixative and stained with alcian blue (0.1% w/v) or crystal violet. Alcian blue selectively stains extracellular acidic mucopolysaccharide (slime) whereas crystal violet uniformly stains adhering bacterial cells regardless of the presence or absence of slimy materials.

Quantification of the microbial film

A variety of methods may be used to determine the nature and extent of the biofilm produced. Examination of the biofilm may be made directly by scanning electron microscopy or the various light microscopic methods described above. Other methods involve indirect examination. These include conventional microbiological culture techniques to estimate the number of viable bacteria present in the film. Although this is relatively easy to perform, the need to homogenize the biofilm to disperse clusters of cells may result in a loss of viability.

The biofilm may be quantified by measurement of biomass. Direct measurement of biomass on the substrate is difficult, although an indication of its extent may be obtained from microscopic examination. An indirect method of determination is often more suitable and one such approach is by measurment of microbial ATP. This requires removal of the biofilm from the substrate or sampling device, as described for example by McCoy & Costerton (1982) for the Robbins device. The test surfaces with biofilm are placed in a test tube containing 2 g of coarse metallic tumbling abrasive in 5 ml distilled water and vortexed for 2 min. A Millipore filter (0.45 μm pore size) is used to filter 3 ml of the exudate through followed by 3 ml of Tris buffer (20 mmol/l, pH 7.75). The filter is placed in 0.5 ml of ice-cold 1 mol/l phosphoric acid and sonicated for 2 min. After 10 min on ice, the solution is neutralized with 0.5 ml 1 mol/l NaOH. Test surfaces are examined microscopically to ensure that all of the biofilm has been removed. The amount of ATP/cm^2 is subsequently determined by the luciferin−luciferase bioluminescence reaction.

Other indirect methods available for determination of biomass are reviewed by Gilbert & Herbert (1987). These authors also detail an indirect method employing radio-respirometric techniques to determine microbial activity within the biofilm. This has the advantage of examining the biofilm *in situ* on the substrate.

Effects of Biocides on the Determinants of Adherence

Bacterial adhesins are often located on the surface of the micro-organism in the form of fimbriae or discrete surface antigens (Fig. 4). Fimbriae are very common in Gram-negative genera though only a few Gram-positive genera (*Corynebacterium, Actinomyces*) have been found to carry such structures. Recently, a new type of fibrillar appendage has been described on strains of *Streptococcus salivarius* and *Strep. sanguis* (Handley *et al.* 1985). Bacteria may also exhibit non-specific adherence related to general physico-chemical characteristics.

It has been noted that several antibiotics, including ampicillin and nitrofurantoin (Sandberg *et al.* 1979), at subMIC levels *in vitro*, produce abnormal forms such as elongated filaments in *E. coli*. The majority of the bacteria that retained their adhesive capacity after treatment were not elongated. The possibility exists therefore that from a structural viewpoint:

1   the elongated forms may have a lower statistical chance of adhering to epithelial cells in solution due to awkward movement;

2   they may not align so readily on the epithelial cell surface; or

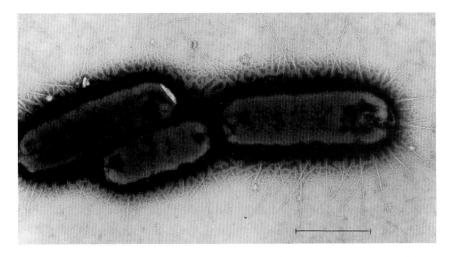

FIG. 4. Electron micrograph of *E.coli* showing peritrichous fimbriae. (Bar marker=1.0 μm.)

3   they may not bind with sufficient force to resist mechanical removal.

Ampicillin may also interfere specifically with the bacterial fimbriae. This type of interference is observed with the non-antibiotic agent taurolidine (Gorman *et al* 1987b). Taurolidine exerts an anti-adherence activity that may be linked to the observed loss of fimbriae from *E. coli* and elongation of the organism following treatment with the agent. A further generalized effect on the bacterial cell surface affecting the cell hydrophobicity also may be responsible for decreased adherence of the micro-organism.

Cell surface hydrophobicity measurement

A number of factors have been investigated for their effect on bacterial adhesion e.g. wettability (Pringle & Fletcher 1983), surface energy (Absolom *et al*. 1983), critical surface tension (Dexter *et al*. 1975), surface texture (Pomerat & Weiss 1946) and hydrophobicity (Rosenberg *et al*. 1980). The indication is that bacterial adherence cannot be explained by a single parameter but may be a multi-factor phenomenon. Several methods are employed to determine cell surface hydrophobicity.

Bacterial adherence to hydrocarbons (BATH) or phase distribution

This test, developed by Rosenberg and colleagues (Rosenberg *et al*. 1980), is frequently applied to hydrophobicity studies. The distribution ratio of microbial cells between an aqueous phase (PUM buffer, pH 7.1 consisting of (g): $K_2HPO_4.3H_2O$; 22.2; KH_2PO_4, 7.26; Urea, 1.8; $MgSO_4.7H_2O$, 0.2, in glass distilled water to 1 l) and an organic solvent (hydrocarbon) such as hexadecane, cyclohexane or xylene, is determined at ambient temperature. The cells may be treated with the drug prior to introduction to the system. To round-bottom test tubes containing 1.2 ml of washed bacterial suspension (approximate absorbance or 0.8 at 540 nm) are added various volumes, up to 0.2 ml, of test hydrocarbons (larger volumes may be used though in the same ratios). The mixtures are vortexed for 2 min and then allowed to stand for 15 min during which time the two phases separate completely.

Occasionally separation is incomplete and gentle centrifugation (150 g) may be required. The lower aqueous phase is then carefully pipetted off and its absorbance measured and compared with that of the cell suspension before addition of the solvent. Rosenberg (1984), as a result of work with the BATH test in many laboratories, has described several important aspects of the test in some detail to improve reproducibility:
1 The aqueous bacterial suspension must be free of surfactants and the test tubes preferably acid-washed.
2 Microscopic examination should be made of the hydrocarbon—water interface to ensure that cells are present and that a decrease in turbidity is not due to other factors such as clumping or lysis.
3 The assay may be overloaded if the bacterial suspension has too high an absorbance.
4 Insufficient mixing may not allow for maximum bacterial adherence to hydrocarbon.
5 The ionic strength and composition of the buffer may influence results.

Salt aggregation test (SAT)

Cell floculation is induced by increasing salt concentration in this test as proposed by Lindahl et al. (1981). The order in which cells are precipitated is a measure of their hydrophobicity, the most hydrophobic being precipitated at lowest salt concentration. Dilutions of ammonium sulphate (pH 6.8) are made in 0.002 mol/l sodium phosphate buffer (pH 6.8) over the range of 0−4.0 mol/l in 0.2-mol/l increments. A 25-μl volume of bacterial suspension (5×10^9 cells/ml) is mixed with an equal volume of salt solution on a glass microscope slide for 2 min at 20°C. The results are expressed as the lowest molarity of ammonium sulphate which gives visual cell aggregates.

An improved salt aggregation test (ISAT) was developed by Rozgonyi et al. (1985) for the sensitive determination of bacterial cell surface hydrophobicity. In this method, incorporation of methylene blue dye in the sodium phosphate buffer and ammonium sulphate solutions renders the aggregates more easily visible when viewed against a white background.

Hydrophobic interaction chromatography (HIC)

This test measures the amount of bacterial cells retained by a hydrophobic gel. As hydrophobic interactions are promoted by using solutions of high ionic strength; 4 mol/l sodium chloride or 1 mol/l ammonium sulphate is used as a suspending medium for the bacteria. Short-ended glass Pasteur pipettes (internal diameter 5 mm, length 85 mm) are used as columns. These are plugged with glass wool and packed with Sepharose (phenyl or octyl) to a height of 30 mm. The columns are washed extensively with the salt solutions buffered to pH 7.0 with 0.01 mol/l sodium phosphate. Bacterial cell suspensions in buffered salt solution are applied in 5-ml volumes to the tops of the columns and allowed to drain into the gel beads. The eluate is collected and the absorbance measured and compared with the optical density of the original applied cell suspension. A modification of this method has been developed to accommodate bacteria which are prone to clumping (e.g. staphylococci) which then may be removed from suspension by simple seiving within the column. In this modified approach, sepharose beads are vortex-mixed with the bacterial suspension and subsequently separated by centrifugation before the absorbance is read (S.P. Denyer, personal communication).

The BATH, ISAT and HIC methods are frequently employed for determination of cell surface hydrophobicity. Personal experience in the application of these methods to investigation of the effects of antimicrobial agents on this cell surface characteristic leads one to advise caution in the interpretation of data obtained. To illustrate this point, Table 3 presents a comparison of results obtained using the three aforementioned methods of cell surface hydrophobicity measurement. Uniformity of results on treatment of the micro-organisms with antimicrobial agent is not always apparent.

Microbial surface charge can be measured in a similar way, using a technique described as electrostatic interaction chromatography by Pedersen (1981). An anion exchange resin such as QAE Sephadex having a quaternary ammonium functional group or a cation exchanger such as CM Sephadex having a sulphonic acid functional group (Pharmacia Fine Chemicals Milton Keynes, UK), is packed as a column into a Pasteur pipette. Bacterial cells washed and suspended in various concentrations of NaCl in 0.01 mol/l phosphate buffer are applied in 0.1-ml volumes to the tops of the columns and eluted with 2 ml of suspending medium. Absorbance is measured and compared with that of the applied suspension.

Zeta potential and contact angle measurements

Quantitative data on the surface charge and hydrophobic properties of bacterial cells are obtained most readily from zeta potential measurements and from

TABLE 3. *Comparison of the BATH, ISAT and HIC methods for determination of cell surface hydrophobicity following microbial cell contact with antimicrobial agents*

| Antimicrobial agent | Micro-organism | Increase (>) or decrease (<) in cell hydrophobicity as indicated by the following methods | | |
		BATH	HIC	ISAT
Chlorhexidine	*Escherichia coli*	>	<	<
	Staphylococcus saprophyticus	<	<	<
	Staphylococcus epidermidis	>	<	=
	Candida albicans	>	=	=
Povidone-iodine	*Escherichia coli*	=	=	>
(0.075% av.I₂)*	*Staphylococcus saprophyticus*	<	<	<
	Staphylococcus epidermidis	=	<	>
	Candida albicans	<	<	>
Taurolidine	*Escherichia coli*	<	<	<
(2.0%)	*Staphylococcus saprophyticus*	<	<	<
	Staphylococcus epidermidis	<	<	>
	Candida albicans	<	=	<

The bacteria (urine isolates) and *Candida* sp. (oral isolate) were grown to stationary phase and treated with the antimicrobial agent or water (control) for 30 min at 37°C. Comparative results are expressed in relation to control. (= Indicates no change.)
* av.I₂ = available iodine.

contact angle measurements on bacterial layers, respectively. In the former, the surface charge is characterized by determining the electrophoretic mobility of the microbial cells in a suitable apparatus (Mozes *et al.* 1987). The cells are suspended at a given concentration in distilled water, the pH of which may be adjusted with buffer prior to the determination. Zeta potentials are calculated from cell velocity.

Contact angle measurement involves the deposition of a drop of water on to a film of bacterial cells on membrane filters. The angle between the film surface and the tangent to the drop at the solid−liquid−air interface is then determined (Busscher *et al.* 1984). The bacteria are suspended in demineralized water and drawn by negative pressure through a cellulose acetate membrane (0.45 μm pore diameter). The membrane plus bacteria (10^8 cells/mm^2) are placed in a Petri dish over 1% agar in 10% glycerol for 1−3 h to maintain a constant moisture content and then mounted with double-sided adhesive to a flat rigid support. Dehydration is allowed to occur under controlled conditions of temperature and humidity before contact angles are measured by the sessile drop technique.

Hydrophobicity of bacterial lawns — direction of spreading (DOS)

Methods such as BATH and HIC measure the hydrophobic properties of individual suspended cells which do not necessarily indicate the properties of the colony from which those cells originated. Contact angle determinations measure the hydrophobicity of cell layers but are quite complex and require special equipment. The direction of spreading method (Sar 1987) provides a rapid measurement of relative hydrophobicity values of bacterial lawns. A small drop of water (5 µl) is placed at the interface between the bacterial lawn and a particular surface (the growth medium solidified with 2% agar, a microscope glass cover slip, or polystyrene cover slip). The direction to which the water drop spreads is noted and a scoring system applied.

Non-ionic surfactant determination of hydrophobicity

As the bacterial cell surface is recognized to contain hydrophilic sites (charged groups such as carboxyl, amino and phosphate and the non-charged hydroxyl group) and hydrophobic sites (lipids and lipopolysaccharides) it is to be expected that a non-ionic surfactant containing a hydrophobic alkyl group and a hydrophilic polyethyleneoxide chain will combine with the cell surface. The alkyl group can combine with the hydrophobic sites such as lipopolysaccharide and the polyethyleneoxide chain will remain in water (Noda & Kanemasa 1986). This principle can be applied to give a quantitative measurement of hydrophobicity of Gram-positive and Gram-negative bacteria. An excess amount of surfactant is added to the bacterial suspension and agitated. After centrifugation, the excess of surfactant in the supernatant fluid is reacted with potassium ion to form a cation complex. This is extracted into dichlorobenzene as an ion pair with tetrabromophenolphthalein ethylester potassium salt. The A_{620} of the resulting ion in the solvent is measured and used to determine the surfactant concentration from which the adsorbed surfactant in the cell surface is calculated.

Conclusion

Bacteria may be clearly demonstrated to adhere to biomaterials and human tissue suggesting that the adherent mechanisms and the glycocalyces of biofilm-enrobed bacteria are important factors in sepsis. The role of adherence in industrial situations is also well established. Antimicrobial agents chosen on the basis of the results from traditional experimental methods using planktonic bacteria may not always be effective against bacteria in biofilm. At the other end of the antimicrobial spectrum, potential or existing antimicrobial agents should always be examined for anti-adherent activity to obtain a true measure of the overall antimicrobial potential of such an agent.

References

ABSOLOM, D.R., LANBERTH, F.V., POLICOVA, Z., ZINGG, W., VAN OSS, C.J. & NEUMANN, A.W. 1983. Surface thermodynamics of bacterial adhesion. *Applied and Environmental Microbiology* **46**, 90−97.

BOLTON, K.J., DODD, C.E.R., MEAD, C.G. & WAITES, W.M. 1988. Chlorine resistance of strains of *Staphylococcus aureus* isolated from poultry processing plants. *Letters in Applied Microbiology* **6**, 31−34.

BUSSCHER, H.J., WEERKAMP, A.H., VAN DER MEI, H.C., VAN PELT, A.W.J., DE JONG, H.P. & ARENDS, J. 1984. Measurement of the surface free energy of bacterial cell surfaces and its relevance for adhesion. *Applied and Environmental Microbiology* **48**, 980−983.

CHRISTENSEN, G.D., SIMPSON, W.A., BISNO, A.L. & BEACHEY, E.H. 1982. Adherence of slime-producing strains of *Staphylococcus epidermidis* to smooth surfaces. *Infection and Immunity* **37**, 318−326.

CHRISTENSEN, G.D., SIMPSON, W.A., YOUNGER, J.J., BADDOUR, L.M., BARRETT, F.F., MELTON, D.M. & BEACHEY, E.H. 1985. Adherence of coagulase-negative staphylococci to plastic tissue culture plates: a quantitative model for the adherence of staphylococci to medical devices. *Journal of Clinical Microbiology* **22**, 996−1006.

COSTERTON, J.W., IRWIN, R.T. & CHENG, K.J. 1981. The bacterial glycocalyx in nature and disease. *Annual Reviews in Microbiology* **35**, 299−324.

COSTERTON, J.W. & LASHEN, E.S. 1984. Influence of biofilm on efficacy of biocides on corrosion-causing bacteria. *Materials Performance* **23**, 34−37.

COWAN M.M. & FLETCHER, M. 1987. Rapid screening method for detection of bacterial mutants with altered adhesion abilities. *Journal of Microbiological Methods* **7**, 241−249.

DEXTER, S.C., SULLIVAN, J.D., WILLIAMS, J. & WATSON, S.W. 1975. Influence of substrate wettability on the attachment of marine bacteria to various surfaces. *Applied Microbiology* **30**, 298−308.

DOUGLAS, J.L. 1987. Adhesion of *Candida* species to epithelial surfaces. *CRC Critical Reviews in Microbiology* **15**, 27−43.

EDWARDS, P.J. & JEFFRYES C.A. 1987. Application of the GTGO−AD procedure in the scanning electron microscopy of streptococci adhered to pellicle-coated dental enamel. *Journal of Microscopy* **148**, 219−221.

FLETCHER, M. 1976. The effects of proteins on bacterial attachment to polystyrene. *Journal of General Microbiology* **94**, 400−404.

FUNFSTUCK, R., STEIN, G., FUCHS, M., BERGNER, M., WESSEL, G., KEIL, E. & SUSS, J. 1987. The influence of selected urinary constituents on the adhesion process of *Escherichia coli* to human uroepithelial cells. *Clinical Nephrology* **28**, 244−249.

GAMLIEL, H., GURFEL, D., LIEZEROWITZ, R. & POLLIAK, A. 1983. Air-drying of human leucocytes for scanning electron microscopy using the GTGO procedures. *Journal of Microscopy* **131**, 87−95.

GILBERT, P.D. & HERBERT, B.N. 1987. Monitoring microbial fouling in flowing systems using coupons. In *Industrial Microbiological Testing*, ed. Hopton, J.W. & Hill, E.C. pp. 79−98 Society for Applied Bacteriology Technical Series No.23. Oxford: Blackwell Scientific Publications.

GORMAN, S.P., MCCAFFERTY, D.F. & ANDERSON, L. 1986. Application of an electronic particle counter to the quantification of bacterial and *Candida* adherence to mucosal epithelial cells. *Letters in Applied Microbiology* **2**, 97−100.

GORMAN, S.P., MCCAFFERTY, D.F., WOOLFSON, A.D. & JONES, D.S. 1987a. A comparative study of the microbial anti-adherence capacities of three antimicrobial agents. *Journal of Clinical Pharmacy and Therapeutics* **12**, 393−399.

GORMAN, S.P., MCCAFFERTY, D.F., WOOLFSON, A.D. & JONES, D.S. 1987b. Electron and light microscopic observations of bacterial cell surface effects due to taurolidine treatment. *Letters in Applied Microbiology* **4**, 103−109.

HANDLEY, P.S., CARTER, P.L., WYATT, J.E. & HESKETH, L.M. 1985. Surface structures (peritrichous fibrils and tufts of fibrils) found on *Streptococcus sanguis* may be related to their ability to coaggregate with other genera. *Infection and Immunity* **47**, 217−227.

HUGO, W.B., PALLENT, L.J., GRANT, D.J.W., DENYER, S.P. & DAVIES, A. 1986. Factors contributing to the survival of a strain of *Pseudomonas cepacia* in chlorhexidine solution. *Letters in Applied Microbiology* **2**, 37−42.

HUMPHRIES, M., JAWORZYN, J.F., CANTWELL, J.B. & EAKIN, A. 1987. The use of non-ionic ethoxylated and propoxylated surfactants to prevent the adhesion of bacteria to solid surfaces. *FEMS Microbiology Letters* **42**, 91−101.

JACQUES, M., TURGEON, P.L., MATHIEU, L.G. & DE REPENTIGNY, J. 1985. Effect of subminimal inhibitory concentrations of antibiotics on adherence of *Neisseria gonorrhoeae* in an experimental model. *Experimental Biology* **43**, 251−256.

KHAN, M.A., DENYER, S.P., DAVIES, M.C. & DAVIS, S.S. 1988. Adhesion of *Staphylococcus epidermidis* to modified polystyrene surfaces. *Journal of Pharmacy and Pharmacology* **40**, 17P.

KIMURA, L.H. & PEARSALL, N.N. 1980. Relation between germination of *Candida albicans* and increased adherence to human buccal epithelial cells. *Infection and Immunity* **28**, 462−468.

KOLAWOLE, D.O. 1984. Resistance mechanisms of mucoid-grown *Staphylococcus aureus* to the antibacterial action of some disinfectants and antiseptics. *FEMS Microbiology Letters* **25**, 205−209.

KOZODY, N.L., HARDING, G.K.M., NICOLLE, L.E., KELLY, K. & RONALD, A.R. 1985. Adherence of *Escherichia coli* in the pathogenesis of urinary tract infection. *Clinical and Investigative Medicine* **8**, 121−125.

LAMBERTS, B.L., PEDERSON, E.D. & SIMONSON, L.G. 1985. The effects of basic and acidic synthetic polypeptides on the adherence of the oral bacteria *Streptococcus mutans* and *Streptococcus sanguis* to hydroxyapatite. *Archives of Oral Biology* **30**, 295−298.

LA TOURETTE PROSSER, B., TAYLOR, D., DIX, B. & CLEELAND, R. 1987. Method for evaluating effects of antibiotics on bacterial biofilm. *Antimicrobial Agents and Chemotherapy* **31**, 1502−1506.

LINDAHL, M., FARIS, A., WADSTROM, T. & HJERTEN, S. 1981. A new test based on 'salting out' to measure relative surface hydrophobicity of bacterial cells. *Biochimica et Biophysica Acta* **677**, 471−476.

LUDWICKA, A., SWITALSKI, L.M., LUNDIN, A., PULVERER, G. & WADSTROM T. 1985. Bioluminescent assay for measurement of bacterial attachment to polyethylene. *Journal of Microbiological Methods* **4**, 169−177.

MCCOURTIE, J., MACFARLANE, T.W. & SAMARANAYAKE, L.P. 1986. A comparison of the effects of chlorhexidine gluconate, amphotericin B and nystatin on the adherence of *Candida* species to denture acrylic. *Journal of Antimicrobial Chemotherapy* **17**, 575−583.

MCCOY, W.F. & COSTERTON, J.W. 1982. Fouling biofilm development in tubular flow systems. *Developments in Industrial Microbiology* **23**, 551−558.

MACKENZIE, A.M.R. & RIVERA-CALDERON, R.L. 1985. Agar overlay method to measure adherence of *Staphylococcus epidermidis* to four plastic surfaces. *Applied and Environmental Microbiology* **50**, 1322−1324.

MARCUS, H. & BAKER, N.R. 1985. Quantitation of adherence of mucoid and non-mucoid *Pseudomonas aeruginosa* to hamster tracheal epithelium. *Infection and Immunity* **47**, 723−729.

MARRIE, T.J. & COSTERTON, J.W. 1981. Prolonged survival of *Serratia marcescens* in chlorhexidine. *Applied and Environmental Microbiology* **42**, 1093−1102.

MARSHALL, K.C., STOUT, R. & MITCHELL, R. 1971. Mechanism of the initial events in the sorption of marine bacteria to surfaces. *Journal of General Microbiology* **68**, 337–348.

MOZES, N., MARCHAL, F., HERMESSE, M.P., VAN HAECHT, J.L., REULIAUX, L., LEONARD, A.J. & ROUXHET, P.G. 1987. Immobilization of microorganisms by adhesion: interplay of electrostatic and non-electrostatic interactions. *Biotechnology and Bioengineering* **30**, 439–450.

NICKEL, J.C., RUSESKA, I. & COSTERTON, J.W. 1985. Tobramycin resistance of cells of *Pseudomonas aeruginosa* growing as a biofilm on urinary catheter material. *Antimicrobial Agents and Chemotherapy* **27**, 619–624.

NODA, Y. & KANEMASA, Y. 1986. Determination of hydrophobicity on bacterial surfaces by nonionic surfactants. *Journal of Bacteriology* **167**, 1016–1019.

OLSSON, J., JONTELL, M. & KRASSE, B. 1980. Effect of macromolecules on adherence of *Streptococcus mutans. Scandinavian Journal of Infectious Diseases* **24**, 173–178.

PARSONS, C.L., ANWAR, H., STAUFFER, C. & SCHIMDT, J.D. 1979. *In vitro* adherence of radioactively labelled *Escherichia coli* in normal and cystitis prone females. *Infection and Immunity* **26**, 453–457.

PAUL, J.H. & JEFFREY, W.H. 1985. The effect of surfactants on the attachment of estuarine and marine bacteria to surfaces. *Canadian Journal of Microbiology* **31**, 224–228.

PEDERSEN, K. 1981. Electrostatic interaction chromatography, a method for assaying the relative surface charges of bacteria. *FEMS Microbiology Letters* **12**, 365–367.

POMERAT, C.M. & WEISS, C.M. 1946. The influence of texture and composition of surface on the attachment of sedentary marine microorganisms. *Biological Bulletin* **91**, 57–65.

PRATT-TERPSTRA, I.H., WEERKAMP, A.H. & BUSSCHER, H.J. 1987. Adhesion of oral streptococci from a flowing suspension to uncoated and albumin-coated surfaces. *Journal of General Microbiology* **133**, 3199–3206.

PRINGLE, J.H. & FLETCHER, M. 1983. Influence of substrate wettability on attachment of fresh water bacteria to solid surfaces. *Applied and Environmental Microbiology* **45**, 811–817.

REID, G. & BROOKS, H.J.L. 1982. The use of double staining techniques for investigating bacterial attachment to mucopolysaccharide-coated epithelial cells. *Stain Technology* **57**, 5–9.

REID, G. & BROOKS, H.J.L. 1985. A fluorescent antibody staining technique to detect bacterial adherence to urinary tract epithelial cells. *Stain Technology* **60**, 211–217.

RIDGWAY, H.F., RIGBY, M.G. & ARGO, D.G. 1984. Adhesion of *Mycobacterium* sp. to cellulose diacetate membranes used in reverse osmosis. *Applied and Environmental Microbiology* **47**, 61–67.

ROSENBERG, M. 1984. Bacterial adherence to hydrocarbons: a useful technique for studying cell surface hydrophobicity. *FEMS Microbiology Letters* **22**, 289–295.

ROSENBERG, M., GUTNICK, D. & ROSENBERG, E. 1980. Adherence of bacteria to hydrocarbons: a simple method for measuring cell-surface hydrophobicity. *FEMS Microbiology Letters* **9**, 29–33.

ROSENSTEIN, I.J., GRADY, D., HAMILTON-MILLER, J.M.T. & BRUMFITT, W. 1985. Relationship between adhesion of *Escherichia coli* to uroepithelial cells and the pathogenesis of urinary infection: problems in methodology and analysis. *Journal of Medical Microbiology* **20**, 335–344.

ROZGONYI, F., SZITHA, K.R., LUNGH, A., BALODA, S.B., HJERTEN, S. & WADSTROM, T. 1985. Improvement of the salt aggregation test to study bacterial cell-surface hydrophobicity. *FEMS Microbiology Letters* **30**, 131–138.

RUTTER, P.R. & ABBOTT, A. 1978. A study of the interaction between oral streptococci and hard surfaces. *Journal of General Microbiology* **105**, 219–226.

SANDBERG, T., STENQVIST, K. & SVANBORG-EDEN, C. 1979. Effects of subminimal concentrations of ampicillin, chloramphenicol and nitrofurantoin on the attachment of *Escherichia coli* to human epithelial cells *in vitro*. *Reviews of Infectious Diseases* **1**, 838–844.

SAR, N. 1987. Direction of spreading (DOS): a simple method for measuring the hydrophobicity of bacterial lawns. *Journal of Microbiological Methods* **6**, 211–219.

SCHAEFFER, A.J., JONES, J. & DUNN, J.K. 1981. Association of *in vitro Escherichia coli* adherence to vaginal and buccal epithelial cells with susceptibility of woman to recurrent urinary tract infections. *New England Journal of Medicine* **304**, 1062–1066.

SHARMA, A.P., BATTERSBURY, N.S. & STEWART, D.J. 1987. Techniques for the evaluation of biocide activity against sulphate-reducing bacteria. In *Preservatives in the Food, Pharmaceutical and Environmental Industries*, ed. Board, R.G., Allwood, M.C. & Banks, J.G. pp. 165–175. Society for Applied Bacteriology Technical Series No. 22. Oxford: Blackwell Scientific Publications.

SHIBL, A.M. 1985. The effect of antibiotics on adherence of microorganisms to epithelial cell surfaces. *Reviews of Infectious Diseases* **7**, 51–65.

SVANBORG-EDEN, C. 1978. Attachment of *Escherichia coli* to human urinary tract epithelial cells. *Scandinavian Journal of Infectious Diseases Supplement* **15**, 1–69.

SVEUM, R.J., CHUSED, T.M., FRANK, M.M. & BROWN, E.J. 1986. A quantitative fluorescent method for measurement of bacterial adherence and phagocytosis. *Journal of Immunological Methods* **90**, 257–264.

TYLEWSKA, S.T. & GIBBONS, R.J. 1987. Application of Percoll density gradients in studies of the adhesion of *Streptococcus pyogenes* to human epithelial cells. *Current Microbiology* **16**, 129–135.

VALENTIN-WEIGAND, P., CHHATWAL, G.S. & BLOBEL, H. 1987. A simple method for quantitative determination of bacterial adherence to human and animal epithelial cells. *Microbiology and Immunology* **31**, 1017–1023.

VERRAN, J., DRUCKER, D.B. & TAYLOR, C.J. 1980. Feasibility of using automatic image analysis for measuring deposition of *Streptococcus mutans* onto glass, in terms of percentage coverage and mean clump size. *Microbios* **29**, 161–169.

VERRIER, D., MORTIER, B. & ALBAGNAC, G. 1987. Initial adhesion of methanogenic bacteria to polymers. *Biotechnology Letters*, **9**, 735–740.

VOSBECK, K., HANDSCHIN, H., MENGE, E.B. & ZAK, O. 1979. Effects of subminimal inhibitory concentrations of antibiotics on adhesiveness of *Escherichia coli in vitro*. *Reviews of Infectious Diseases* **1**, 845–851.

WOOLFSON, A.D., GORMAN, S.P., McCAFFERTY, D.F. & JONES, D.S. 1987. On the statistical evaluation of adherence assays. *Journal of Applied Bacteriology* **63**, 147–151.

ZUFFEREY, J., RIME, B., FRANCIOLLI, P. & BILLE, J. 1988. Simple method for rapid diagnosis of catheter-associated infection by direct acridine orange staining of catheter tips. *Journal of Clinical Microbiology* **26**, 175–177.

Detection and Measurement of Combined Biocide Action

N.A. HODGES AND G.W. HANLON

Department of Pharmacy, Brighton Polytechnic, Moulsecoomb, Brighton, E. Sussex
BN2 4GJ, UK

The potential benefits arising from the use of combinations of biocides have long been recognized. It is now well over 50 years ago that Sabalitschka (1932) recommended the use of a mixture of parabens and suggested a potentizing action, and 30 years since it was demonstrated that such mixtures had antimicrobial activity greater than the sum of the individual components (Littlejohn & Husa 1955). This finding, however, did not stimulate the same level of published research in biocide combinations as that seen with mixtures of antibiotics, and of the literature available on biocides, most of it is confined to preservatives used in the food, cosmetic or pharmaceutical industries, rather than biocides in the broader sense, which may include antiseptics, disinfectants and industrial agents.

The high level of research interest in antibiotic combinations compared with that in biocides is somewhat surprising, because the justifications for the use of their respective combinations are similar. In both cases one or more of the following effects might arise: a broader spectrum of antimicrobial activity; delayed resistance; synergy; or diminished toxicity resulting from the use of lower concentrations. Indeed it may be argued that with respect to delayed resistance and synergy, the results of *in vitro* tests on biocides are more likely to be of predictive value for the 'in-use' situation than those with antibiotics, because the former are not complicated by the problems of drug absorption and distribution and the protection of pathogens located at relatively inaccessible sites within the body.

The purpose of this present paper is to give an account of the laboratory methods which may be used to assess the interactions resulting from the use of biocide combinations; thus it is primarily concerned with techniques for detecting and quantifying the degree of synergy that may be obtained. Consideration will also be given to the prediction of likely interactions between biocides based upon a knowledge of their mechanism of action. The other possible benefits of the use of biocide combinations are not within the scope

Mechanisms of Action of
Chemical Biocides

297

of the paper, nor will it include an account of the published work describing synergistic combinations which have previously been identified; this aspect has recently been reviewed comprehensively by Denyer *et al.* (1985).

Many of the laboratory methods which are appropriate for the study of biocide mixtures are equally valid for antibiotics, thus there is much valuable technical information in the reviews by Beale & Sutherland (1983) and Krogstad & Moellering (1985). Probably the major difference between the two situations is that in the case of antibiotics there is the need for both microbiocidal and microbiostatic tests because some antibiotics fail to produce any significant killing effect even at high concentrations. This is less likely with biocides, of which disinfectants and antiseptics must be rapidly bactericidal at 'in-use' concentrations and preservatives may exhibit a somewhat slower, but nevertheless significant bactericidal action.

Qualitative and Quantitative Effects

The potential exists for the effects of biocide combinations to extend from antagonism at one extreme, through indifference or a merely additive effect, to synergy at the other extreme. Although antagonism exists, it appears to be relatively rare among biocides, and it has been reported far less frequently than have additive or synergistic effects (Denyer & King 1988).

Experimental procedures which quantify the degree of synergy existing in a combination are likely to be far more useful than a qualitative method which simply demonstrates that the phenomenon occurs. Unfortunately quantitative experiments are more laborious and except for the chessboard method, usually suffer from the disadvantage that the biocides are present together in predetermined fixed concentration ratios, rather than the spectrum of concentrations which may be achieved by some qualitative tests. An obvious prerequisite of a quantitative method is a definition of synergy, a subject upon which there is not unanimous agreement (Beale & Sutherland 1983).

Synergy between mixtures of two antimicrobial agents is considered to be exhibited when an effect greater than that to be expected from the simple addition of the effects of the two agents is found. The term 'potentiation', which is sometimes used synonymously with synergy, is probably best used, as by Hart (1984), to describe the situation in which the antimicrobial activity of a recognized biocide is enhanced by the addition of a second substance, e.g. ethylenediaminetetraacetic acid (EDTA) which may have little or no antibacterial activity in its own right.

Synergy is most conveniently quantified in terms of the reduction in biocide concentrations required to achieve a fixed end-point as a result of their use in combination. The end-point selected is usually inhibition of visible growth in liquid or solid media. The time required to kill a standardized inoculum may be the chosen parameter, but here careful selection of sampling times is required. If the sampling interval is long, the results, although perhaps demonstrating markedly improved activity, may not lend themselves to quantification.

The concept of fractional inhibitory concentrations (FIC) is that most commonly employed for quantitative purposes. The FIC for each antimicrobial compound in a combination is usually calculated from minimum growth inhibitory concentration (MIC) determinations and is the ratio of the MIC for the substance in combination to that for the substance alone. The sum of the FIC values (FIC index) for the components of the most effective combination is indicative of the nature of their interaction. If, for example, the most effective combination of two biocides A and B was found to be 10 mg/l A plus 25 mg/l B and their respective MICs when used alone were 100 mg/l and 75 mg/l, respectively, the FIC index would be:

$$\frac{10}{100} + \frac{25}{75} = 0.1 + 0.33 = 0.43.$$

A value of 0.43 would normally be regarded as synergistic because this is less than the value of 0.5 which is generally accepted to be definitive for synergy, although an alternative value of 0.7 has been proposed (Kerry et al. 1975). The two compounds are additive if their FIC index approximates to 1.0 and antagonistic if it significantly exceeds that value. This method may readily be adapted to measure bactericidal activity rather than merely growth inhibition, simply by subculturing from those tubes or wells in a microtitre plate which show no growth. It was used by Hugbo (1977) for example, for measuring the concentrations of biocides which, in combination, killed standard inocula in specified times.

Experimental Methods

By far the most common techniques used for the detection and evaluation of synergy are those based on agar diffusion, or on MIC determinations. The latter is of value because it can easily be quantified, whilst the former, although only qualitative, is easy to perform. Other methods, based on spiral plating or measurement of growth inhibition or death by turbidity or viable counting, have also been described, but these are probably less convenient for routine use than those detailed above.

Although no ideal method for the determination of synergy exists, it is useful to identify the characteristics of a hypothetical ideal method in order to permit a better appreciation of the relative merits of the techniques to be described subsequently. Obviously speed and ease of operation are desirable features, as is readily available, and inexpensive equipment which is capable of automatic or semi-automatic operation. The selected method should be precise and sufficiently sensitive to detect minor degrees of synergy; usually improved precision and reduction in error can only be achieved at the expense of speed and by greater preparative effort. A good method would be one that would permit the prediction or experimental determination of the concentrations at which synergy occurs. This is important because the quantitative or even the qualitative nature of the interaction may be crucially concentration-dependent; King & Krogstad (1983) demonstrated that synergy between gentamicin and sodium azide changed to antagonism as the ratio of the two components was altered. The rate and extent of kill in the microbial population is useful information which is not provided by the most commonly employed methods. It is conceivable that a biocide combination may achieve a more rapid microbiocidal action without permitting a significant reduction in concentration of the two components. Thus such a combination would not be regarded as synergistic if it were assessed on the basis of change in MIC, but would be synergistic by other criteria.

Agar diffusion methods

There are various agar diffusion methods described, particularly in the antibiotic literature, but they are all based upon the same principle. The biocides which constitute the combination of interest are made to diffuse through inoculated agar to give a continuous spectrum of concentration ratios, and the nature of the interaction is based upon the interpretation of the pattern of resulting growth inhibition. The biocides are most commonly contained on paper strips which are placed on the inoculated agar at right angles (Fig. 1) or in the form of a cross. It is usual, although not absolutely necessary, to use concentrations of the two agents which both give inhibition zones of several mm when used alone; these concentrations must be determined by preliminary experimentation if necessary. Although it is possible for an inhibition zone to result from the interaction of two agents which, alone, are not at sufficient concentration to cause inhibition, a marked degree of synergy would be necessary to achieve this effect, and the principle of using individual sub-inhibitory concentrations in this way is unsatisfactory, because minor degrees of synergy may be overlooked. Where there is doubt about the concentrations, the use of three strips in each direction with the concentration differing by a factor of 5 or 10 from one to the next probably avoids the necessity of repeating the whole procedure. Best results arise from the use of relatively long thin paper strips from which surplus liquid has been drained or blotted prior to application to the plate.

The various results which might arise from this method are illustrated in Fig. 1. The degree of synergy occurring in biocide combinations is frequently

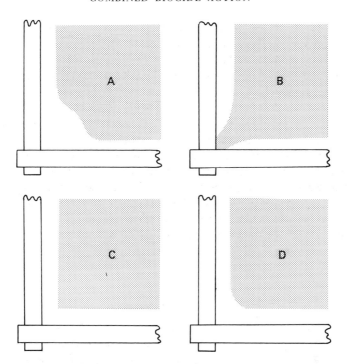

FIG. 1. Patterns of growth inhibition by agar diffusion methods: shaded areas represent growth. A, synergy; B, antagonism; C, indifference; D, additivity.

low and it may be difficult to distinguish between indifferent, additive and synergistic effects. Although species variation in response to combinations of agents is well established amongst antibiotics, it is less common amongst biocides where the mechanism of action is less subtle and the existence and distribution of resistance plasmids is less extensive. It is possible, therefore, that only a small number of microbial species may be needed to examine the behaviour of biocide mixtures. If the purpose of the work is to assess the suitability of a wide range of preservative mixtures, in the development of a new product for example, it may be convenient to conduct the tests on a large plate of the type used for antibiotic assays (Mast Laboratories Bootle, UK or Gibco Plastics Paisley, UK) rather than on a standard Petri dish; an example is shown in Fig. 2 which shows synergy between phenylmercuric nitrate and benzalkonium chloride. Here the agar was inoculated throughout to give *c.* 10^6 cells/ml of *Escherichia coli*. An obvious limitation of this method is that the concentrations in the agar which exhibit synergy are unknown. The counter argument, however, is that the technique does at least permit the whole

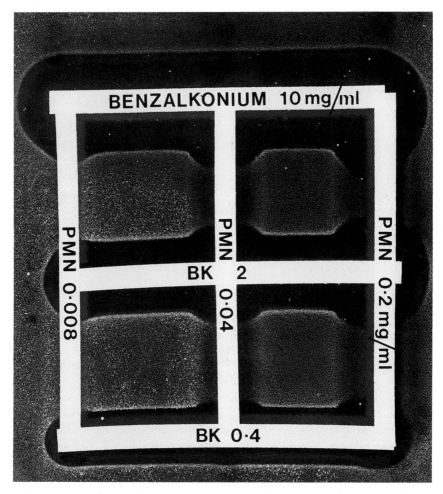

FIG. 2. Synergy between phenylmercuric nitrate (PMN) and benzalkonium chloride. Isosensitest agar inoculated with *E. coli*.

spectrum of biocide ratios to exist at different positions in the agar, and methods which utilize fixed concentration ratios are, themselves, limiting.

This agar diffusion method may be modified in various ways. It is possible to omit the filter paper strips and incorporate the biocides in the agar to give two-dimensional gradients in a 10-cm square Petri dish. This method, based on the Szybalski technique, involves pouring the agar in four separate aliquots, with the plate being raised by 3 mm on one side whilst the medium incorporating the first biocide is poured in. When this is set as a wedge the dish is levelled and the second layer of medium alone is poured. The plate is then turned through 90° and the third (+ second biocide) and fourth (plain) aliquots of agar are poured; a surface inoculum is spread after the plate has been left for 24 h to permit biocide diffusion (Wimpenny & Waters 1984). One problem with this method is detecting the exact boundary of growth. McClure & Roberts (1986) have demonstrated the benefits of using buffers and pH indicators such as phenol red and bromocresol purple for acid-producing organisms, but even better visualization of the growth resulted from the use of a tetrazolium salt which is reduced by respiring bacteria and stains the cells red.

A variant of the agar diffusion technique which is claimed (Hammond & Lambert 1978) to be more sensitive for the purpose of detecting synergy employs a single paper strip soaked in biocide solution laid on the surface of inoculated agar containing a concentration gradient of a second agent; this is known as the filter paper gradient plate. The strip is placed in the same direction as the biocide gradient in the agar and any synergy resulting from the combination will give the inhibition pattern shown in Fig. 3.

Chessboard method

The name arises from the pattern of test tubes, or of wells on a microtitre plate, which are used for the determination of MIC values for the two agents in combination. Usually between six and 10 doubling-dilutions are prepared for each biocide from concentrations slightly above the MICs for the two agents used alone, and these are mixed together; thus the test organism is exposed to every possible combination of concentrations. The test may be carried out in liquid media or by uniform incorporation of the biocides in the agar in Petri dishes. Microtitre plate methods obviously result in savings on space and materials, and are more amenable to automation. Petri dishes, when used with a multi-point inoculator allow the test to be performed on several organisms simultaneously and may permit the detection, by their macroscopic appearance, of contaminants that would be overlooked in liquid culture. The dilution increment does not have to be a factor of 2 but doubling-dilutions are particularly convenient from a preparative point of view. Precision is related to the dilution increment; if doubling-dilutions are used the determination of the end-point is subject to a twofold error, thus the use of a smaller dilution increment may be beneficial. The results may be represented as an isobologram on which either the MIC values in concentration units or FIC values may be plotted for each drug alone and in combination. The isobols, which are lines connecting points of equivalent biological activity, have a negative slope (Fig. 4) and the shape of the plot indicates the nature of the interaction. If there is a straight line which joins the MIC values for the two agents when used alone

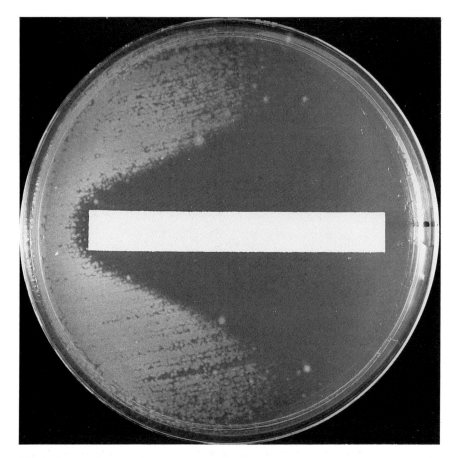

FIG. 3. Pattern of growth inhibition indicative of synergy on a filter paper gradient plate. The first biocide is in the agar and increases in concentration; the second biocide is in the paper strip.

they are additive in effect; if the line is concave the combination is synergistic, if convex, antagonistic. This method, although more laborious, is certainly more sensitive than agar diffusion. The potentiation of benzalkonium chloride by EDTA, which was determined by the chessboard method (see Fig. 4), was undetectable by agar diffusion despite efforts to optimize the experimental conditions.

Spiral plating

Schalkowsky (1982) has developed the equations required to detect and evaluate synergy by a spiral plating technique. This involves the application of a solution of antimicrobial agent at a decreasing concentration on a spiral track

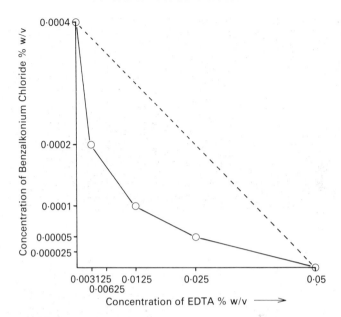

F<small>IG</small>. 4. Isobologram showing potentiation of benzalkonium chloride activity against *Staph. aureus* by EDTA.

on the surface of a seeded Petri dish. The geometry of the spiral can be varied to alter the concentration of the agent in a predetermined manner between the centre and periphery of the dish. This technique requires the use of three dishes of which the first two are used to determine the inhibitory concentrations for the individual components, and the third is used to plate out a combination of the two agents in proportion to their inhibitory concentrations. Alternatively, one antimicrobial compound is incorporated uniformly thoughout the medium whilst the second is added in decreasing concentration along the spiral.

Growth inhibition and lysis

The decline in growth rate or increase in rate of kill have been used to assess antimicrobial activity in biocide combinations (Richards & McBride 1971; Denyer & King 1988). A reduced growth rate is most readily measured by a turbidimetric technique, but this is obviously limited to testing organisms that will grow as a uniform suspension; it could not be applied to moulds or to bacteria which clump in shaken cultures. The alternative methods of measuring the growth of such organisms, e.g. dry weight determinations, are probably less convenient than other methods of measuring combined action.

A further problem with turbidimetric techniques is that they may not be appropriate for certain concentrations. As a result of adsorption and charge neutralization on the cell surface, quaternary ammonium compounds, for example, may cause aggregation of the test organism.

Turbidimetric methods are ideal when death of the test organism results in lysis, but if this does not arise there is scope only for a reduction from the normal growth rate to an apparent rate of zero. If biocide concentrations are selected which, individually and in combination, still give positive growth rates, this inevitably means that the test is being conducted using concentrations lower than those employed in practice, because in use, a killing effect, albeit a slow one, is now required in all cosmetic and pharmaceutical preservative efficacy tests.

The turbidimetric measurement of growth inhibition or lysis provides information on the kinetics of the antimicrobial activity of a biocide combination which cannot be obtained from agar diffusion or chessboard methods, but the technique is laborious in the absence of an instrument such as the Abbott MS2 which will monitor multiple cultures at frequent intervals.

If death rate is to be the criterion of assessment for combinations of non-lytic biocides, then viable counts must be used. This is usually regarded as less convenient than turbidimetric monitoring, and, because of the incubation time, slower to give results. The first of these problems may be reduced by measuring, not death rate, but the time required to kill a standard inoculum, and there are numerous reports in the literature where the results are expressed as the presence or absence of surviving cells in samples removed at suitable time intervals. This procedure, however, suffers from the well-rehearsed argument that the mere recording of growth or no growth on subculture may result in a dramatic initial killing rate being overlooked because of the presence of a small number of atypically resistant cells persisting in the inoculated biocide mixture.

Recently Drugeon et al. (1987) have described a composite chessboard/viable count (killing curve) method which, the authors claim, combines the advantages of both techniques, and may help to eliminate the poor correlation which has been reported when antimicrobial combinations are assessed by different methods (Norden et al. 1979).

The Prediction of Synergy

The prediction of synergy from a knowledge of action mechanisms is an objective which has yet to be achieved even in the well-researched field of antibiotics. The problem is more difficult amongst the (predominantly bactericidal) antiseptics and preservatives because the guidelines often used for antibiotics, which are based on interactions of bactericidal and bacteriostatic agents, are of no use. Thus, the prediction of biocide synergy must be based either upon the empirically accumulated knowledge of the use of combinations from particular chemical classes or modes of action, or on a logical assessment of the likely consequences of one biocide-induced cellular change on another. Perhaps the best example of the former approach, which comes from the antibiotic field, is the expectation that the combination of a β-lactam antibiotic with an aminoglycoside is likely to be synergistic, simply from the large number of reported examples in the literature. An example of the second approach is the anticipated potentiation of many antibiotics and biocides by EDTA, phenylethanol or other agents which permeabilize the cell and facilitate the antibiotic or biocide entry. This particular phenomenon has been well documented elsewhere (Hart 1984; Parker 1984; Denyer & King 1988) and will not be considered further here.

Any convenient analysis of the reported cases of biocide synergy which are not attributable to permeabilization requires the grouping of biocides either by chemical class or by site of action in the cell. Although, for this particular purpose, the latter might be the method of choice, the former is still generally favoured, probably for the reasons suggested by Parker (1984); namely that in practical terms, the success or failure of a preservative system involves so many formulation factors that physico-chemical characteristics are probably of greater predictive value.

It has frequently been suggested that synergy is most likely to occur between chemicals which have dissimilar modes of action (Hugbo 1977; Parker 1984; Denyer et al. 1985), and an additive action is the most probable result of combinations of agents having the same mechanism. Even this straightforward guideline, however, is complicated by the fact that several agents act at more than one site in the microbial cell depending upon concentration. Phenols, for example, have variously been reported to cause bacterial lysis (which indicates an action on the cell wall), membrane damage as shown by leakage of potassium and 260 nm absorbing materials, and, in high concentrations to cause protein precipitation in the cytoplasm (Hugo 1982).

Denyer et al. (1985) have recently reviewed the reported cases of synergy in biocide combinations. If these are used as a basis for analysis of the frequency of synergy which is not attributable to permeabilization, i.e. cases in which EDTA or phenylethanol are part of the combination are ignored, then the 28 examples they identified are reduced to 17, which is barely sufficient for the purpose and is in marked contrast to the 126 examples of antibiotic synergy tabulated by Krogstad & Moellering (1985). Of these 17, the most frequently reported synergistic combinations are parabens together with a formaldehyde producer or a weak organic acid, sulphite with organic acids and phenylmercuric derivatives with phenols. It is interesting to note that the first case, parabens plus a formaldehyde donor, is similar to the combination recommended by Hugo & Russell (1982) after consideration of the data on frequency of use of various preservatives in the cosmetic products marketed in the USA. Not surprisingly most of the reports reviewed by Denyer *et al.* (1985) deal with the longer established preservatives with little work having been published on the relatively recently introduced types, e.g. the imidazolidinyl urea and *iso*thiazolidone derivatives which are becoming of increasing importance in the cosmetic field. This absence does not, of course, mean that such synergistic combinations do not exist.

Caution is required in the interpretation of certain of the reports on synergy. In some, a broad definition is adopted which encompasses a widening of the spectrum of activity by combining a bactericide with a fungicide or a water-soluble preservative with a lipid-soluble preservative so that adequate concentrations are achieved in both phases of an emulsion. In others, synergy has been claimed to be evident from experiments in which the activity of one of the biocides alone was not examined.

Predicting synergy on the basis of a knowledge of the mode of action of one agent and the likely consequences of the addition of a second has been most successful in the general area of uncoupling agents which dissociate transmembrane proton gradients from energy-requiring processes. Corner (1981) correctly predicted that there should be an interactive response between a lipophilic weak acid which reversibly inhibits growth by this means, and any lipophilic companion molecule that can shield the charge on the dissociated acid. In this respect he demonstrated synergy between octanoic acid and octanol and hexachlorophene and octanol. A more recent detailed investigation of synergy for which permeabilization was not the proposed mechanism was that by Denyer *et al.* (1986) on the interaction between phenylethanol and chlorocresol. The effects were examined of the two preservatives alone and in combination on *Staphylococcus aureus* growth rate, respiration, glucose uptake, active transport of glutamate, ATP synthesis and Mg^{2+} ATP-ase activity. Here again, the mechanism of synergy appeared to be inhibition of proton gradient-supported transport processes, and the authors concluded that the combination simultaneously affects several interrelated energy-creating and energy-dependent functions of the cell.

With these exceptions, the reports on synergy between biocides of dissimilar mode of action and chemical group have generally contained little that would explain the experimental findings, and proposed synergistic mechanisms have tended to be of a speculative, rather than of a factually based, nature. Thus it is clear that there is ample scope for further work designed to detect true synergy, which embodies experimental designs that will illuminate the detailed biochemical lesions which result from the combination of biocides.

References

BEALE, A.S. & SUTHERLAND, R. 1983. Measurement of combined antibiotic action. In *Antibiotics: Assessment of Antibiotic Activity and Resistance*, ed. Russell, A.D. & Quesnel, L.B. pp. 299–316. Society for Applied Bacteriology Technical Series No. 18. London: Academic Press.

CORNER, T.R. 1981. Synergism in the inhibition of *Bacillus subtilis* by combinations of lipophilic weak acids and fatty alcohols. *Antimicrobial agents and Chemotherapy* 19, 1082–1085.

DENYER, S.P. & KING, R.O. 1988. Development of new preservative systems. In *Microbial Quality Assurance in Non-Sterile Pharmaceuticals, Cosmetics and Toiletries*, ed. Bloomfield, S.F., Baird, R., Leak, R.E. & Leech, R. pp. 156–170. Chichester: Ellis Horwood Ltd.

DENYER, S.P., HUGO, W.B. & HARDING, V.D. 1985. Synergy in preservative combinations. *International Journal of Pharmaceutics* 25, 245–253.

DENYER, S.P., HUGO, W.B. & HARDING, V.D. 1986. The biochemical basis of synergy between the antibacterial agents chlorocresol and 2-phenylethanol. *International Journal of Pharmaceutics* 29, 29–36.

DRUGEON, H.B., CAILLON, J., JUVIN, M.E. & PIRAULT, J.L. 1987. Dynamics of ceftazidime-perfloxacin interaction shown by a new killing curve – chequer board method. *Journal of Antimicrobial Chemotherapy* 19, 197–203.

HAMMOND, S.M. & LAMBERT, P.A. 1978. *Antibiotics and Antimicrobial Action*, p. 18. London: Edward Arnold.

HART, J.R. 1984. Chelating agents as preservative potentiators. In *Cosmetic and Drug Preservation: Principles and Practice*, ed. Kabara, J.J. pp. 323–337. Cosmetic Science and Technology Series, Vol. I. New York: Marcel Dekker Inc.

HUGBO, P.G. 1977. Additivity and synergism *in vitro* as displayed by mixtures of some commonly employed antibacterial preservatives. *Cosmetics and Toiletries* 92, 52–56.

HUGO, W.B. 1982. Disinfection mechanisms. In *Principles and Practice of Disinfection Preservation and Sterilisation*, ed. Russell, A.D., Hugo, W.B. & Ayliffe, G.A.J. pp. 158–185. Oxford: Blackwell Scientific Publications.

HUGO, W.B. & RUSSELL, A.D. 1982. Types of antimicrobial agents. In *Principles and Practice of Disinfection Preservation and Sterilisation*, ed. Russell, A.D., Hugo, W.B. & Ayliffe, G.A.J. pp. 8–196. Oxford: Blackwell Scientific Publications.

KERRY, D.W., HAMILTON MILLAR, J.M.T. & BRUMFITT, W. 1975. Trimethoprim and rifampicin: *in vitro* activities separately and in combination. *Journal of Antimicrobial Chemotherapy* 1, 417–427.

KING, T.C. & KROGSTAD, D.J. 1983. Spectrophotometric assessment of dose-response curves for single antimicrobials and antimicrobial combinations. *Journal of Infectious Diseases* 147, 758–764.

KROGSTAD, D.J. & MOELLERING, R.C. 1985. Antimicrobial combinations. In *Antibiotics in Laboratory Medicine*, ed. Lorian, V. pp. 537–595. Baltimore: Williams and Wilkins.

LITTLEJOHN, O.M. & HUSA, W.J. 1955. The potentising effect of antimolding agents in syrups. *Journal of the American Pharmaceutical Association* 44, 305–308.

MCCLURE, P.J. & ROBERTS, T.A. 1986. Detection of growth of *Escherichia coli* on two-dimensional diffusion gradient plates. *Letters in Applied Microbiology* 3, 53–56.

NORDEN, C.W., WENTZEL, H. & KELETI, E. 1979. Comparison of techniques for measurement of *in vitro* antibiotic synergism. *Journal of Infectious Diseases* 140, 629–633.

PARKER, M.S. 1984. Design and assessment of preservative systems for cosmetics. In *Cosmetic and Drug Preservation: Principles and Practice*, ed. Kabara, J.J. pp. 389–402. Cosmetic Science and Technology Series Vol. I. New York: Marcel Dekker Inc.

RICHARDS, R.M.E. & McBRIDE, R.J. 1971. Phenylethanol enhancement of preservatives used in ophthalmic preparations. *Journal of Pharmacy and Pharmacology* 23, 141S–146S.

SABALITSCHKA, T. 1932. Cited by Littlejohn, O.M. & Husa, W.J. 1955. The potentising effect of antimolding agents in syrups. *Journal of the American Pharmaceutical Association* **44**, 305–308.

SCHALKOWSKY, S. 1982. *Spiral End Point Test for Synergy Determination*. Bethesda, Maryland: Spiral System Instruments, Inc. Available in UK through Don Whitley Scientific, Shipley, W. Yorkshire.

WIMPENNY, J.W.T. & WATERS, P. 1984. Growth of microorganisms in gel stabilized two dimensional diffusion gradient systems. *Journal of General Microbiology* **130**, 2921–2926.

Microcalorimetric Investigations of Mechanisms of Antimicrobial Action

A.E. BEEZER

Chemistry Department, Royal Holloway and Bedford New College, University of London, Egham Hill, Egham, Surrey TW20 0EX, UK

Microcalorimetry has, for a long time been cited as a rapid, sensitive, discerning, non-destructive technique for the investigation of biological systems, both intact and sampled (see for example, Beezer 1980; James 1987). In this respect, the capacity of a microcalorimeter to handle suspended material, coloured material and heterogeneous systems is of considerable advantage. The principal application of the microcalorimetric technique in biology has been in the study of microbial metabolism. It depends on the fact that when bacteria metabolize heat is produced. This heat is measured by sensitive microcalorimeters. The heat generated per unit time is a measure of the power output of the system. Microbiological studies have investigated the effects of medium composition, strain variation, environmental factors (for example, pH, oxygen tension, temperature and trace element concentration) upon metabolism. Studies have also examined the effect of metabolic modifiers, for example uncouplers, and other antimicrobial agents on the microbial microcalorimetric response.

Microcalorimetry can be employed in both qualitative and quantitative studies of metabolic activity. One commercially available instrument (Thermal Activity Monitor, Thermometric AB, Järfälla, Sweden) is capable of measuring a power signal of as little as $1\,\mu W$ (i.e. $1\,\mu J/s$). In operation it therefore functions as a sensitive power meter recording power output (W) as a function of time (t), where power is given by the rate (dq/dt) of thermal energy (q) generation. With this level of sensitivity ($1\,\mu W$), and assuming an enthalpy (heat) of reaction of $40\,kJ/mol$ (a reasonable value for a biological reaction), then a reaction rate of $2.5 \times 10^{-11}\,mol/s$ can be followed. Thus the microcalorimeter can be used to yield precise and very accurate measurements of rates of reaction.

Present address: Chemical Laboratory, University of Kent, Canterbury CT2 7NH, UK.

The equations describing the output of a calorimeter have been discussed in detail by Beezer & Tyrell (1972). By appropriate mathematical manipulation the calorimetric signal can be shown to be proportional to:

1 the concentration, when the instrument may be used purely analytically;
2 the heat of reaction; and
3 the reaction rate constant.

It is in furnishing this latter information that the microcalorimeter may be most successfully used to illuminate mechanisms of antimicrobial action.

Despite the quantitative potential of microcalorimetry, disappointingly little has been achieved other than mainly qualitative observations of differences in modes of antimicrobial action. This chapter will of necessity therefore, concentrate on qualitative approaches but where possible, will draw attention to those quantitative studies which do exist. It is important, however, to appreciate the potential of the technique, its present range of application being more a consequence of limited analytical information relating to the complex systems under study than to any inherent limitation of the method.

Factors Influencing Microcalorimetric Response

A typical power–time $(p-t)$ curve for an organism incubated in growth medium will show, initially, an exponential increase followed by, in the case of the exhaustion of the carbon source, a decline to the baseline. In a complex medium, where several utilizable carbon sources exist, a series of peaks and troughs representing interchange between them, and growth on another substrate is revealed. Thus, in mechanism of antimicrobial action studies, the microcalorimetric response of the organism toward added drug will be influenced by the nature of the organism, the composition and complexity of the medium, and environmental factors. Effective use of microcalorimetry in analysing biocide action must therefore involve careful control of experimental conditions.

Microcalorimetry and Antibacterial Agents

Frequently, antibacterial agents are studied over concentration ranges which are directly related to minimum growth inhibitory concentration (MIC) values. It has been shown that MICs and minimum bactericidal concentrations (MBCs) can be determined from microcalorimetric data (Beezer et al. 1980); in general no power generation represents the absence of viable metabolizing microbes (with the lower limits for detection of an exponential phase organism in growth medium being c. 10^4 organisms/ml).

Mårdh et al. (1976a, b) have investigated the action of tetracyclines on Escherichia coli. All the tetracyclines studied, when added in the exponential growth phase, caused an immediate decrease in the power output, the extent and duration of which varied with the drug used. Thus, doxycycline had a more pronounced bacteriostatic effect over a longer time than did tetracycline. Similar accounts can be found of the interaction of tetracyclines with *Staphylococcus aureus* (Semenitz & Tiefenbrunner 1977; Semenitz 1978). The many references that exist describing the effects of drugs upon bacteria have been exhaustively reviewed (Beezer 1980; Chowdhry *et al.* 1983; James 1987).

The effects of some platinum group metal complexes (PGMC) have been investigated for their antibacterial action against a range of organisms growing in different nutrient media (Bunker 1985). Figure 1 shows the microcalorimetric output from these studies. From the curves it was concluded that the

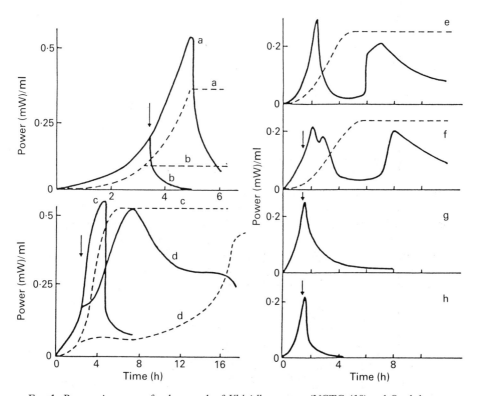

FIG. 1. Power–time traces for the growth of *Klebsiella aerogenes* (NCTC 418) and *Staphylococcus aureus* (13137) when PGMC 1 is added during exponential growth (after Bunker 1985): – – – –, growth curve; ↓, introduction of complex. *Klebsiella aerogenes* growing in glucose-limited medium: (a) control; (b) after the addition of complex (final concentration, 10^{-4} mol/l). *Klebsiella aerogenes* growing in glucose-limited medium supplemented with Oxoid Nutrient Broth (5% w/v): (c) control; (d) after the addition of complex (10^{-4} mol/l). *Staphylococcus aureus* growing in Oxoid Nutrient Broth: (e) control; and after the addition of PGMC 1 at various final concentrations; (f) 10^{-4}; (g) 10^{-3}; (h) 10^{-2} mol/l. Redrawn with permission from the publisher.

complex reacted with some component(s) present in the nutrient broth so producing an apparent reduction in bioactivity.

Microcalorimetry and Antifungal Agents

Kinetic equations can be described for organism growth in either complete medium or for metabolism without growth in, for example, glucose buffer. In this latter situation, provided that the substrate (glucose) is present in excess, then the metabolic rate can be accurately described by a zero-order kinetic equation. This simple respiration reaction produces $p-t$ curves as shown in Fig. 2. Here, it can be seen that simple rectangular displacement of the

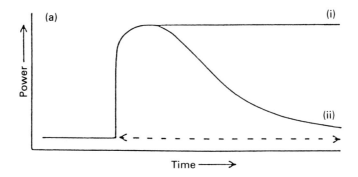

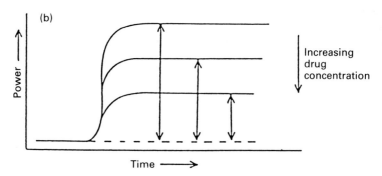

FIG. 2. Types of $p-t$ curves obtained for the interaction of antifungal drugs with respiring cultures of *Saccharomyces cerevisiae*: a(i) represents the response of yeast cells alone; a(ii) the response of yeast cells in the presence of nystatin, filipin, candicidin, amphotericin B and lucensomycin (the latter at concentrations 5 µg/ml); b represents the types of $p-t$ curves obtained with pimaricin, clotrimazole and lucensomycin (the latter at concentrations of 5 µg/ml). Redrawn with permission from the publishers.

baseline results from the zero-order process. The addition of drugs can therefore be easily studied, particularly in bioassay, via interference with this simple experimental variable. This was the method adopted in the assay of nystatin, a polyene antifungal antibiotic (Beezer *et al.* 1977 a,b). However, study of several antifungals has led to the observation that the drugs may be divided into two groups in terms of their mode of action. The first group appears to 'kill' the target organism (*S. cerevisiae*) and includes nystatin, candicidin, amphotericin B, filipin and lucensomycin (at concentrations > 5 μg/ml). The second group contains pimaricin, clotrimazole and lucensomycin (at concentrations < 5 μg/ml). At low concentrations, nystatin has the effect of increasing the power above control levels for a short period of time. This increase over controls is believed to be due to the increased permeability of the membrane brought about by the action of the nystatin thus allowing temporarily an increased influx of glucose and a greater metabolic activity. With pimaricin, clotrimazole and lucensomycin at low concentration the reaction observed appears like that seen for enzyme/inhibitor reactions. It has been shown that miconazole sequentially inactivates peroxidase and then catalase in *Candida albicans* grown aerobically (Denollin *et al.* 1977). It is, therefore, tempting to explain the results obtained with clotrimazole on the basis of a similar enzyme inhibition reaction.

Microcalorimetric experiments allow the measurement of the rates of chemical reactions as noted above. At equimolar concentrations, the polyene antibiotics appear to have the potency order described in Table 1. The judgement used was 'time-to-kill', (i.e. no energy observed in a microcalorimetric experiment: no metabolism is equivalent to death), the most potent antibiotic being the one which, at equal molar concentration, inhibits the

TABLE 1. *Comparison of potency ranking of polyene antibiotics*

| | | | Microcalorimetric potency ranking | |
Antibiotic	MIC (μg/ml)	Assumed mol. wt	$\frac{1}{2}$ MIC*	Equimolar concentrations
Candicidin	0.03	1200	1	2
Amphotericin B	0.09−0.5	924	2	1
Nystatin	0.8−3.1	926	5	5
Filipin	5.0	654	3	4
Pimaricin	0.9−15.0	665.7	4	3
Lucensomycin	—	707.7	—	3−4

* Half MIC concentration taken was half the lowest value in the quoted range. Note the wide variation in MICs. This is characteristic of interlaboratory results for the assay of polyenes.

metabolism of the yeast cells in the shortest time. The order for equal molar concentrations of the antifungal agents is different from that obtained when half the MICs were applied, and both differ substantially from the conventional MIC poteney ranking. The differences between the microcalorimetric and conventional rank orders is, no doubt, the consequence of the inherent differences in the techniques compared. However the free solution conditions employed in the microcalorimeter are, in the author's opinion, a more realistic basis for such a comparative potency ranking than is a conventional tube or plate assay. The observation of the time course of interaction is more informative than is the single end-point of growth/no growth.

Microcalorimetry and Combined Antimicrobial Agents

It is in the realm of antagonism and synergy, i.e. interactions between sensitive organisms and combinations of agents, that microcalorimetry has a potentially wide application. Initially the observation was made by Cosgrove *et al.* (1978) that amphotericin B was more effective alone than when presented in combination with either clotrimazole or miconazole implying that the combinations were antagonistic. Microcalorimetric studies (Joslin 1984) of the responses of sensitive challenge organisms (*Bacillus pumilis, Micrococcus luteus, Bordetella bronchiseptica*) to individual and combined drugs (polymyxin B, neomycin, zinc bacitracin) showed that the proportion of each was important in determining efficacy.

Figure 3 shows the microcalorimetrically observed consequences of the addition of amoxycillin (AMX) or clavulanic acid (CA) to ampicillin-resistant *E. coli*. These separate additions produced no variation from control incubations. When added together (i.e. AMX + CA or Augmentin^R) the $p-t$ curves showed a marked fall in power and indicated evidence of cell lysis. The extent of the events was found to be dependent upon the concentration of AMX. In the above experiments, AMX-sensitive strains of *E. coli* showed considerable reductions in power and again the effects of cell lysis.

Quantitative Structure Activity Relationships

Finally it is possible to derive from microcalorimetric data a group response parameter for the biological activity of series of hydroxybenzoates and alkoxyphenols (Beezer *et al.* 1986, 1987, 1988) leading to a quantitative structure activity relationship (QSAR). This has been achieved by plotting a measure of biological response (the logarithm of the maxium dose which can be applied without eliciting a response: this is, therefore, equal to the intercept value on extrapolation of the log dose−response line to zero response) against carbon number in the homologous series (hydroxybenzoates and alkoxyphenols). A linear relationship has been observed in microcalorimetric data derived from

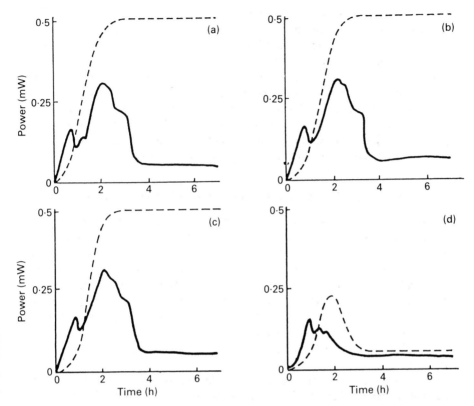

FIG. 3. Power–time traces for the growth of *E. coli* JT39 (β-lactamase-producing strain) in Columbia broth in the presence of antibacterial agents (after Semenitz & Casey 1983, redrawn with permission from Elsevier) (– – – –, growth curve). (a) Control; (b) clavulanic acid 10 μg/ml; (c) amoxycillin 40 μg/ml; (d) amoxycillin 20 μg/ml + clavulanic acid 10 μg/ml.

the interaction of the hydroxybenzoates with both *E. coli* and *Staph. aureus*. The slope and intercept of such plots clearly carry information on the relative sensitivity of these organisms, and their mechanism of interaction with a series of hydroxybenzoates and alkoxyphenols. It is, as yet, not known how general these findings are but if they are repeated elsewhere using other techniques and similar relationships are discovered for other, structurally quite different compounds then an interesting area of biocide design and mechanistic investigation will be established.

References

BEEZER, A.E. (ed.) 1980. *Biological Microcalorimetry*. London: Academic Press.
BEEZER, A.E., CHOWDHRY, B.Z., NEWELL, R.D. & TYRRELL, H.J.V. 1977b. Bioassay of antifungal antibiotics by flow microcalorimetry. *Analytical Chemistry* **49**, 1781–1784.

BEEZER, A.E., FOX, G.G., GOOCH, C.A., HUNTER, W.H., MILES, R.J. & SMITH, B.V. 1988. Microcalorimetric studies of the interaction of m-hydroxybenzoates with *E. coli* and with *Staph. aureus*. Demonstration of a Collander relationship for biological response. *International Journal of Pharmaceutics* 45, 153–155.

BEEZER, A.E., GOOCH, C.A., HUNTER, W.H., LIMA, M.C.P. & SMITH, B.V. 1987. Quantitative structure–activity relationships: a group additivity scheme for biological response of *E. coli* to the action of o-, m- and p-alkoxyphenol. *International Journal of Pharmaceutics* 38, 251–254.

BEEZER, A.E., MILES, R.J., SHAW, E.J. & VICKERSTAFF, L. 1980. Antibiotic bioassay by flow microcalorimetry. *Experientia* 36, 1951–1053.

BEEZER, A.E., NEWELL, R.D. & TYRRELL, H.J.V. 1977a. Bioassay of nystatin bulk material by flow microcalorimetry. *Analytical Chemistry* 49, 34–37.

BEEZER, A.E. & TYRRELL, H.J.V. 1972. Applications of flow microcalorimetry to biological problems. Part I. Theoretical aspects. *Science Tools* 19, 13–16.

BEEZER, A.E., VOLPE, P.L.O., GOOCH, C.A., HUNTER, W.H. & MILES, R.J. 1986. Quantitative structure–activity relationships: microcalorimetric determination of a group additivity scheme for biological response. *International Journal of Pharmaceutics* 29, 237–242.

BUNKER, J. 1985. The effects of some platinum group metal complexes on bacterial growth. *PhD Thesis*, University of London.

CHOWDHRY, B.Z., BEEZER, A.E. & GREENHOW, E.J. 1983. Analysis of drugs by microcalorimetry, isothermal power conduction calorimetry and thermometric titrimetry. *Talanta* 30, 209–243.

COSGROVE, R.F., BEEZER, A.E. & MILES, R.J. 1978. *In vitro* studies of amphotericin B in combination with the imidazole antifungal compounds clotrimazole and miconazole. *Journal of Infectious Diseases* 138, 681–686.

DENOLLIN, S., VANBELLE, H., GOOSENS, F. & BORGERS, M. 1977. Cytochemical and biochemical studies of yeasts after *in vitro* exposure to miconazole. *Antimicrobial Agents and Chemotherapy* 11, 500–513.

JAMES, A.M. (ed.) 1987. *Thermal and Energetic Studies on Cellular Biological Systems*. Bristol: Wright.

JOSLIN, N. 1984. Bioassay and interaction of antibiotics with sensitive cells. *PhD Thesis*, University of London.

MÅRDH, P.A., ANDERSSON, K.-E., RIPA, T. & WADSÖ, I. 1976a. Microcalorimetry as a tool for evaluation of antibacterial effects of doxycycline and tetracycline. *Scandinavian Journal of Infectious Diseases Supplement* 9, 12–16.

MÅRDH, P.A., RIPA, T., ANDERSSON, K.-K. & WADSÖ, I. 1976b. Kinetics of action of tetracyclines on *Escherichia coli* as studied by microcalorimetry. *Antimicrobial Agents and Chemotherapy* 10, 604–609.

SEMENITZ, E. 1978. Mikrokalorimetrische Untersuchungen zur Charakterisierung der antibakteriellen Wirksormkeit von Chemotherapeutika. *Immunität und Infektion* 6, 220–226.

SEMENITZ, E. & CASEY, P.A. 1983. Microcalorimetric and turbidimetric investigation of the actions of amoxycillin, clavulanic acid and augmentin on amoxycillin-resistant strains of *Escherichia coli*, *Klebsiella* and *Staphylococcus aureus*. Augmentin: clavulante-potentiated amoxycillin. In *Proceedings of the European Symposium*, Scheveningen, The Netherlands, June 1982. ed. Croydon, E.A.P. & Michel, M.F. pp. 68–76. Amsterdam: Elsevier. (See also *Excerpta Medica* (1983) pp. 68–76.)

SEMENITZ, E. & TIEFENBRUNNER, F. 1977. Mikrokalorimetrische Untersuchungen zur Bestimmung der antibacteriellen Aktivität von Chemotherapeutika. *Azneimittel–Forschung/Drug Research* 27, 2247–2251.

Mechanisms of Action and Rapid Biocide Testing

G.S.A.B. Stewart,[1] S.A.A. Jassim[2] and S.P. Denyer[2]

[1] *Department of Applied Biochemistry and Food Science, School of Agriculture, University of Nottingham, Sutton Bonington, Loughborough, Leicestershire LE12 5RD, UK; and* [2] *Department of Pharmaceutical Sciences, University of Nottingham, University Park, Nottingham NG7 2RD, UK*

Biocides employed for microbiological control can suffer depletion through chemical decomposition, dilution and inactivation. Recent events, in particular regarding *Legionella* contamination of cooling tower waters, have highlighted the importance of continually monitoring and maintaining adequate biocide levels in systems prone to contamination or requiring disinfection (EACB 1989). Frequently such assessments are retrospective in nature, relying entirely upon conventional microbial challenge methodologies and subsequent culture of surviving cells. Where chemical analytical techniques are available, little account can be taken of the influence of organic soil and other factors affecting biocide efficacy. Tests designed to monitor biocidal potential in a system must therefore seek to establish the available activity and not the mere presence of a biocidal agent. The ideal test method would thus employ a biological rather than chemical monitor, and would seek to provide a rapid* answer to ensure that remedial action were taken quickly.

There is, therefore, a current impasse in biocide testing; efficient monitoring demands evaluation in terms of biological efficacy but detecting microbial growth following biocide challenge requires a time-scale that is incompatible with on-site testing. A 'rapid' biocide monitoring device/system must therefore move away from a traditional cultural method to an indirect method for determining microbial survival. This may be achieved by monitoring some aspect of metabolic activity in surviving cells following biocide treatment. A knowledge of biocide mechanism of action can thus assists in determining a

---

* It is important to remember that the term 'rapid' is variously applied to techniques of 5 min to overnight duration, the definition often reflecting the expectations of the user. In biocide testing, a test time of a few hours or less might be suitable for immediate on-site analysis by a visiting or resident engineer while an overnight or longer method would often entail sample despatch to a central laboratory facility.

suitable event(s) that can be monitored, always assuming that the event(s) does not reflect an interaction with a uniquely sensitive target showing poor correlation with cell death.

The purpose of the following discussion is to present two indirect methods for following antimicrobial effects − tetrazolium salt reduction, and bioluminescent sensors − as possible approaches to rapid biocide testing. Recent reports have also shown the potential for indirect radiometric (Cutler *et al.* 1989) and conductrimetric (Dale & Edwards 1989a,b) techniques to follow antibacterial activity and elucidate mechanisms of action, respectively.

Tetrazolium Salt Reduction

A wide range of actively metabolizing bacteria reduce colourless soluble tetrazolium salts to their respective coloured water-insoluble formazan derivatives, the transformation being effected by dehydrogenase enzyme action. This transformation can take place in the presence of a variety of substrates (Hugo 1954), and a specificity towards certain dehydrogenase enzyme systems in the respiratory chain can be achieved by the selection of a tetrazolium salt with an appropriate redox potential (Altman 1972; Gilbert *et al.* 1977). Any biocide influencing the metabolic activity of bacteria may have the potential to affect tetrazolium salt reduction. At bacteriostatic levels the effect may be incomplete (Table 1), unless dehydrogenase enzymes represent the prime target.

The influence of a biocide on dehydrogenase activity can be simply tested using the following reaction system:

2,3,5-triphenyltetrazolium bromide (0.1% w/v)
solution　　　　　　　1.0 ml;
Staphylococcus aureus or *Escherichia coli*
(4 × 10^{10} cells/ml) washed suspension　　0.5 ml;
Buffer containing biocide　　　　2.5 ml.

All solutions are prepared in 0.01 mol/l HEPES (or Sorensen's phosphate) buffer (pH 7.0) and the experiment is initiated by the addition of 1.0 ml of

TABLE 1. *Effect of three antibacterial agents at their MIC on dehydrogenase activity in* Staph. aureus *(4 × 10^9 cells/ml) energized with 0.02 mol/l glucose*

Biocide	Minimum growth inhibitory concentration (MIC) (%w/v)	Inhibition of formazan production (%)
Phenylmercuric acetate	0.0005	85
Chlorocresol	0.035	61
2-phenylethanol	0.485	39

substrate (0.02 mol/l glucose solution). The reaction mixture is incubated at 37°C and samples are removed at 10-min intervals for analysis. Absorbance readings can be read directly at 480 nm or the insoluble formazan can first be extracted from the reaction mixture by partitioning into butanone (Hurwitz & McCarthy 1986). The reductive power of biocide-treated cells should be compared to an untreated control suspension.

Tetrazolium salt reduction has been successfully employed as a novel method for examining bactericidal action against *E. coli* (Hurwitz & McCarthy 1986) and this suggests a suitable methodology for 'rapid' biocide testing. In this approach, *E. coli* cells previously challenged with bactericidal levels of preservative agents have been separated from the biocide by filtration, washed with an appropriate neutralizer of the agent, and the filter transferred to a liquid growth medium containing 2,3,5-triphenyltetrazolium chloride (TCC). The mixture is then incubated at 37°C and colour development measured at 480 nm following butanone extraction of the formazan. Through incubation, surviving cells become metabolically active and thus reduce the TCC, the process being significantly enhanced as the population multiplies. An incubation period of 4.5 h provides a minimum detection level of *c.* 1×10^5 c.f.u./ml, thus, starting from an initial challenge inoculum of $10^7 - 10^8$ c.f.u./ml a $2-3$ log cycle reduction can be followed. By this method, kill kinetics can be rapidly established; biocide characteristics derived in this way compare closely with those obtained using conventional viable counting methods (Table 2).

The combination of tetrazolium salt reduction with conventional, but modified, challenge methodology ensures the generation of results within a

TABLE 2. *Comparison of biocide characteristics derived from tetrazolium salt reduction (TSR) with those obtained by conventional surface plate counts (SPC)*

| | | Biocide characteristics | |
| | | Concentration exponent | Extrapolated *D*-value at 1% (w/v) concentration (h) |
Biocide	Method		
Bronopol	TSR	1.13	0.12
	SPC	0.92	0.29
Germall II	TSR	1.06	0.33
	SPC	0.96	0.20
Benzylalcohol	TSR	7.50	12.21
	SPC	7.06	10.53
2-phenylethanol	TSR	10.45	0.36
	SPC	9.00	0.32

Data taken from Hurwitz & McCarthy (1986).

working day. Sensitivity can be increased by using larger inoculum sizes or increased incubation periods, the latter approach having been applied by Mattila in a microtitre plate version of the Kelsey–Sykes disinfectant test (Mattila 1987). Recently a commercial product has been developed, incorporating *Bacillus* spores and based on the dye-reduction principle, for use in on-site biocide testing (EACB 1989). While an overnight incubation period is usually required to demonstrate the survival of micro-organisms (and hence the extent of biocidal activity) the 'dipstick' technology associated with the product offers significant advantages in convenience for on-site analysis.

Bioluminescent Biosensors

Many marine bacteria from the genus *Photobacterium* have the biochemical facility to emit light. Light emission, or bioluminescence, does not result from previous light absorption but from an exergonic reaction converting chemical energy to light energy via an excited intermediate. In 1983, Engebrecht *et al.* (1983) isolated from *Photobacterium fischeri* a segment of DNA which when cloned into *E. coli* provided this new host with a bioluminescent phenotype. The clear implication from this was that only a relatively few genes are required to confer, on a normally dark micro-organism, the ability to emit light. In fact there are five structural genes encoded on a 9-kb DNA operon. Three provide components of a fatty acid reductase (necessary for the production of an aldehyde) and two provide the α and β subunits of bacterial luciferase. (Meighen (1988) has reviewed the expression of these genes in their parental organisms.)

In practice, the genetic system for prokaryotic bioluminescence can be simplified still further. It is possible to supply cells with the aldehyde component exogenously (typically as dodecanal). Although the apparent K_m for aldehyde is increased by some 1000-fold over an *in vitro* enzyme assay, the compound can be supplied in sufficient excess to ensure that it is non-limiting in the bioluminescent pathway. With this addition, the genetic components necessary for bioluminescence are reduced to only 2 kb of DNA, comprising the *lux* A and *lux* B genes. Providing that these genes are expressed and that the luciferase product is sufficiently stable, the potential exists to confer a bioluminescent phenotype on any prokaryotic organism.

Since *in vitro* bioluminescence requires functional intracellular biochemistry, bioluminescence necessarily provides a direct measure of cell viability (Stewart *et al.* 1989). Given the exquisite sensitivity of detection (in the extreme, light from a single cell may be detected) it follows that viability could be monitored in real time, in complex environments and during or after the imposition of an environmental stress. With this bioluminescent approach rapid on-site biocide testing becomes feasible.

Feasibility testing using a model bioluminescent organism

In principle, any micro-organism can be converted to a bioluminescent pheno-type and so, clearly, those organisms which form the current basis for biocide evaluation tests (e.g. Table 3) could be genetically engineered accordingly. Such a development, however, would be a long-term project first requiring the design of efficient expression systems for each individual host and then the stabilization of any recombinant construct by, for example, chromosome integration. The principle of using bioluminescent bacteria as a biocide monitor can, however, be demonstrated using any bioluminescent derivative. We have, therefore, explored this avenue using a strain of *E. coli* K12 (designated *E. coli* pSB100) harbouring a plasmid termed pBTK5 (Carmi *et al.* 1987) which requires the addition of aldehyde for functional bioluminescence.

Figure 1 shows the bioluminescence profile for the detection of *E. coli* in an Amerlite Microtitre Plate Luminometer (Amersham International plc, Little Chalfont, Bucks, UK). The response is linear over the four orders of magnitude tested and has an effective detection limit of 6×10^2. Such a detection limit would allow a 5-log reduction in bioluminescence to be measured from

TABLE 3. *Examples of biocide test organisms as employed in disinfectant assay Anon. (1987)*

Escherichia coli NCTC		8196
Pseudomonas aeruginosa NCTC	6749	
Proteus vulgaris NCTC		4635
Staphylococcus aureus NCTC		4163

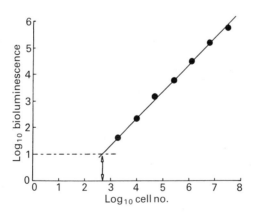

FIG. 1. The relationship between bioluminescence (arbitrary units) and cell number for *E. coli* pSB100. The arrow indicates where the Amerlite instrument background and sensitivity determine the limit of detection.

an initial inoculum of 10^8 cells with ease but it still needs to be determined whether there is a direct relationship between the current use of the term viability and the immediate impact of a biocide on bacterial bioluminescence. To explore this, the bioluminescence of *E. coli* containing pBTK5 was compared with viable counts after treatment with selected levels of phenol.

Portions of a washed cell suspension of *E. coli* pSB100 (25-μl) (grown overnight at 30°C in L-broth (yeast extract, 0.5%; tryptone, 1%; NaCl, 0.5%; pH 7.0) supplemented with 30 μg/ml ampicillin), containing *c.* 2.5×10^8 cells, were distributed into duplicate sterile 96-well microtitre plates containing 25 μl of appropriate double-strength phenol solutions. Each solution was present in eight wells in each microtitre tray, giving final concentrations of 0.2, 0.3, 0.4, 0.5 and 1.0% (w/v) upon the addition of bacteria. Control reaction mixtures were prepared using 25 μl of distilled water. The microtitre trays were well mixed and maintained at 22°C. After 15-min contact, 25-μl portions were withdrawn from one tray and serially diluted in 0.1% peptone water containing 2% (v/v) Tween 80 (as a neutralizer of phenol action) for viable counting (Miles *et al.* 1938). To the wells of the second tray were added 200-μl samples of aldehyde solution (sodium azide, 2%; polymyxin B sulphate, 40 μg/ml; Triton X100, 1%; dodecanal, 0.5%) supplemented with 0.25% (w/v) glucose and 2% (v/v) Tween 80, and the bioluminescence was measured in an Amerlite Microtitre Plate Luminometer. The experiment was repeated for contact times of 30, 60 and 120 min.

From the time course of biocidal action, survivor curves were prepared based on viable count (Fig. 2) and bioluminescence (Fig. 3). From these curves, the decimal reduction time (*D*-value) was determined for each concentration and a graph of *D*-value against phenol concentration was prepared on a logarithmic scale for both viable counts and bioluminescence (Fig. 4). The concentration exponents derived from each method were identical (5.7) and within the range expected for phenol (Hugo & Denyer 1987). In this experiment, therefore, bioluminescence gave a rapid measure of biocide efficiency and, of equal importance, this measure could be correlated to existing mechanisms of evaluation, thus providing reasons for optimism for the likely suitability of such a technology in the field.

In addition to its potential in the direct measurement of biocide activity, bioluminescence can facilitate more subtle approaches to biocide monitoring. Given that in many cases commercial biocides are adversely affected by dilution (Hugo & Denyer 1987) an important aspect of biocide testing is to ensure that a safe margin exists in terms of residual bioactivity. Failure to ensure a safe margin can lead to biofouling which will not necessarily be combated by a subsequent increase in biocide concentration. Thus a biocide dilution test could be used to compare an on-site dilution profile with a standard profile presented as part of a commercial biocide description. If, in

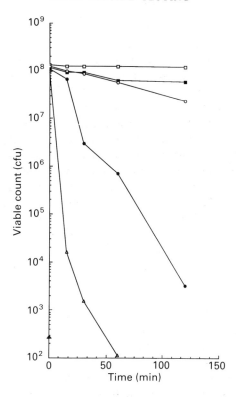

FIG. 2. The effect of contact time and concentration of phenol on the viability of *E. coli* pSB100. Phenol concentrations (% w/v): (□) 0; (■) 0.2; (○) 0.3; (●) 0.4; (△) 0.5; (▲) 1.0.

the test sample, biocide activity titrated out earlier than the standard then this would provide a clear indication that the effective biocide concentration in the test system was below the manufacturer's recommended level.

Figure 5 shows the result of using a model bioluminescent system to evaluate the effect of biocide dilution. Nine commercial biocides of differing chemical nature were employed with significantly different dilution tolerances. *Escherichia coli* containing the plasmid pBTK5 was mixed directly with the biocides in distilled water at concentrations representing 2-fold, 20-fold and 200-fold dilution of the manufacturer's recommended level.

It is not our intention here to present a league table of commercial biocides and hence we will simply refer to these as biocides 1−9. It is, however, interesting to observe that in one case even a 2-fold dilution was sufficient to allow residual bioluminescence in the test system.

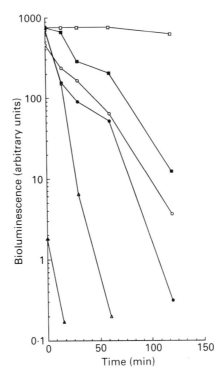

FIG. 3. The effect of contact time and concentration of phenol on the bioluminescence produced by *E. coli* pSB100. Phenol concentrations (% w/v): (□) 0; (■) 0.2; (○) 0.3; (●) 0.4; (△) 0.5; (▲) 1.0.

From Fig. 5 the potential for monitoring biocide efficiency as a function of dilution is clearly evident and there seems little doubt, therefore, that this procedure could form the basis of an industrially relevant evaluation and monitoring system. By definition, such a test must be simple, rapid and require unsophisticated instrumentation so that it can be carried out by an engineer on-site. Just such a system is possible using bioluminescent bacteria and a polaroid camera luminometer (Dynatech Laboratories Ltd, Guernsey UK) and a typical photographic image is given in Fig. 6.

Further developments in bioluminescent bacterial testing of biocides

Bacillus subtilis spores containing the genetic elements required for expressing a bioluminescent phenotype have been developed. These are dark in the dormant state (G.S.A.B. Stewart, unpublished observations), a phenomenon

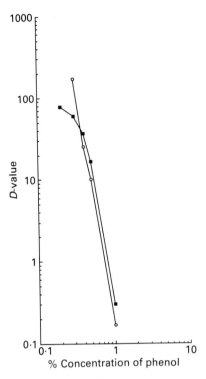

FIG. 4. The relationship between D-value for *E. coli* pSB100 and phenol concentration as described by viable count (○) and bioluminescence (■).

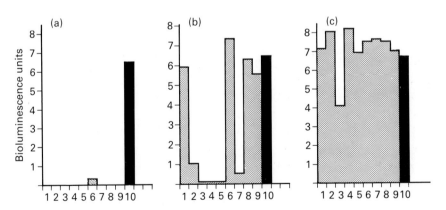

FIG. 5. Histogram profiles for the bioluminescence (arbitrary units) produced when *E. coli* pSB100 was incubated with nine different biocides. Column 10 represents the control bioluminescence in the absence of biocide. Sets a, b and c represent the results obtained with 2-, 20- and 200-fold dilutions of biocide, respectively, in relation to the manufacturer's recommended concentration.

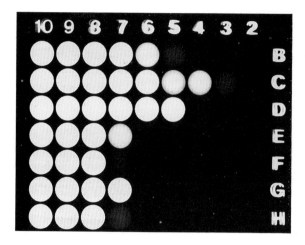

FIG. 6. Biocide dilution profiles derived from bioluminescence measurements in a camera luminometer following exposure of 10^8 cells/ml of *E. coli* pSB100 to doubling-dilutions (lanes 2−10) of biocides B−H. Wells containing viable bacteria produced a white image on the film after a 5-min exposure.

entirely consistent with the total absence of intracellular biochemistry in the dormant bacterial spore. On germination of such spores, however, the appearance of bioluminescence is rapid, correlating with the onset of energy production and metabolism occurring in the first minutes after addition of germinants. The sporicidal activity of biocidal agents can thus be followed by these organisms. If such spores are damaged in their germination mechanism by biocide activity they will remain in the dormant state and hence remain dark. Failure of a biocide would result in spore germination and consequently in the emission of light which could form the basis of a rapid detection system. It would represent a significant advance in rapidity over the commercial spore−dye-reduction system described earlier.

Conclusion

The ability of a microbial population to reduce colourless tetrazolium salts to a coloured formazan has been shown to provide an efficient method by which microbial survival can be established. A challenge test based on this principle can be used to determine biocide efficacy within the working day. A particularly promising further approach employs genetically engineered bioluminescent test organisms which demonstrate luminescence only in the metabolically active 'viable' state. Such a genetically manipulated system would be entirely compatible with a 'dipstick' approach provided that the luminescence detection can be made simple and relatively inexpensive. Fortunately, rapid developments in luminometer design are being driven by parallel interests in ATP measurement, which already has a firm commercial base. It is reasonable to assume that fibreoptic solid-phase sensors with disposable bio-optic transducers will be developed in the future, perhaps along the lines described by Freeman & Sietz (1978) for a chemiluminescence monitor.

References

ALTMAN, F.P. 1972. *An Introduction to the Use of Tetrazolium Salts in Quantitative Enzyme Cytochemistry*. Colnbrook: Koch-Light Laboratories Ltd.

ANON. 1987. *Estimation of concentration of disinfectants used in 'dirty' conditions in hospitals by the modified Kelsey–Sykes test*. British Standard No. 6905. London: British Standards Institution.

CARMI, O.A., STEWART, G.S.A.B., ULITZUR, S. & KUHN, J. 1987. Use of bacterial luciferase to establish a promoter probe vehicle capable of nondestructive real-time analysis of gene expression in *Bacillus* spp. *Journal of Bacteriology* 169, 2165–2170.

CUTLER, R.R., WILSON, P. & CLARKE, F.V. 1989. Evaluation of a radiometric method for studying bacterial activity in the presence of antimicrobial agents. *Journal of Applied Bacteriology* 66, 515–521.

DALE, L.D. & EDWARDS, D.I. 1989a. Determination of conductance of the cytotoxic effects of bioreductive antimicrobial and radiosensitizing agents. *Letters in Applied Microbiology* 9, 53–56.

DALE, L.D. & EDWARDS, D.I. 1989b. Application of conductance measurements to drug mode of action studies. *Letters in Applied Microbiology,* 9, 57–59.

EACB 1989. *Report of the Expert Advisory Committee on Biocides*, Chairman Wright, A.E. London: HMSO.

ENGEBRECHT, J., NEALSON, K. & SILVERMAN, M. 1983. Bacterial bioluminescence: isolation and genetic analysis of functions from *Vibrio fischeri*. *Cell* 32, 773–781.

FREEMAN, T.M. & SIETZ, W.R. 1978. Chemiluminescent fibre optic probe for hydrogen peroxide based on the luminol reaction. *Analytical Chemistry* 50, 1242–1246.

GILBERT, P., BEVERIDGE, E.G. & CRONE, P.B. 1977. Inhibition of some respiration and dehydrogenase enzyme systems in *Escherichia coli* NCTC 5933 by phenoxyethanol. *Microbios* 20, 29–37.

HUGO, W.B. 1954. The use of 2,3,5-triphenyltetrazolium bromide in determining the dehydrogenase activity of *Bact. coli. Journal of Applied Bacteriology* 17, 31–37.

HUGO, W.B. & DENYER, S.P. 1987. The concentration exponent of disinfectants and preservatives (biocides). In *Preservatives in the Food, Pharmaceutical and Environmental Industries*, ed. Board, R.G., Allwood, M.C. & Banks, J.G. pp. 281–291. Oxford: Blackwell Scientific Publications.

HURWITZ, S.J. & McCARTHY, T.J. 1986. 2,3,5-triphenyltetrazolium chloride as a novel tool in germicide dynamics. *Journal of Pharmaceutical Sciences* 75, 912–916.

MATTILA, T. 1987. A modified Kelsey–Sykes method for testing disinfectants with 2,3,5-triphenyltetrazolium chloride reduction as an indicator of bacterial growth. *Journal of Applied Bacteriology* 62, 551–554.

MEIGHEN, E.A. 1988. Enzymes and genes from the *lux* operons of bioluminescent bacteria. *Annual Reviews in Microbiology* 42, 151–176.

MILES, A.A., MISRA, S.S. & IRWIN, J.O. 1938. The estimation of the bactericidal power of the blood. *Journal of Hygiene, Cambridge* 38, 732–749.

STEWART, G.S.A.B., SMITH, A.J. & DENYER, S.P. 1989. Genetic engineering for bioluminescent bacteria. *Food Science & Technology Today* 3, 19–22.

Mechanisms of Antibacterial Action – A Summary

S.P. DENYER[1] AND W.B. HUGO[2]

[1] Department of Pharmaceutical Sciences, University of Nottingham, University Park, Nottingham NG7 2RD, UK; and [2] 618 Wollaton Road, Nottingham NG8 2AA, UK

There is a growing awareness of the need to establish mechanisms of action for antibacterial agents. This information assists in the design of new compounds or combinations of compounds and in the understanding of resistance mechanisms, and provides a focus for toxicological attention. Certainly, mechanism of action studies have shown that biocidal agents (preservatives, disinfectants, industrial biocides) can no longer be considered under a crude umbrella as general cell poisons; furthermore their activity may be optimized by design.

Target regions for antibacterial agents can be classified very conveniently as the cell wall, cytoplasmic membrane and cytoplasm. Within these broad areas of the cell a further division of targets can be made (Fig. 1). It should be remembered that these divisions are accepted for convenience only and do not represent mutually exclusive areas for biocide interaction. Indeed, many of the antibacterial agents currently in use will have more than one target within the bacterial cell, and it is axiomatic that the vital interdependence of cellular functions must not be ignored.

Experimental Approach to Mechanism of Action Studies

Before attempting an assessment of the mechanism of action of an antimicrobial agent, quantitative measurements of minimum growth inhibitory concentration (MIC) and minimum bactericidal concentration (MBC) must be made; consideration should also be given to establishing rates of action.

MIC and MBC values give reference points when looking at other dose-related effects described in this volume and enable an assessment to be made of possible significant relationships between these effects and growth inhibition or death. In the whole-cell system, a causal relationship between antibacterial action and a particular effect or effects can only be presumed if both responses

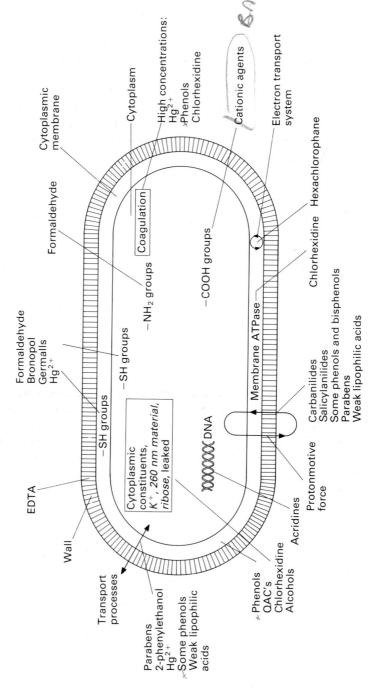

FIG. 1. Diagram showing major targets for some preservative agents. (Modified with permission from Hugo & Russell 1987.)

are achieved at a similar concentration level. Clearly, however, when studies are performed on isolated cell components a greater sensitivity may be anticipated than would be realized in the intact cell. Under these circumstances, confirmatory evidence of the proposed lesion must be sought in a whole-cell experimental system.

Success in mechanism of action studies depends greatly upon careful attention to detail. If experimental conditions are not optimized or carefully controlled, biocide-induced responses can be supplemented or altered by experimentally induced effects. Comparisons with biocide-free experimental systems should always be made.

Variation in Mechanism of Action

It is important to remember that the activity of compounds may well result from effects on several cell functions and the relative importance of each effect may vary depending upon the value of that function to the species of organism challenged. Furthermore, an altered sensitivity towards antibacterial agents may reflect changes in the accessibility of targets within the cell and again may alter significantly the principal lesion(s) responsible for antibacterial activity. Such alterations in sensitivity may arise through changes in the physiological state of the organism dependent upon growth phase, environment and selective pressures.

Most importantly, mechanism of action studies can usually only determine the bulk population behaviour. It should never be assumed that every cell in that population is suffering the same type, and degree of, damage at the same time. Observed effects are an average of the whole population and do not necessarily reflect the sensitivity of all cells; this is undoubtedly the basis by which surviving fractions in a treated population sometimes remain, possibly to emerge more adequately equipped to deal with a subsequent biocide challenge.

Consequences of Biocide Interaction

Antibacterial agents may exert both bacteriostatic and bactericidal effects. The mechanisms of action responsible for each effect may not necessarily be the same. Bacteriostatic effects can be considered generally to represent some form of metabolic inhibition which is released upon removal of the biocide, while bactericidal action is caused by irreversible or irreparable damage to a vital structure or function of the cell. Quite possibly, damage arising from interactions with biocides may, in many instances, be repairable but, because of inhibition at another metabolic site, appropriate repair processes cannot be initiated and cell death occurs.

With this in mind, it is essential that any study of mechanisms of action consider the most suitable approaches for cell recovery and biocide inactivation. A completely false impression of the prime lesion(s) may be gained if inadequate opportunity is given to the cells to recover from induced damage.

Finally, in the search for specific antibacterial reactions it is important to remember that some agents have such high chemical reactivity that they have a wide spectrum of cell interactions and it is difficult to pin-point the fatal reaction. In fact, it is reasonable to say that with these compounds there is no single fatal reaction but that death results from the accumulated effects of many reactions. Examples of compounds in this category include β-propriolactone, ethylene oxide and sulphur dioxide.

Bibliography

DENYER, S.P. 1990. Mechanisms of action of biocides. *International Biodeterioration* **26**, 89–100.

GILBERT, P. & WRIGHT, N. 1987. Non-plasmid resistance towards preservatives of pharmaceutical products. In *Preservatives in the Food, Pharmaceutical and Environmental Industries*, ed. Board, R.G., Allwood, M.C. & Banks, J.G. pp. 255–279. Society for Applied Bacteriology Technical Series No. 22. Oxford: Blackwell Scientific Publications.

HUGO, W.B. 1982. Disinfection mechanisms. In *Principles and Practice of Disinfection, Preservation and Sterilisation*, ed. Russell, A.D., Hugo, W.B. & Ayliffe, G.A.J. pp. 158–185. Oxford: Blackwell Scientific Publications.

HUGO, W.B. & RUSSELL, A.D. (eds) 1987. *Pharmaceutical Microbiology*, 4th edn. Oxford: Blackwell Scientific Publications.

Index

335

THE SOCIETY FOR APPLIED BACTERIOLOGY TECHNICAL SERIES

General Editor: F.A. Skinner